IMMUNOPOWER

FULL SPECTRUM NUTRITION PROTECTION

HARNESSING THE INCREDIBLE HEALING POWER OF NATURE AND SCIENCE THROUGH NUTRITIONAL SYNERGISM

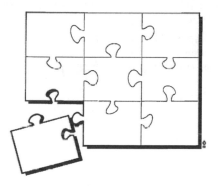

Patrick Quillin, PhD,RD,CNS

NUTRITION TIMES PRESS, INC.
TULSA, OKLAHOMA

Other books by Patrick Quillin (website: www.4nutrition.com)
available at your local bookstore or health food store, or Bookworld 1-800-444-2524,
or on the Internet at www.amazon.com
-BEATING CANCER WITH NUTRITION, Nutrition Times Press, Tulsa,1998;
now translated into Japanese and Chinese and used in the U.S. as a continuing
education course for R.N.s
-THE HEALING POWER OF CAYENNE PEPPER, Leader Co., Canton, 1998
-KITCHEN HEALTH TIPS (video), Nutrition Times Press, Tulsa, 1997
-HEALING SECRETS FROM THE BIBLE, Nutrition Times Press, Tulsa, 1996
-HONEY, GARLIC & VINEGAR, Leader Co., N. Canton, OH, 1996
-HEALING POWER OF WHOLE FOODS, Vitamix, Cleveland, 1994
-ADJUVANT NUTRITION IN CANCER TREATMENT, Cancer Treatment
Research Foundation, Arlington Heights, IL, 1994
-AMISH FOLK MEDICINE, Leader Co., N.Canton, OH, 1993
-SAFE EATING, M.Evans, NY, 1990
-THE LA COSTA BOOK OF NUTRITION, Pharos Books, New York, 1988
-HEALING NUTRIENTS, Contemporary Books, Chicago, 1987, in paperback by
Random House, NY, 1988; also published in paperback in Europe and Australia
through Penguin Press, London
-THE LA COSTA PRESCRIPTION FOR LONGER LIFE, Ballantine, NY, 1985

Copyright 1999 Patrick Quillin
ISBN 0-9638372-6-5

Printed in the United States of America

How to order this book:
Visit your bookstore or call BOOKWORLD 1-800-444-2524

Nutrition Times Press, Inc., Box 700512, Tulsa, OK 74170
phone & fax 918-495-1137

TELL US YOUR STORY
We want to hear your experiences about using nutrition as part of your
cancer treatment. Please send us your personal experience with an
address or phone number on how to contact you. Your story may
provide hope and inspiration for others suffering from the same
condition. Thank you.

CONTENTS

Dedication
To the many cancer patients that I was privileged to work with. For your privacy, you are anonymous here. Yet, your names and faces are permanently etched in the gallery of my mind. Thank you for sharing your courage, your wisdom, your insight on priorities and your souls with me. For the many ImmunoPower users who have stuck with us through good times and "developmental times". Thanks for your belief in us.

Acknowledgements
To the many brilliant and creative physicians and scientists whose courage in the face of scorn helped us to improve outcome for cancer patients the world over, especially: Weston Price, DDS, Linus Pauling, PhD, Abram Hoffer, MD, PhD, John Prudden, MD, PhD, and Stan Burzynski, MD, PhD. Nobody ever said that being an ice breaker is an easy job. But someone has to do it.

IMPORTANT NOTICE!!! PLEASE READ!!!

CAUTION!! Cancer is a life-threatening disease. The program and products outlined in this book are designed to be used in conjunction with, not instead of, your doctor's program. All of the foods and supplements described in this book will work synergistically with your oncologist's program. Do not use this information or the ImmunoPower product as sole therapy against cancer. If you cannot agree to these terms, then you may return this book in new condition for a full refund. This information has not been evaluated by the Food and Drug Administration. ImmunoPower is not intended to diagnose, treat, cure or prevent any disease.

PREFACE: RE-ENGINEERING CANCER TREATMENT

"If everyone is thinking alike, then no one is thinking." Ben Franklin

A well nourished cancer patient can better manage and beat the disease. And today's cancer patient needs more help than ever before. After spending $39 billion in research in the 28 year "war on cancer" at the National Cancer Institute and over $1 trillion in therapy at hospitals around the country, we now have a 13% increase in the incidence and 7% increase in the death rate from cancer. Five year survival is virtually unchanged at around 50%. The reason for this lack of progress in beating cancer is our inability to use good judgment in both research and treatment. Blasting the cancer with the cytotoxic therapies of chemotherapy, radiation, and surgery can reduce tumor burden INITIALLY; but they do not change the underlying causes of the disease. And when the cancer returns, it is much more ferocious the second time, now having developed "drug resistance" or "hormone independence" to make medical intervention ineffective.

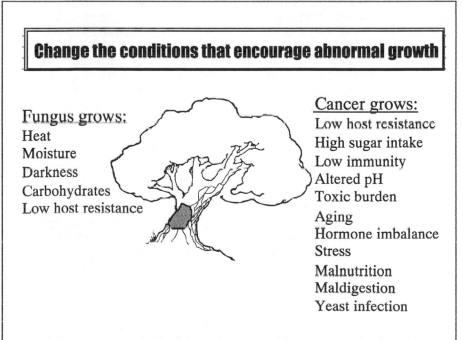

Change the conditions that encourage abnormal growth

Fungus grows:
Heat
Moisture
Darkness
Carbohydrates
Low host resistance

Cancer grows:
Low host resistance
High sugar intake
Low immunity
Altered pH
Toxic burden
Aging
Hormone imbalance
Stress
Malnutrition
Maldigestion
Yeast infection

We need to re-think the cancer battle plan. Fungus grows on the bark of a tree because of the underlying conditions of heat, moisture and darkness. You could cut on the fungus with an axe, or burn with a blow torch, or poison with bleach; yet the fungus would return as long as the underlying conditions of heat, moisture and darkness are present. Similarly, cancer grows in a human body because of one or more underlying conditions; including lack of oxygen (cancer is an anaerobic organism), sugar feeding, immune suppression, toxin overload, and so on. If all you do is "cut, burn and poison" with surgery, radiation and chemotherapy; then there is a very good chance that the cancer will return and the patient's defense mechanisms, like the immune system, will be so compromised that the patient will be consumed by the cancer.

In order to improve outcome in cancer treatment, it is essential that the patient and physician address the underlying causes of the cancer, which are briefly discussed later in this book, and in more detail in BEATING CANCER WITH NUTRITION. ImmunoPower is the most complete, clinically-tested, convenient and economical means of using nutrition to improve the body's ability to heal itself. ImmunoPower should not be considered sole therapy against cancer.

THE IMMUNOPOWER STORY: how it came to be

In 1993, after working with hundreds of cancer patients at a major cancer hospital, I saw the "bewildered look" too often. The "bewildered look" was when I would provide the cancer patient with some insight regarding foods and nutrition supplements that may improve outcome in cancer treatment. I would recite a list of vitamins, minerals, herbals, glandulars, fatty acids, and accessory factors that may help bolster this vague but all important "non-specific host defense mechanisms", which help us to beat cancer. The patient would get increasingly "bug eyed" and finally ask: "Do you really expect me to take all of those vitamin pills? And if I could swallow them and not choke, who could afford all of that?" I began my quest to find a manufacturer who could produce the ImmunoPower.

In 1994, my book, BEATING CANCER WITH NUTRITION, was first released. In that book, I listed many nutrition factors that may help the cancer patient, and rated them on a *** or ** or * start basis, depending on the level of credibility behind that nutrient. To my surprise, a few of our patients who were "poor prognostic", meaning they were very sick and not expected to recover, showed me their dresser drawers full of nutrition supplement bottles, saying: "I took all of the 3 star nutrients in your book, and now I'm well." I then began a fervent quest for information regarding nutritional synergism, or "1 plus 1 equals more than 2." I still could not find a vitamin manufacturer willing to take on this project, which would be the "Panama Canal" for the manufacturer, given the complexity and potential for failure in the project.

In 1995, I had a fruitful discussion with the President and Founder of Metabolic Maintenance, Inc. in Sisters, Oregon. Ed Fitzjarrell had watched his mother use nutrition and psychoneuroimmunology to beat her leukemia 20 years ago. This wonderful recovery for his mother led Ed back to nutrition school, where he eventually became a production manager for a large vitamin company in Los Angeles. Then Ed had made the big leap by starting his own nutrition supplement facility. When I approached him with the possibility of creating this ridiculously complex product, he was sympathetic, given the experiences of his mother, still healthy 20 years after her diagnosis of leukemia.

Together, we made the first product, called the Advanced Nutrition Composite (ANC), with nearly 70 ingredients. Given the 4 million cancer patients being treated in the U.S. today and the huge number of these patients who are "poor prognostic", there was no shortage of people willing to try this pilot project. We had some major successes, in tolerance of the ANC, improvement of health, and ability to "sail through" chemo and radiation therapies. See the "clinical highlights" sections in this book for encouraging news about what can happen when the cancer patient provides his or her body with the raw ingredients necessary to help fight the cancer. We were encouraged.

We then added some nutrients to the ANC product, including the sulfur-bearing tripeptide, glutathione, which gave an unpleasant odor and flavor to the product for about 10% of our users. Fortunately, many of our users forgave us and continued with their usage of the product as we switched the glutathione from the powder to the pills.

In September of 1997, we changed the name to ImmunoPower, created a website: www.immunopower.com, wrote a book to explain the concept and the scientific backing behind the individual ingredients. This new ImmunoPower product, version 4.0, offers significant improvements in taste, odor, and potency of formula over the preceding formulas.

There is no question that ImmunoPower is one of the most complicated nutrition supplements in the world and that ImmunoPower will continue to evolve as new information becomes available to make it more potent and tolerable. We will never "arrive" at a destination with respect to this formula and project. It is a journey that we continue to take together. We look forward to your input.

EXECUTIVE SUMMARY

If you have been recently diagnosed with cancer and are too tired to read much, then please do the following:

⇒ **Bolster your spirits**. Millions before you have beat cancer. So can you.

⇒ **Get educated**. Find out all of your options for cancer treatment. Unless you have an extremely aggressive form of cancer, you can take 2 weeks to get a second opinion and do some serious investigation before you leap into a therapy that may be irreversible or, worse yet, ineffective. See chapters 14, 15, and 16 for more information regarding doctors and cancer information referral agencies who can point you in the right direction.

⇒ **Avoid any sweet foods**. Sugar feeds cancer. Don't eat any white sugar. Seriously curtail your intake of anything that tastes sweet, including fruit, or any foods with a high glycemic index, including carrot juice and rice cakes.

⇒ **Go for the color in vegetables**. Eat all the colorful and fresh vegetables that your bowels can tolerate. Leafy greens (like spinach and collards), beets, tomatoes, peppers, squash, carrots and broccoli are some examples.

⇒ **Get adequate protein**. While the average healthy adult can subsist on 30-50 grams of protein each day, the cancer patient needs more protein; maybe 80-120 grams per day, depending on patient size and potential for weight loss. The backbone of your immune system is built from dietary protein. Without adequate protein, your immune system becomes the Three Stooges trying to round up King Kong.

⇒ **Work with your health care professional** to change the underlying causes of your cancer. This can be an easy or complex process, but it usually requires professional guidance. See chapter 11 for more on this subject.

⇒ **Take some form of restrained cancer-killing therapy**. The most common traditional therapies are chemotherapy, radiation, and surgery. There are many other useful cancer therapies which are more selectively toxic to cancer. See chapter 11 for more information and chapter 16 for referral agencies to help you.

⇒ **Take ImmunoPower**. If you ignore the first 7 guidelines just mentioned, then ImmunoPower will be much less effective against your condition. Use all of these guidelines and you are bringing maximum force to reverse the cancer.

Best wishes for a long, healthy and happy life.

Patrick Quillin, PhD,RD,CNS
Tulsa, Oklahoma, February 1999

CHAPTER 1
★
IMPORTANT FACTS ABOUT IMMUNOPOWER

WHO SHOULD NOT USE THIS PRODUCT

ALLERGIES. Anyone with an allergy or intolerance to soy products or any of the other ingredients listed on the label should not use this product.

PREGNANT WOMEN. Since pregnancy is such a vulnerable phase of life, it is best not to use higher than normal nutrients during this crucial phase of fetal development. While thalidomide is a relatively harmless drug in healthy adults, it can induce permanent birth defects if taken by a pregnant women. While a couple of alcoholic drinks may not do harm to most healthy adults, alcohol consumed during pregnancy can induce Fetal Alcohol Syndrome, a common form of birth defect. While all nutrients in ImmunoPower are provided in safe levels, do not use ImmunoPower if pregnant.

BRAIN CANCER. Anyone being treated for brain cancer (glioblastoma or astrocytoma) should not use this product, since a proper immune attack on the cancer may involve inflammation of the tumor, which cannot be tolerated in brain cancer patients with no room for the inflammation to occur. In these brain cancer patients, swelling, edema and severe headaches can result after the use of immune-stimulating products. If you or a loved one has brain cancer, then I recommend that you contact:
Stanislaus R. Burzynski, MD, PhD; 12000 Richmond Ave. #260, Houston, TX 77082, ph. 713-597-0111

Or consult with the cancer referral agencies listed in chapter 16.

WHO MAY BENEFIT FROM THE USE OF THIS PRODUCT?

ImmunoPower is designed to be used as a general high dose supplement for people being treated for immune-suppressive disorders, especially cancer.

PREVENTION: If used for preventive measures and as part of a comprehensive lifestyle wellness program, then take 1 scoop of powder and 1 packet of pills per day, preferably in divided dosages and with meals.

REMISSION: If used for persons in remission from cancer (i.e. no measurable disease), and used in conjunction with a comprehensive program structured by your health care professional, then take 2 scoops of powder and 2 packets per day until you have been disease-free for 6 months; then back the dosage down to the preventive level of 1 scoop of powder and 1 packet of pills daily.

THERAPEUTIC: For people who are being actively treated for cancer, chronic fatigue or AIDS, take up to 3 scoops of powder and 3 packets of pills daily, working under the direct supervision of your health care professional. If you experience any gastric distress, such as nausea or diarrhea, then reduce dosage to 1/3 scoop of powder and 1 packet of pills daily and increase dosage slowly as tolerance permits. If symptoms persist, then discontinue use of ImmunoPower and consult your physician.

WHAT IS SO SPECIAL ABOUT IMMUNOPOWER?

Imagine if you went to a car dealership and wanted to buy a car. The salesperson shows you a picture of what you want, and then proceeds to tell you to order the transmission from Mexico, the engine from Canada, the seats from Florida, and many of the parts "we don't know where you can get them." What would you think?? Pretty poor customer service, right?? Well, that's exactly what most people are told to do when they develop a health challenge and are confronted with the daunting prospects of assembling a long list of valuable nutrition factors. That is an outdated and customer-insensitive approach to providing nutrition support. ImmunoPower changes all of that by providing a condition-specific formula.

ImmunoPower is the world's most comprehensive, clinically-proven, cost-effective, convenient, and bioavailable method for taking nutrition support. ImmunoPower sets itself apart from the rest of nutritional supplements by originating the future of naturopathic healing: condition specific products. No more "life and death scavenger hunts" to find a lengthy grocery list of different supplements. No more opening dozens of jars of vitamin pills at each meal to try to mix the right amount and ratio of nutrients. No more hoping that the long list of vitamin manufacturers that you patronize all have the same concept of integrity, purity of ingredients, and Good Manufacturing Practices (GMP). No more filling up your stomach with gelatin capsules, excipients, impurities and blending agents. ImmunoPower has done all of the work for you and saved you about 75% of the cost of buying these ingredients individually, or "a la carte" while also cutting the number of pills taken by 90%.

ImmunoPower provides the top 77 nutrition ingredients in their purist, most bioavailable, most economical and most convenient form to bolster host defense mechanisms when your immune system is not fully protecting you. Welcome to the future of nutritional supplements.

QUALITY CONTROL ON INGREDIENTS

All ingredients in ImmunoPower come from the finest raw ingredient distributors with a Certificate of Analysis (CA) from an independent laboratory that is certified by the Food and Drug

Administration. The ingredient must be what it says it is and with no bacterial contamination.

All fatty acids (shark liver oil, fish oil, primrose oil) in the product are packed and shipped in liquid nitrogen, which reduces lipid peroxidation (oxidation of fats) to a negligible level. These products are then taken from liquid nitrogen containers to a special soft gelatin encapsulation process where they are hermetically sealed against the presence of oxygen. There are minimal lipid peroxides in the fatty acids found in ImmunoPower.

The Cat's claw concentrate (3 to 1) comes from the Peruvian rainforest and is the tested and safe variety of Uncaria Tomentosa.

IMMUNOPOWER: SAFE AND EFFECTIVE IF USED AS DIRECTED

ImmunoPower was developed and used in a major cancer hospital. Over 300 cancer patients over the course of 3 years have used this product with results varying from "improvement in energy levels while going through chemotherapy" to "complete remission from cancer" when used as part of a comprehensive cancer treatment program.

GASTRO-INTESTINAL SYMPTOMS

The only side effects noted in these advanced cancer patients was that about 10% of the patients could not tolerate full strength dosage of 3 scoops of powder and 3 packets of pills each day. GI symptoms were more likely to be pronounced with:

* the more advanced and aggressive the cancer
* the more involvement in the gastro-intestinal tract
* the smaller the person
* the more weight loss (cachexia)
* older and more frail women.

Each of the above conditions increases the chances that GI tolerance to ImmunoPower will be less than ideal. Best approach to this problem is to reduce dosage to 1/3 scoop per meal and 1/3 packet per meal, and increase dosage as tolerance permits.

Many of the patients who were initially unable to tolerate full strength ImmunoPower, were able to increase dosage as their condition improved. Indeed, many people with malnutrition experience atrophy of the gut mucosa or microvilli. Sometimes the starving babies in Third World countries must be carefully fed with small amounts of easily digested food initially, or the nutrition that they so desperately need can induce diarrhea in their compromised smooth gut. Cancer patients can follow this same path, starting slowly with ImmunoPower and building dosage as tolerance permits.

WHAT ABOUT THE COLOR OF IMMUNOPOWER?

As you will read through this book, many valuable therapeutic nutritional products are pigments in Nature. Some of these pigments work with chlorophyll to capture the sun's energy in the process called photosynthesis. Others are "sunscreen" to protect the plant from the damaging effects of excess solar radiation. Others have color because that is the nature of that molecule or atom.

ImmunoPower powder contains betatene, or mixed carotenoids from algae, which give a red and orange color, many minerals which have various colors, B vitamins which have a yellowish color, and so on. Also, the bulk ingredients in the ImmunoPower powder are soy protein, bovine cartilage, and vitamin C , which are white. When all of the ingredients are thoroughly mixed together, the various pigments are overwhelmed by the white ingredients. However, shortly after the product has been packaged, the various pigments may begin to detach from the white ingredients, which means that there is a gradual changing of colors as these once-hidden pigments begin to appear. Imagine if you had a red car, but covered it with chalk dust. Or a white cue ball from billiards, then cover it with various colored chalk. As the chalk dust begans to fall off of the car or the cue ball, the colors will change. That is what is happening with the ImmunoPower powder. Do not be alarmed. This color change is perfectly normal and to be expected.

WHEN CAN I EXPECT RESULTS?

In 8 to 12 weeks, if all goes well, then you should notice some difference in your well being and condition. Remember, nutrition products work on the underlying cause of the problem, but they do not work quickly. A person with angina (pain in the heart) might take a tablet of nitroglycerin under the tongue and feel relief within a minute. Nutrients, on the other hand, must be absorbed into the cell matrix and become part of the structure and function of your body before you will notice a change in overall health status.

Please be patient and continue taking ImmunoPower for 2-3 months, at which time you should notice a significant change in your health status.

WHY IS SOME OF THE PRODUCT IN PILLS AND SOME IN POWDER?

In the beginning, all of these products were available in pill form only. But few people had the determination or strong stomach to take over 200 pills per day, with all of the inherent gelatin capsules and excipients (blending ingredients) that are part of the tabletting process. The purpose of ImmunoPower was to make the consumption of many different nutritional products as convenient as possible. Therefore, any ingredient that was palatable or neutral in flavor was moved into the powdered ingredients.

There are some nutritional ingredients that cannot be made palatable to the average American taste buds, including herbal agents, like astragalus and echinacea, garlic, glandular extracts of spleen and thymus, special fatty acids of fish, evening primrose and shark oil.

These ingredients had to be put in capsule form to be included in the complete formula. Every effort has been made to reduce the number of pills and excipients in ImmunoPower.

HOW CAN ONE FORMULA HELP MANY PEOPLE?

Modern medicine uses the "one symptom-one drug" model of treating disease, such as aspirin for headache and Tagamet for ulcers. Natural healing forces work with a very different paradigm: "non-specific host defense mechanisms". Whether your body is attacking an invading bacteria or a virus, a wooden splinter, an organ transplant, or any form of cancer; there are many common features in the immune system that apply to all sorts of invading disease states. Macrophages, neutrophils, cytokines, Natural Killer cells all work equally well against a wide assortment of infectious diseases and cancers. Whether you have the flu or lung cancer, your liver makes acute phase proteins, like Complement C9, and other cells manufacture cytokines, like interferon and interleukin, to fight off the invaders. ImmunoPower is designed to bolster these non-specific host defense mechanisms.

HOW TO PREPARE IMMUNOPOWER

ALWAYS TAKE PILLS AND POWDER AT MEALTIME-- NEVER TAKE ON AN EMPTY STOMACH. The powdered product is best used when mixed with fruit juice or water in an electric or manual blender.

◊ **BASIC RECIPE:** Mix 1 cup of fruit juice (like apple, grape, grapefruit, pineapple, tomato, orange) with up to one scoop of powdered ImmunoPower and blend for 10 seconds.

◊ **ADVANCED RECIPE:** For some extra flavor and texture, do the above mixture with ImmunoPower powder, then blend in a frozen banana in your high speed electric blender.

◊ **COMBINED RECIPE:** You can mix in other powdered nutrition products with ImmunoPower for additional nutrient intake. Mix the BASIC RECIPE, then add a scoop of powdered protein, such as whey, rice protein, rice bran, or powdered egg white.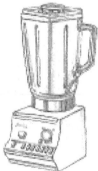

◊ **DRAGON SLAYER SHAKE:** Pour 4 ounces of fruit juice into a high speed blender. Add 1/2 cup to 1 cup of vegetables (i.e. peeled carrots, cooked beets) and blend until smooth. Add your dosage of ImmunoPower powder (1/3 to 1 scoop), then blend. Add 1/2 frozen banana, then blend. This is the best recipe of all; providing a great taste, nice smooth texture and cool feel on the tongue which is very helpful for patients undergoing chemotherapy.

◊ **INSTRUCTIONS:** Drink with meal and as soon as possible after blending to avoid settling of dissolved ingredients. Take the packet of pills at mealtime and in divided dosages. If you are taking 3 packets of pills per day, then take 1 packet at each meal. If you are taking only 1 packet of pills, then divide the pills out over the course of the 3 meals.

CHAPTER 2

✰
ACCESSORY FACTORS:

GARLIC, COENZYME Q, GLANDULARS, ENZYMES, PROBIOTICS, LIPOIC ACID, MSM, LYCOPENE, ELLAGIC ACID, QUERCETIN, CARNITINE

The following list of ingredients in ImmunoPower is complete. The list of scientific references to support the use of that ingredient is only representative of the peer-reviewed data used to develop ImmunoPower. This book does not provide a complete review of the literature on any particular ingredient; but merely good examples. Each ingredient in ImmunoPower is included for one or more of the following reasons:

⇒ **1) Reverse the malnutrition** that is common among many Americans, especially cancer patients. Over 40% of cancer patients actually die from malnutrition.
⇒ **2) Reduce the toxic side effects** of chemotherapy and radiation, while enhancing the tumor-killing capacity of these medical therapies.
⇒ **3) Bolster immune functions** to help recognize and destroy cancer cells.
⇒ **4) Help to regulate blood sugar** levels. Sugar feeds cancer. By lowering and stabilizing blood sugar levels while reducing circulating insulin, the cancer patient can help to deprive the cancer of its primary fuel.
⇒ **5) Using nutrients as "biological response modifiers"** to help the body reverse the cancer process. More on this in chapter 10.

Garlic, (Kyolic, 1 capsule) 600 mg
Immune stimulant[1], detoxifying agent, antioxidant[2], powerful anti-fungal compound[3], protects[4] and rebuilds the liver[5], controls blood sugar levels, reduces the toxic effect of chemotherapy and radiation[6] on healthy cells, increases energy.

First mentioned as a medicine about 6000 years ago, garlic has been a major player in human medicines throughout the world. In the tomb of the Egyptian king, Tutankhamen, were found gold ornaments and garlic bulbs. Slaves who built the Great Pyramids relied heavily on the energizing power of garlic for their work. Hippocrates, father of

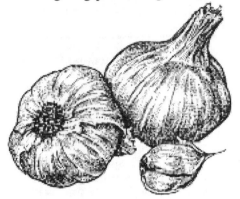

modern medicine, used garlic to heal infections and reduce pain. Although garlic has been a medical staple of many societies for over 4000 years, only in the past few decades when over 2000 scientific studies have proven its healing value, has garlic received the respect and attention that it deserves.

Garlic grown on selenium-rich soil, such as found in ImmunoPower, may be directly toxic to tumor cells.[7]

ImmunoPower contains aged-deodorized garlic from Kyolic, which has unique properties not found in other garlic supplements. Garlic may be able to impact the cancer process[8] by inhibiting:

◊ carcinogen formation in the body (i.e. nitrosamines)
◊ the transformation of normal cells to pre-cancerous cells[9]
◊ the promotion of pre-cancerous cells to cancer[10]
◊ spreading (metastasis) of cancer cells to the surface of blood vessels
◊ formation of blood vessels in tumor mass, i.e. anti-angiogenesis

The debate continues regarding the active ingredients in garlic, but they may include amino acids (like the branched chain amino acids of leucine and isoleucine), S-allyl cysteine, allicin, and organically-bound selenium. In a double blind trial in humans with high serum cholesterol, aged deodorized garlic with no allicin content was able to lower serum cholesterol by 7%.[11] While garlic, in general as either aged, fresh, cooked or in supplement form, is a healthy addition to anyone's nutrition program; aged garlic extracts were effective at protecting animals from liver damage.[12] An extensive review of the literature on garlic and its influence on the cancer process shows the impressive and multiple ways that garlic can help the cancer patient.[13] In a Chinese study, people who ate more garlic had a 60% reduction in the risk for stomach cancer.[14]

Aged garlic was effective at preventing the initiation and promotion phase of esophageal cancer in animals.[15] In one animal study, garlic was more effective against bladder cancer than the drug of choice in human bladder cancer, BCG (bacillus Calmette-Guerin).[16] Garlic grown on selenium-rich soil was more effective than selenium supplements at inhibiting carcinogen-induced tumors in animals.[17] A study published in the Journal of the National Medical Association referred to garlic as "...a potent, non-specific biologic response modifier."[18] Garlic protects against the DNA-damaging potential of DMBA[19] and the liver carcinogen, aflatoxin.[20] Stimulates immune functions by activating macrophages and spleen cells.[21] Enhances Natural Killer cell activity.[22]

> **Probiotics (friendly bacteria), 1.5 billion active bacteria (Lactobacillus acidophilus, Bifido bifidum and Bifido longum) per capsule**
> Reduces Candida overgrowth in the intestines, assists in immune regulation and detoxification via the colon.

It was the Nobel laureate from Russia, Dr. Eli Metchnikoff, who told us at the turn of the century: "Death begins in the colon." Metchnikoff isolated the bacteria in yogurt, Lactobacillus, that ferments milk sugar and spent much of his illustrious career shedding light on the function of bacteria in the gut.

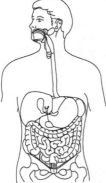

In order to better appreciate the importance of probiotics for cancer patients, we need to rewind the video cassette recorder to Louis Pasteur's deathbed confession in 1895: "I have been wrong. The germ is nothing. The terrain is everything." Pasteur was the famous French chemist who developed pasteurization, or the killing of bacteria with heat. Pasteur spent much of his life trying to figure out how to kill all the bacteria in the universe. Didn't work. By "terrain", Pasteur was referring to the land that bacteria grow on--your body. We now find that some bacteria are helpful, such as those which manufacture biotin and vitamin K in the gut. Many bacteria are relatively harmless, unless we have compromised immune functions. Many bacterial infections are called "opportunistic" because they only happen when the bacteria seizes the opportunity while the host is weakened. Many bacteria in the gut can produce carcinogens and estrogens, to further a cancer process.[23] To finally give long overdue respect to an important area of human nutrition, the classical textbook MODERN NUTRITION IN HEALTH AND DISEASE now contains a chapter on intestinal microflora.[24]

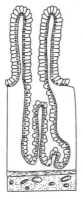

Oncologists have toiled for 3 decades trying to isolate cancer patients from all external bacteria, since death from infections is so common in cancer patients, especially those treated with chemotherapy. Oncologist working in bone marrow transplant (BMT) units will isolate cancer patients from family members and tell the patient to avoid fruits and vegetables, hoping to prevent an infection in the immune-compromised patient. Some BMT units would even autoclave the food to try to reduce exposure to bacteria. Meanwhile, we have more bacteria in our gut than all the cells in our body. There is an ongoing struggle in your gut between bifidobacteria (good guys) and putrefactive bacteria and yeast (bad guys). The typical American diet of too much fat, sugar, beef and not enough whole grains, fruits, and vegetables will often create a very lethal mixture of bacteria and yeast in the gut. One pound of fecal matter contains over 50 billion bacteria.

What happens in too many cancer patients is that the infection comes from the inside, called bacterial translocation, not from the outside.[25] Only one of three factors needs to be present for disease-causing bacteria from the intestines to slide through the intestinal wall and create a life-threatening infection in the blood (sepsis):

⇒ Disruption of the ecological balance of the normal intestinal microflora, resulting in overgrowth of certain harmful bacteria or yeast

⇒ Impairment of host immune functions

⇒ Physical disruption of the gut mucosal barrier.

Over 40% of our immune system is clustered around the gastro-intestinal tract. Lymph nodes sit on the intestinal wall like international border guards, keeping dangerous bacteria inside the gut from migrating into the bloodstream. Friendly bacteria in the human gut can decompose undigestible plant matter into butyric acid, a potent anti-cancer agent.

Probiotics include a wide assortment of favorable bacteria, including Lactobacillus acidophilus from yogurt. When comparing the dietary habits of 1000 women with and 1000 women without breast cancer, yogurt was found to be the most protective of all foods analyzed.[26] Yogurt also helped to prevent the normal intestinal side effects caused by radiation therapy in women undergoing radiation for ovarian and cervical cancer.[27] There are soil-based organisms that are equally intriguing as means of rectifying an imbalanced collection of bacteria in the human gut.

When friendly bacteria are killed, usually by antibiotics, then unfriendly yeast can take over. There is an epidemic of yeast, or Candida, infections in this country.[28] Based upon copious intake of unnecessary antibiotics (which wipe out the friendly competitive bacteria), and the excessive consumption of sugar (which feeds the unfriendly yeast), and the prevalence of toxins (which allow the yeast to mutate beyond the friendly stage), and the lack of probiotics in the American diet; yeast is taking a mighty toll on our health. I have worked closely with many cancer patients who suffer blatant yeast infections, including thrush (yeast overgrowth in the mouth) and stomach bloating. Probiotics help to re-establish the normal environment in the gut and to compete with the yeast that can become lethal. When yeast are allowed to thrive, they generate by-products, like alcohol and acetyaldehyde, which cause fatigue, immune problems, nerve and muscle dysfunctions and more.

Probiotics may help the cancer patient via:

➢ Regularity. A healthy gut is more likely to offer regular elimination of waste products, which is one of the more important routes of detoxification in the human body. When the liver is trying to neutralize dead cancer cells, they are ejected from the body via the gallbladder and intestines to go out with the feces. If the cancer patient gets constipated, then a bad situation becomes worse.

➢ Compete with yeast. Candida overgrowth can become the final burden on the cancer patient's immune system that allows the cancer to win. Probiotics help to keep Candida in check.

➢ Regulating immune functions. When unhealthy bacteria and yeast are allowed to attach to the microvilli in the intestines, then allergic reactions, autoimmune problems, and general distractions for the immune system take place. By occupying the "parking spaces" along the intestinal microvilli, probiotics help to keep the castle moat in place.

Mixed Digestive Enzymes, 520 mg
    Improves digestion, reduces nausea.

Without enzymes, life would be impossible. **Enzymes** are organic catalysts that speed up the rate of a biochemical reaction. Enzymes either put things together, called conjugases, or take things apart, called hydrolases. There are literally millions of enzymes produced by your body each second. Without hydrolase enzymes in your gut, the digestion of food could not occur. Our body makes digestive enzymes to break down large food particles into usable molecules:
◆ proteins are digested into amino acids by the action of proteases
◆ starches are digested into simple sugars by the action of amylase
◆ fats are digested into fatty acids and glycerol by the action of lipase.
    Our ancestors ate a diet high in uncooked foods. Cooking food denatures enzymes, like changing the white on an egg from waxey to white when it is cooked. All living tissue contains an abundance of hydrolase enzymes as part of the lysosomes, or "suicide bags", which are there to mop up cellular debris and destroy invading organisms. When our ancestors ate this diet high in uncooked food, they were receiving a regular infusion of "enzyme therapy" as a lucky by-product. These hydrolytic enzymes would help to digest the food, and about 10% of the unused enzymes would end up crossing through the intestinal wall into the blood stream.
    It is clear that people who are undernourished without being malnourished live a longer and healthier life. Why this occurs is less obvious. Many good European studies support the use of digestive enzymes as a critical component of cancer treatment. Your mouth, stomach and intestines will make a certain amount of enzymes to digest your food into smaller molecules for absorption through the intestinal wall into the bloodstream.

Enzymes absorbed into the bloodstream help to:
❖ break up immune complexes
❖ expose tumors to immune attack
❖ assist in cell differentiation.

People who eat less food may live longer because they are able to absorb a certain percentage of their unused digestive enzymes, which then have many therapeutic benefits. Indeed, as far back as 1934, an Austrian researcher, Dr. E. Freund found that cancer patients do not have the "solubilizing" tumor-destroying enzymes in their blood that normal healthy people have.

One of the founders of alternative cancer treatment, Donald Kelley, DDS, felt that cancer was caused by a deficiency of digestive enzyme production, just as diabetes is caused by a deficiency of insulin production. Both the diabetic and cancer patient have some genetic predisposition that makes he or she vulnerable to the disease. The symptoms of diabetes and cancer may be controlled with proper lifestyle, but the underlying genetic vulnerability will never go away. This enzyme theory may help to explain why the vast majority of cancer patients are older people, who have demonstrated a reduced output of digestive enzymes; and also explains why raw foods, which are high in hydrolytic enzymes, may sometimes help cancer patients.

There is twenty years of good research from Europe showing that enzyme therapy helps many types of cancer patients. Digestive enzymes absorbed into the bloodstream can:

* reduce tumor growth and metastasis in experimental animals.[29]
* prevent radon-induced lung cancer in miners.[30]
* improve 5 year survival in breast cancer patients. Stage I at 91%, stage II at 75% and stage III at 50%.[31]
* bromelain (enzyme from pineapple) inhibited leukemic cell growth and induced human leukemia cells in culture to revert back to normal (cytodifferentiation).[32]
* reduce the complications of cancer, such as cachexia (weight loss), pain in joints, and depression.
* reduced the secondary infections that result from certain chemo and radiation methods, especially bleomycin-induced pneumotoxicity.[33]

Digestive enzymes are included in ImmunoPower primarily to assist in digestion. Many cancer patients have problems with nausea, gas, bloating, constipation, or diarrhea. Enzymes can help break up foods before unfriendly fermentative bacteria can do so. Enzymes can help prevent the sense of fullness and nausea that many cancer patients experience. If some of these digestive enzymes are absorbed into the bloodstream and help in the immune attack on the cancer, then all the better. But the main goal of including these enzymes is to encourage healthy digestion and to prevent or reduce nausea.

Lipoic acid 33 mg

Alpha lipoic acid (a.k.a. thioctic acid) is involved in energy metabolism, but also works as a potent antioxidant, regulator of blood sugar metabolism, chelator (remover) of heavy metals, improves memory, discourages the growth of cancer, prevents glycation (sugar binding to cell membranes) that can change the flexibility of cell membranes and blood vessels.

Lipoic acid works with pyruvate and acetyl CoA in a critical point in energy metabolism.[34] Partly because of this pivotal job in generating ATP, lipoic acid becomes an incredibly multi-talented nutrient. Though lipoic acid is not considered an essential nutrient yet, as humans age we produce less and less of lipoic acid internally.[35] Because of its unique size and chemical structure, lipoic acid works as an antioxidant that can penetrate both fat soluble (like vitamin E) and water soluble (like vitamin C) portions of the body.[36] This gives lipoic acid access to virtually the entire body, whereas most antioxidants only protect isolated areas of the body.

Lipoic acid prevents "glycation" or glycosylation, which means the binding of sugar molecules to important proteins in the bloodstream, cell membrane, nerve tissue, etc. Glycation is a disastrous "tanning" that occurs, not unlike turning soft cow skin into hard leather in the tanning process. These new proteins that are bound to sugars do not have the same abilities as before the glycation process. Supplements of lipoic acid have been found to reverse the peripheral neuropathy from diabetes in as little as 3 weeks.[37] Lipoic acid improves blood flow to the nerves, which then improves nerve conduction.[38] Many cancer patients suffer peripheral neuropathy as a by-product of the damaging effects of chemotherapy. Lipoic acid may prevent and reverse this destruction of nerve tissue. Because of its role in aerobic metabolism, lipoic acid supplements in animals provided an increase in the amount of oxygen reaching the heart by 72% and the liver by 128%. Since cancer is an anaerobic growth, enhancing aerobic metabolism in a cancer patient is like shining daylight on a vampire.

Lipoic acid increases the available levels of other antioxidants in the body, like vitamin E[39] and glutathione.[40] While there are many antioxidants found in a healthy diet and produced in the body (like uric acid), lipoic acid is the only antioxidant that meets the "wish list" of Dr. Lester Packer of the University of California at Berkeley. That "perfect" antioxidant should:

⇒ neutralize free radicals
⇒ be rapidly absorbed and quickly utilized by the body cells
⇒ be able to enhance the action of other antioxidants
⇒ be concentrated both inside and outside cells and cell membranes
⇒ promote normal gene expression
⇒ chelate metal ions, or drag toxic minerals out of the body.[41]

Because of its role as an antixoxidant and the critical need for immune cells to be protected from their own cellular poisons, lipoic acid has been shown to improve antibody response in immunosuppressed animals.[42]

Lipoic acid also works to improve the efficiency of insulin by allowing blood glucose into the cells. Animal studies showed that supplements of lipoic acid increased insulin sensitivity by 30-50% and reduced plasma insulin and free fatty acids by 15-17%.[43]

SAFETY ISSUES. In over 30 years of extensive use and testing in European clinical trials there have been no serious side effects reported from the use of lipoic acid.

Lycopene 3 mg
    Potent antioxidant and immune stimulant.

Lycopenes are one of the most potent antioxidants yet tested, having double the protective capacity of betacarotene.[44] Lycopenes are reddish pigments from the carotenoid family. Most fruits and vegetables

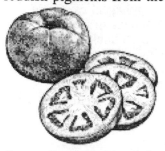

contain little to no lycopenes. Tomatoes are the richest source of lycopenes, with watermelon, and red grapefruit containing appreciable amounts of lycopenes.[45] 100 grams of raw tomatoes, or about 1 cup, contains about 3 milligrams of lycopenes. Lycopenes made headlines around the world, and cheers in many college dorms, in December of 1995 when a scientific study published in the Journal of the National Cancer Institute found that men who ate more PIZZA experienced less prostate cancer.[46] Pizza is obviously not a "nutrient dense" healthy food with all the fat, difficult-to-digest cheese and white flour. Yet lycopenes from tomatoes are such potent antioxidants, immune stimulants and regulators of cancer gene expression; that a little tomato sauce on the pizza could neutralize the otherwise unhealthy meal of pizza and offer significant protection against the second most common cancer in American men.

As little as one serving per week of tomatoes could reduce esophageal cancer risk by 40% and other sites by 50%.[47] In another study, blood samples from 25,000 people were frozen for 15 years. Of the people in this study who developed cancer, those with the highest levels of lycopenes had the lowest incidence of pancreatic cancer.[48]

Ellagic acid, 100 mg
    Potent antioxidant, protects DNA against potential harm, potent detoxifier, protects healthy cells against radiation damage, helps to deter the growth of pathogenic bacteria, helps to induce "suicide" or apoptosis in cancer cells.

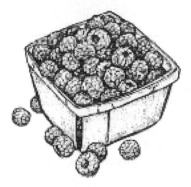

One of my few "sound bite" dietary recommendations for all cancer patients is to: "Go for the color." In the 20,000 bioflavonoids and 800 different carotenoids found in richly pigmented fruits and vegetables lie a myriad of potent anti-cancer compounds. Ellagic acid is one of the colorful phytochemicals found in strawberries, grapes, blueberries, raspberries, blackberries and boysenberries.

Ellagic acid may be able to help cancer patients:

➤ Protects DNA. Since cancer patients have demonstrated a genetic vulnerability toward cancer, and since radiation and chemo both can induce further DNA damage to cause secondary malignancies, it is encouraging to note that ellagic acid exhibits anti-mutagenic and anti-carcinogenic activity both in vitro and in vivo in a wide range of toxins tested.[49]

➤ Anti-cancer. Ellagic acid was able to inhibit esophageal cancer in animals exposed to carcinogens.[50] Ellagic acid binds to DNA to protect from methylating carcinogens, while also inducing critical Phase II detoxification enzymes, thus explaining some of its anti-cancer activity.[51] Ellagic acid may defuse cancer through gene expression, perhaps apoptosis, or programmed cell death.[52]

➤ Radio-protective. In animals given oral ellagic acid, curcumin, vitamin E, and bixin (antioxidant) then exposed to whole body radiation, there was a significant reduction in abnormal blood cells (micronucleated polychromatic erythrocytes).[53]

➤ Antioxidant. In animal studies measuring fetal damage from toxins and protection against prooxidants, ellagic acid was superior to vitamin E succinate.[54]

➤ Detoxifier. Ellagic acid protected cells in culture from the normally disastrous exposure to a potent carcinogen, aflatoxin B.[55] Ellagic acid protected animals exposed to carbon tetrachloride from the liver damage (fibrosis) that usually follows.[56] In animal studies, ellagic acid was able to block the malformations caused by cocaine exposure in utero.[57]

➤ Heart protector. When animals were exposed to excess epinephrine to cause heart problems (neoepinephrine myocarditis), ellagic acid was able to restore normal functions to the disturbed heart.[58] Since many chemo drugs can damage the heart, ellagic acid may help protect the heart.

➤ Anti-bacterial activity. Ellagic acid killed the Helicobacter pylori from peptic ulcer patients in vitro.[59]

Quercetin 167 mg
   Bioflavonoid with unique immune stimulating and anti-neoplastic activity.

While a review paper from 1983 estimated that about 500 varieties of bioflavonoids existed in nature[60], more current estimates go as high as 20,000 different bioflavonoid compounds. Bioflavonoids are basically accessory factors used by plants to assist in photosynthesis and reduce the damaging effects from the sun. Best sources of bioflavonoids are citrus, berries, onions, parsley, legumes, green tea and bee pollen. The average Western diet contains somewhere between 150 mg/day[61] and 1000 mg/day[62] of bioflavonoids, with about 25 mg/day of quercetin. Best source of quercetin is the white rind in citrus fruits. Of all the nutrition factors discussed in this book, only a few, including quercetin, have shown the potential to revert a cancerous cell back to a normal healthy cell, called prodifferentiation.[63]

Quercetin has many talents that may help the cancer patient:[64]

◊ Induces apoptosis, or programmed cell death in otherwise "immortal" cancer cells

◊ Inhibits inflammation, by reducing histamine release

◊ Inhibits tumor cell proliferation

◊ Competes with estrogen for binding sites, thus defusing the damaging effects of estrogen

◊ Helps to inhibit drug resistance in tumor cells[65]

◊ Potent antioxidant

◊ May inhibit angiogenesis (making of blood vessels from the tumor)

◊ Inhibits capillary fragility which protects connective tissue against breakdown by tumors

◊ Has anti-viral activity

◊ Reduces the "stickiness" of cells, or aggregation, thus slowing cancer metastasis

◊ Reduces the toxicity and carcinogenic capacity of substances in the body[66] YET at the same time may enhance the tumor killing capacity of cisplatin[67]

◊ Helps to eliminate toxic metals through chelation[68]

◊ Increases the anti-neoplastic activity of hyperthermia (heat therapy) on cancer cells

◊ May revert cancer cells back to normal cells (prodifferentiation), possibly by repairing the defective energy mechanism in the cancer cells[69]

Quercetin has taught scientists a great lesson. "In vitro", literally "in glass", means doing an experiment on cells growing in a Petri dish or test tube. There are certain merits in doing in vitro studies, including ease and cost. Most chemotherapy drugs originated by "passing" the in vitro test for killing cancer cells in culture. The "gold standard" for the National Cancer Institute is the in vitro test. Since few nutrition factors kill cancer cells on contact and none of them are patentable, research on nutrition factors at the NCI has been disappointing. Quercetin was considered a possible carcinogen based upon the Ames in vitro test in 1977, since it caused mutagenic changes to cells. Yet, new studies show that quercetin is not a carcinogen, but may be one of the most potent anticarcinogens in nature.[70]

Another area of debate surrounding quercetin is bioavailability. One study gave a 4 gram oral dose once of quercetin to 6 healthy volunteers, then measured for quercetin in the blood. No quercetin could be found in the blood or urine and 53% of the dose ended up in the stools, giving suspicions that quercetin is not well absorbed from the diet.[71] However, since then many studies giving oral doses of quercetin to animals and humans have found major therapeutic benefits, indicating that it is somehow absorbed into the bloodstream, according to world reknowned experts in the field, Elliott Middleton, MD and Chithan

Kandaswami, PhD. Quercetin may travel through the bloodstream as a similar structure molecule (called an analog), making it difficult to detect in bioavailability studies.

In animals fed 5% of their diet as quercetin, there was a 50% reduction in the incidence of tumors after exposure to carcinogens, while animals fed 2% quercetin had a 25% reduction in tumor incidence.[72] Quercetin has been shown to inhibit estrogen dependent tumors by occupying the critical estrogen receptor sites on the tumor cell membranes.[73] Quercetin, at relatively low concentration, has been shown to inhibit the proliferation of squamous cancer cells.[74] Quercetin and other bioflavonoids have shown the ability to inhibit metastasis in cultured cells.[75] Quercetin significantly increased the tumor kill rate of hyperthermia (heat therapy) in cultured cancer cells.[76] Head and neck squamous cancers in humans are resistant to most medical therapies and have a high rate of tumor recurrence. Quercetin was selectively toxic in both in vitro and in vivo head and neck cancers in a dose dependent fashion.[77]

One problem for cancer patients can be inflammation, or swelling of tissue. This is a crucial "tightrope walk", in which you want a certain amount of alarm in the immune system, which creates dumping of free radicals and swelling; yet you don't want too much of this or it creates weakness, pain, discomfort, and tissue wasting. Rigdon Lentz, MD is a pioneering oncologist who has developed and patented a device for filtering the factors in the blood of cancer patients (Tumor Necrosis Factor inhibitors) that prevent the immune system from attacking the tumor. Dr. Lentz finds that he must provide a gradual attack on the tumor, or else swelling and tumor lysis (bursting of cancer cells) can actually kill the cancer patient with toxic by-products. Quercetin can help reduce swelling by helping to produce anti-inflammatory prostaglandins.[78] Quercetin inhibits the release of histamine from mast cells, thus reducing allergic reactions.[79] Quercetin also helps to stabilize cell membranes, decrease lipid peroxidation and inhibit the breakdown of connective tissue (collagen) by hyaluronidase (one of the ways that cancer spreads).[80]

SAFETY ISSUES. There has been no demonstrated toxicity of quercetin in humans or animals.

L-carnitine 100 mg
Involved in energy metabolism of fats, thus preventing fatty buildup in heart and liver and encouraging the complete combustion of fats for energy. Cancer cells are less likely to use fat for energy.

Think of carnitine as the "shoveller throwing fresh coals into the furnace" of the cell's mitochondria. Carnitine was first isolated from meat extracts in 1905, hence the "carnitine", refers to animal sources. Indeed, there is virtually no carnitine in plant foods, with red meats having the highest carnitine content.[81] The typical American diet provides from 5-100 mg/day of carnitine. Humans can manufacture carnitine in the liver and kidney from the precursors (raw materials to make) of lysine and methionine, and the cofactors of vitamin C, niacin, B-6 and iron. A deficiency of any of these precursors may lead to a carnitine deficiency, which involves buildup of fats in the blood, liver and muscles and may lead to symptoms of weakness. Since infants require carnitine in their diet and other individuals have been found to have clinical carnitine

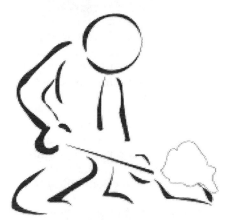

deficiencies, some nutritionists have lobbied to have carnitine included as an essential nutrient, not unlike niacin.[82]

Carnitine may help the cancer patient by:

◊ protecting the liver from fatty buildup[83]

◊ improving energy and endurance[84]

◊ protecting the heart against the damaging effects of adriamycin.[85]

◊ In cultured cells, carnitine supplements provided for bolstering of immune functions

(polymorphonuclear chemotaxis) and reduced the ability of fats to lower immune functions.[86]

Carnitine is probably essential in the diet for people who are very young, or sick, stressed, older, burdened with toxins, etc.

Methyl Sulfonyl Methane (MSM), 250 mg

Provides the crucial mineral sulfur for various reactions, including detoxification, cell membrane stability, immune functions, bowel regularity, blood glucose regulation, fortifying connective tissue against tumor invasion.

Sulfur is one of the most important yet ignored minerals in human nutrition. While the average human body has 6 times more sulfur than magnesium, most nutrition textbooks only give brief and passing reference to sulfur.[87] Sulfur is your "steel rebar" in structural proteins in the body, which is why there is more sulfur in a meat eater's diet of flesh than a vegetarian diet. Sulfur is also a crucial mineral for detoxification and improving cell membrane permeability. Most agri-businesses ignore the need to fertilize the soil with sulfur, hence each time we harvest the crops, we have progressively less sulfur in our food supply. The sulfur provided in ImmunoPower is Methylsulfonylmethane, or MSM, which is an organically bound form of sulfur. Inorganic forms of sulfur, such as the preservative sulfites found in dried fruit and wine can be harmful and do not contribute to the body's need for organically bound sulfur.

DMSO, or dimethylsulfoxide, is one of the more riveting chapters in 20th century healthcare. It all started in the 1950s and 60s when workers in paper mill plants in the Pacific Northwest noticed that their health began to deteriorate when they took a 2 week vacation from work. Coming back to work, these men would dip their hands into the solvent, DMSO, that was produced as a by-product from processing trees into paper. The DMSO seemed to have life-giving properties, which attracted the attention of a Harvard-trained surgeon, Dr. Stanley Jacob and a chemist Robert Herschler at the University of Oregon Medical School.[88] Jacob found that DMSO provided an ideal substance for preservation of organs during transplant procedures. DMSO is still the substance of choice for preserving bone marrow tissue in cancer patients undergoing bone marrow transplantation. In spite of its safety, low cost, and great potential health benefits, DMSO was considered an unapproved drug by the FDA, which only allows its use in interstitial cystitis. Meanwhile, other advanced countries around the world have allowed DMSO to be used widely. Horse breeders can't do without the healing benefits of DMSO on sore muscles and joints for the horses. DMSO is one of the most amazing substances and solvents on earth, since it dissolves water soluble and fat soluble substances with ease and transports many different compounds across the human skin membrane when applied topically. The DMSO story reads like a fascinating and frustrating mix of Watergate and the Marx Brothers.

However, DMSO is an integral part of the food chain. Algae and phytoplankton in the ocean and ponds everywhere take in inorganic sulfur and release a volatile vapor, dimethyl sulfide, which rises in the atmosphere and is converted into DMSO by the action of the sun's ultra-violet light. Add an oxygen atom to DMSO and you have DMSO2, which is MSM.[89] These sulfur-bearing compounds then mix with rain clouds and scatter over the world to provide organic sulfur for plants. On an ecological note, sulfites and sulfates from cars and factories can react in the atmosphere to form sulfuric acid, which makes acid rain that has been devastating forests around the world.

MSM is found in small amounts in fresh plant foods, but is easily lost in storage, cooking, and processing. Hence, most of us get very little MSM in the diet. MSM has the health advantages of DMSO without giving the user the characteristic "garlic breath" that is almost immediately apparent when rubbing DMSO on the skin. MSM is very safe, since it is found in small amounts in fresh produce and is, therefore, either used or excreted by the body. Since MSM is a patented compound, it is referred to in scientific literature as "polar solvents" or "dimethyl sulfone".

Sulfur is a critical ingredient in some of the healthiest foods on earth: garlic, beans, eggs, cabbage, broccoli, and red peppers. Sulfur used to be called "brimstone", and was a threat of sorts from the "fire and brimstone" preachers of old. Flowers of sulfur is a yellow powder that our grandparents would sometimes sprinkle in their shoes to help ward off rheumatoid arthritis. Now we use glucosamine sulfate or DMSO, both contributors of sulfur to our connective tissue, to help people with arthritis. The list of nutrients which contain sulfur is a "who's who" of super nutrients: glutathione, cysteine, taurine, glucosamine, homocysteine, lipoic acid, and Coenzyme A. Sulfur has long been the favorite of organic gardeners to prevent bug and fungal infestation in the garden without harming the human who eats the produce.

MSM may help cancer patients in the following ways:

➤ Cancer protection. In animals bred with a tendency for breast cancer, MSM was able to delay the onset of breast cancer after exposure to a carcinogen by 100-130 days compared to the control group.[90] This 100 days in mouse life is comparable to 10 years in human life. MSM provided similar benefits in animal studies on colon cancer.[91]

➤ Detoxification. Sulfur-bearing amino acids, including methionine, cysteine, and the tripeptide glutathione, all have the unique ability to grab heavy metals and other toxins and escort them from the body.

➤ Blood glucose regulation. Insulin contains several sulfur atoms to give it a unique three dimensional shape and function in regulating blood glucose. People who are deficient in sulfur will probably develop diabetic-like symptoms.

➤ Protective barrier. Since sulfur provides the strong bonds in structural proteins, like muscle, tendons, and hair; a low intake of sulfur may make the cell membranes more vulnerable to cancer cell invasion.

➤ Regular bowel movements. According to the "grandfather" of DMSO, Dr. Stanley Jacobs, MSM seems to induce regularity and treat constipation without side effects.[92]

➤ Immune regulation. There is some evidence that DMSO and its metabolite, dimethyl sulfone, may help to downregulate an over reactive immune system in autoimmune diseases.[93]

➤ Parasite protection. Sulfur creates a barrier that makes worms, yeast, and bacteria slide right out of the body.

➤ Membrane fluidity. Since sulfur is a crucial component of every cell membrane in every form of life on earth, some experts have speculated that low intake of sulfur can lead to defective cell membrane functions. Cell membranes are the "gate keepers", with the assignment of expelling toxins and bringing in essential nutrients. If the cell membrane fails in either the intake or output processes, we can have a cell that begins to distance itself from the normal processes of life and become a cancer cell.

Coenzyme Q-10, 100 mg
Improves aerobic metabolism, immune stimulant, membrane stabilizer, improves prostaglandin metabolism.

CoQ is found in the energy transport system of mammals, specifically the mitochondrial membrane. Dr. Peter Mitchell was awarded the Nobel prize for his work in 1975 on CoQ. CoQ is nearly a wonder drug in reversing cardiomyopathy.[94] CoQ is either manufactured in the human body from the amino acid tyrosine and mevalonate or consumed in the diet, with heart and liver tissue being particularly rich in CoQ-10 for humans. Hence, CoQ, along with carnitine, EPA and other nutrition factors are considered "conditionally essential nutrients", since we may not be able to manufacture enough of these nutrients at certain phases of the life cycle. Niacin is an essential vitamin that also is produced within the body (endogenous source) and consumed in the diet (exogenous sources). CoQ is also called ubiquinone, since various forms of this molecule are found everywhere, as in ubiquitous. CoQ may help cancer patients by:

◊   correcting CoQ deficiency states[95], since we don't eat liver or heart and lose the capacity to make CoQ within as we age
◊   radical scavenger (antioxidant) that works with vitamin E in the fat soluble portions of the body and cells[96]
◊   stabilizes cell membranes through interaction with phospholipids[97]
◊   correction of mitochondrial "leak" of electrons during oxidative respiration, which improves aerobic production of ATP[98]
◊   improving prostaglandin metabolism[99]
◊   stabilizing calcium dependent channels on cell membrane receptor sites[100]

CoQ may enhance immune functions.[101] CoQ reduces the damage to the heart (probably by sparing mitochondrial membranes) from the chemotherapy drug adriamycin.[102] Long term users of adriamycin risk cardiac arrest, unless given adequate CoQ, vitamin E, niacin and other nutrients to reduce the damage to the heart. Using 300 mg daily of CoQ as sole therapy, 6 of 32 breast cancer patients (19%) experienced partial tumor regression, while one woman took 390 mg daily and gained complete remission.[103] Given the fact that CoQ probably becomes an essential nutrient as we age and become ill, there is good reasons to include CoQ in ImmunoPower. Best absorbed in the presence of fats, which are found in ImmunoPower from lecithin, fish, shark, and borage oils.

Glandulars

Glandular therapy has been practiced, at least inadvertently, since the dawn of mankind. In the seminal book, NUTRITION AND PHYSICAL DEGENERATION by Weston Price, DDS, he found that Native Americans in the cold regions of northern Canada avoided scurvy in the winter by first eating the raw adrenal gland from any animal captured. Adrenal glands provide the most concentrated depot of vitamin C in the body. Our hunter-gatherer ancestors would offer the liver and heart of the captured animal to the slayer. Liver and heart are among the organs that are rich in CoQ, carnitine, lipoic acid, trace minerals and a variety of nutrients that are missing in our diets.

Today, there are millions of people taking prescription supplements of thyroid gland from animals to bolster a failing thyroid gland. This is glandular therapy. We now use gelatin extracts (which are from connective tissue of hooves and hides) of glucosamine sulfate and chondroitan sulfate to improve connective tissue diseases, like osteo and rheumatoid arthritis. There are peptides in each gland that are specific to that gland, such as thymus and spleen, which will be targeted to that gland once consumed.

As we mature, many of our glandular functions deteriorate.[104] Although our biochemistry textbooks would have us believe that polypeptides, such as found in glandular extracts, are all hydrolyzed in the digestive processes of the gut, in fact many peptides survive this chemical gauntlet. How else do we explain the passage of Immunoglobulin A from mother's milk to bolster the newborn infant's immune system or the food proteins which pass directly into the bloodstream and trigger allergic responses? Glandular replacement therapy, such as thymus and spleen, may be essential for many people who are struggling with life threatening diseases.

Thymic concentrate 300 mg
Bolsters functions of thymus gland, which is crucial to the maturation of immune cells into T-cells.

The thymus gland in humans usually atrophies with aging. Anyone over 30 years of age probably has a thymus gland that is well below optimal in size and functional capacity. There are thymus-derived factors with hormone-like activity, called thymosins, that have long been recognized for their potential at stimulating immune functions.[105] An extract of thymus, thymosin 5, was able to stimulate immune functions in mice with induced tumors.[106] Other researchers found that thymus extract is more of an immune regulator than an immune stimulant. In human lung cancer patients receiving chemotherapy, thymus supplements provided for longer survival time.[107] Other researchers found that thymus extract (TP-1) was able to increase lymphocyte counts in incurable gastro-intestinal cancer patients treated with chemotherapy.[108] Other researchers followed over 1000 patients who had been treated with thymus extract (TFX) over the course of 15 years and found the thymus to be extremely helpful in normalizing immune panels and improving outcome in a wide variety of immune suppressive disorders.[109] Researchers at the University of California isolated a fraction of thymus (thymic protein A) which improved immune parameters in mice.[110] Probably a wide variety of subsets of peptides and glycoproteins in thymus work to improve differentiation of bone marrow (B-cells) lymphocytes into active T-cells that can recognize and destroy cancer cells.

Spleen concentrate   300 mg
Bolsters functions of the spleen gland, a storage and filtering organ for the blood and immune system.

The spleen oftentimes atrophies with aging in humans. Supplements of spleen extract have been used in conjunction with ginseng (also in ImmunoPower) as a clinically tested immune stimulant for cancer and AIDS patients in Europe.

ENDNOTES

[1] . Lau, BHS, et al., Molecular Biotherapeutics, vol.3, p.103, June 1991
[2] . Imai, J., et al., Planta Medica, p.417, 1994
[3] . Tadi, PP, et al., International Clinical Nutrition Reviews, vol.10, p.423, 1990
[4] . Nakagawa, S., et al., Phytotherapy, Research, vol.1,p.1, 1988
[5] . Horie, T., et al.; Planta Medica, vol.55, p.506, 1989
[6] . Lau, BHS, International Clinical Nutrition Reviews, vol.9, p.27, 1989
[7] . Ip, C., et al., Nutr.Cancer, vol.17, p.279, 1992
[8] . Dausch, JG, et al., Preventive Medicine, vol.19, p.346, 1990
[9] . Wargovich, MJ, et al., Cancer Letters, vol.64, p.39, 1992
[10] . Belman, S, Carcinogenesis, vol.4, p.1063, 1983
[11] . Steiner, M., et al., Amer.J.Clin.Nutr., vol.64, p.866, 1996
[12] . Nakagawa, S., et al., Phytotherapy Res., vol.1, p.1, 1988
[13] . Dausch, JG, et al., Preventive Med., vol.19, p.346, 1990
[14] . You, WC, et al., J. Nat.Cancer Inst., vol.81, p.162, 1989
[15] . Wargovich, MJ, et al., Cancer Letters, vol.64, p.39, 1992
[16] . Marsh, CL, et al., J. Urology, vol.137, p.359, Feb.1987
[17] . Ip, C., et al., Nutrition and Cancer, vol.17, no.3, p.279, 1992
[18] . Abdullah, TH, et al., J.Nat.Med.Assoc., vol.80, p.439, 1988
[19] . Amagase, H., et al., Carcinogenesis, vol.14, p.1627, 1993
[20] . Yamasaki, T., et al., Cancer Letters, vol.59, p.89, 1991
[21] . Hirao, Y., et al., Phytotherapy Research, vol.1, p.161, 1987
[22] . Abdullah, TH et al., Onkologie, vol.21, p.53, 1989
[23] . Tomomatsu, H., Food Technology, p.61, Oct.1994
[24] . Goldin, BR, et al., MODERN NUTRITION IN HEALTH AND DISEASE, Shils, ME (eds), p.569, Lea & Febiger, Philadelphia, 1994
[25] . Deitch, EA, Archives Surgery, vol.125, p.403, Mar.1990
[26] . Le, MG, et al., J.Nat.Cancer Inst., vol.77, p.633, Sept.1986
[27] . Salminen, E., et al., Clin.Radiol., vol.39, p.435, 1988
[28]. Truss, O., THE MISSING DIAGNOSIS, Missing Diagnosis, Inc., Birmingham, AL, 1983; see also Crook, WG, THE YEAST CONNECTION HANDBOOK, Professional Books, Jackson, TN 1997; see also Winderlin, C., CANDIDA-RELATED COMPLEX, Taylor Publ., Dallas, 1996
[29]. Ransberger, K, et al., Medizinische Enzymforschungsgesellschaft, International Cancer Congress, Houston 1970
[30]. Miraslav, H., et al., Advances in Antimicrobial and Antineoplastic Chemotherapy, proceedings from 7th international congress of chemotherapy, Urban & Schwarzenberg, Munchen, 1972
[31]. Rokitansky, O., Dr. Med., no.1, vol.80, p.16ff, Austria
[32]. Maurer, HR, et al., Planta Medica, vol.54, no.5, p.377, 1988
[33]. Schedler, M., et al., 15th International Cancer Congress, Hamburg, Germany, Aug.1990
[34] . Budavari, S. (eds), THE MERCK INDEX, p.1591, Merck & Co., Whitehouse Station, NJ 1996
[35] . Packer, L., et al., Free Radical Biol. Med., vol.19, p.227, 1995
[36] . Stoll, S., et al., Ann.NY Acad.Sci., vol.717, p.122, 1994
[37] . Passwater, R., LIPOIC ACID, Keats, New Canaan, CT, 1996
[38] . Nagamatsu, M., et al., Diabetes Care, vol.18, p.1160, Aug.1995
[39] . Podda, M., et al., Biochem.Biophys., Res.Commun., vol.204, p.98, 1994
[40] . Han, D., et al., Biochem.Biophys.,Res.Commun., vol.207, p.258, 1995
[41] . Ou, P., et al., Biochem.Pharmacol., vol.50, p.123, 1995
[42] . Ohmori, H., et al., Jpn.J.Pharmacol., vol.42, p.275, 1986
[43] . Jacob, S., et al., Diabetes, vol.45, p.1024, 1996
[44] . DiMascio, P., et al., Arch.Biochem.Biophysics, vol.274, p.532, 1989
[45] . Mangels, AR, et al., J.Am.Diet.Assoc., vol.93, p.284, 1993
[46] . Giovannucci, E., et al., J.Nat.Can.Inst., vol.87, p.1767, 1995
[47] . Franceschi, S., et al., Int.J.Cancer, vol.59, p.181, 1994
[48] . Comstock, GW, et al., Amer.J.Clin.Nutr., vol.53, p.260S, 1991
[49] . Loarca-Pina, G., et al., Mutation Research, vol.398, no.1, p.183, Feb.1998
[50] . Kaur, S., et al., Cancer Letters, vol.114, no.1, p.113, Mar.1997
[51] . Barch, DH, et al., Carcinogenesis, vol.17, no.2, p.265, Feb.1996
[52] . Ahn, D, et al., Carcinogenesis, vol.17, no.4, p.821, Apr.1996
[53] . Thresiamma, KC, et al., Indian J.Exp.Biol., vol.34, no.9, p.845, Sept.1996
[54] . Hassoun, EA, et al., Toxicology, vol.124, no.1, p.27, Dec.1997
[55] . Loarca-Pina, G., et al., Mutation Research, vol.360, no.1, p.15, May1996
[56] . Thresiamma, KC, Indian J.Physiol.Pharmacol., vol.40, no.4, p.363, Oct.1996
[57]. Bohn, AA, Toxicol.Letters, vol.95, no.1, p.15, Mar.1998
[58] . Iakovleva, LV, et al., Eksp.Klin.Farmakol., vol.61, no.3, p.32, May1998

[59] . Chung, JG, Microbios, vol.93, no.375, p.115, 1998
[60] . Havsteen, B., Biochem.Pharmacol., vo.32, p.1141, 1983
[61] . Murray, MT, ENCYCLOPEDIA OF NUTRITIONAL SUPPLEMENTS, p.321, Prima, Rocklin, CA 1996
[62] . Middleton, E., et al., in ADJUVANT NUTRITION IN CANCER TREATMENT, Quillin, P. (eds), p.319, Cancer Treatment Research Foundation, Arlington Heights, IL 1994
[63] . Middleton, E., et al., in ADJUVANT NUTRITION IN CANCER TREATMENT, Quillin, P. (eds), p.325, Cancer Treatment Research Foundation, Arlington Heights, IL 1994
[64] . Boik, J., CANCER & NATURAL MEDICINE, p.181, Oregon Medical Press, Princeton, MN 1995
[65] . Scambia, G., et al., Cancer Chemother. Pharmacol., vol.28, p.255, 1991
[66] . Wood, AW, et al., in PLANT FLAVONOIDS IN BIOLOGY AND MEDICINE, p.197, Cody, V. (eds), Liss, NY, 1986
[67] . Scambia, G., et al., Anticancer Drugs, vol.1, p.45, 1990
[68] . Afanasev, IB, et al., Biochem.Pharmacol., vol.38, p.1763, 1989
[69] . Suolinna, E., et al., J.Nat.Cancer Inst., vol.53, p.1515, 1974
[70] . Stavric, B., Clin.Biochem., vol.27, p.245, Aug.1994
[71] . Gugler, R., et al., Eur.J.Clin.Pharmacol., vol.9, p.229, 1975
[72] . Berma, AK, et al., Cancer Res., vol.48, p.5754, 1988
[73] . Ranelletti, FO, et al., Int.J.Cancer, vol.50, p.486, 1992
[74] . Kandaswami, C., et al., Anti-Cancer Drugs, vol.4, p.91, 1993
[75] . Bracke, ME, et al., in PLANET FLAVONOIDS IN BIOLOGY AND MEDICINE II, CELLULAR AND MEDICINAL PROPERTIES, p.219, Cody, E. (eds), Liss, NY, 1988
[76] . Kim, JH, et al., Cancer Research, vol.44, p.102, Jan.1984
[77] . Castillo, MH, et al., Amer.J.Surgery, vol.158, p.351, Oct.1989
[78] . Bauman, J., et al., Prostaglandins, vol.20, p.627, 1980
[79] . Middleton, E, et al., Arch.Allergy Appl.Immunol., vol.77, p.155, 1985
[80] . Busse, WW, et al., J.Allergy Clin.Immunol., vol.73, p.801, 1984
[81] . Bremer, J., Physiol.Rev., vol.63, p.1420, 1983
[82] . Borum, PR, et al., J.Am.Coll.Nutr., vol.5, p.177, 1986
[83] . Sachan, DS, et al., Am.J.Clin.Nutr., vol.39, p.738, 1984
[84] . Dragan, GI, et al., Physiologie, vol.25, p.231, 1987
[85] . Furitano, G, et al., Drugs Exp.Clin.Res., vol.10, p.107, 1984
[86] . DeSimone, C., et al, Acta Vitaminol. Enzymol., vol.4, p.135, 1982
[87] . Forbes, GB, in PRESENT KNOWLEDGE IN NUTRITION, p.11, International Life Sciences Institute, Washington, 1996
[88] . McGrady, P., THE PERSECUTED DRUG: THE STORY OF DMSO, Grosset & Dunlap, NY, 1979
[89] . Mindell, EL, THE MSM MIRACLE, p.10, Keats, New Canaan, 1997
[90] . McCabe, D., et al., Arch.Surg., vol.121, no.12,p.1455, Dec.1986
[91] . O'Dwyer, PJ, et al., Cancer, vol.62, no.5, p.944, Sept.1988
[92] . Jacob, SW, et al., Ann.NY.Acad.Sci., vol.441, p.13, 1983
[93] . Morton, JI, et al., Proc.Soc.Exp.Med., vol.183, no.2, p.227, Nov.1986
[94] . Langsjoen, PH, et al., Int. J. Tiss Reac, vol.12, p.163, 1990
[95] . Folkers, K, et al., International Journal of Vitamin and Nutrition Research, vol.40,p.380, 1970
[96] . Sugiyama, S, Experientia, vol.36, p.1002, 1980
[97] . Gwak, S. et al., Biochem et Biophys Acta, vol.809, p.187, 1985
[98] . Turrens, JF, Biochem J., vol.191, p.421, 1980
[99] . Ham, EA, et al., J. Biol Chem, vol.254, p.2191, 1979
[100] . Nakamura, Y, et al., Cardiovasc Res, vol.16, p.132, 1982
[101] . Folkers, K., Med Chem Res, vol.2, p.48, 1992
[102] . Folkers, K., Biomedical and Clinical Aspects of Coenzyme Q, vol.3,p.399, Elsevier Press, 1981
[103] . Lockwood, K., et al., Biochem and Biophys Res Comm, vol.199, p.1504, Mar.1994
[104] . Klatz, R., et al., STOPPING THE CLOCK, Keats, New Canaan, CT, 1996
[105] . Oats, KK, et al., TIPS, p.347, Elsevier Press, Aug.1984
[106] . Wada, A., et al., J.Nat.Cancer Institute, vol.74, no.3, p.659, Mar.1985
[107] . Chretien, PB, et al., NY Acad Sci, vol.332, p.135, 1979
[108] . Shoham, J., et al., Cancer Immunol. Immunother., vol.9, p.173, 1980
[109] . Skotnicki, AB, Med. Oncol. & Tumor Pharmacother., Vol.6, no.1, p.31, 1989
[110] . Hays, EF, et al., Clin Immun. & Immunopath., vol.33, p.381, 1984

CHAPTER 3
★
BOTANICALS

Since the dawn of time, herbs have been the primary healer for the vast majority of mankind. Women have been the "keepers of the flame" in botanical medicine. Herbs have been used throughout the ages as supplements (tinctures, tablets), poultices (applied topically), foods, and seasonings. Many have merit. None are "magic bullets". Let the healing begin.

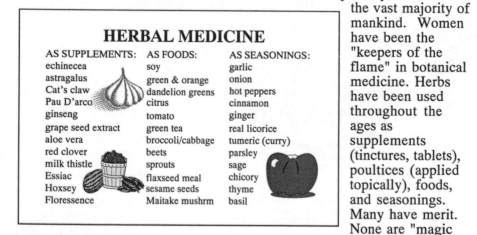

HERBAL MEDICINE

AS SUPPLEMENTS:	AS FOODS:	AS SEASONINGS:
echinecea	soy	garlic
astragalus	green & orange	onion
Cat's claw	dandelion greens	hot peppers
Pau D'arco	citrus	cinnamon
ginseng	tomato	ginger
grape seed extract	green tea	real licorice
aloe vera	broccoli/cabbage	tumeric (curry)
red clover	beets	parsley
milk thistle	sprouts	sage
Essiac	flaxseed meal	chicory
Hoxsey	sesame seeds	thyme
Floressence	Maitake mushrm	basil

Oligomeric proanthocyanidins (OPC) 50 mg
Potent antioxidant, supports vitamin C functions, penetrates the blood brain barrier, reduces capillary fragility, enhances peripheral circulation, protects DNA from damage by radiation and chemotherapy.

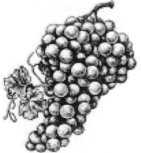

Scurvy (deficiency of vitamin C) has played a huge role in human history. Humans roamed the oceans of the world throughout the 15th through 19th century, often losing up to half of the people on board ship due to scurvy. The English physician, James Lind, discovered that limes cured scurvy in 1747 and began to wind down the death toll from scurvy, while also labelling the English sailors as "limeys". In 1930, Nobel prize winner, Albert Szent-Gyorgy, MD, PhD, isolated pure vitamin C. Ironically, the pure white crystalline vitamin C that Dr. Szent-Gyorgy isolated would not cure bleeding gums, whereas the crude brown mixture of citrus extract would. The difference between these two mixtures was "bioflavonoids", which include over 20,000 different chemical compounds that generally assist chlorophyll in photosynthesis and protect the plant from the harmful effects of the sun's radiation. The rainbow colors of fall foliage are Nature's art exhibit of bioflavonoids and carotenoids.

Some of the main categories of bioflavonoids include:

◊ anthocyanins; deep purple compounds found in black grapes, beets, red onions, and berries
◊ catechins and epigallocatechin, which are polyphenols found in apples and green tea (also included in ImmunoPower)
◊ ellagic acid (also included in ImmunoPower), a true anti-cancer compound found in cranberries, raspberries, and other berries.
◊ flavones, found in citrus fruit, red grapes and green beans
◊ flavanols, such as quercetin (also in ImmunoPower), myricetin, found in kale, spinach, onions, apples, and black tea
◊ flavanones, such as hesperidin and naringen found in citrus fruits of grapefruit, oranges and lemons.

Some of the better known bioflavonoids include rutin, which is defined in the DORLAND'S MEDICAL DICTIONARY as capable of "preventing capillary fragility." Hesperidin, quercetin (also in ImmunoPower and discussed later), pycnogenol from pine bark, and proanthocyanidins are other popular bioflavonoids. While bioflavonoids are known to be essential in the diet of insects, bioflavonoids are not yet considered essential in the human diet.

Proanthocyanidins can exist in a variety of forms, including dimers, trimers, etc.. A collective group of these proanthocyanidins are known as OPC, often referred to as grape seed extract. As the science of nutrition matures, we are finding that some of the "star" nutrients of the past may be just "supporting actors" for the real star nutrients. For instance, tocotrienols and Coenzyme Q may be more important than vitamin E in human health. Eicosapentaenoic acid (EPA from fish oil), though not considered essential, may be more important than alpha-linolenic acid (ALA from flax oil), which is considered essential. And bioflavonoids may be more important than vitamin C. OPC bound to phosphatidylcholine (lecithin) has been shown to improve absorption and cell access to OPC, which is one of the reasons why there are 4.5 grams of lecithin in a full day's supply of ImmunoPower.

Animals with implanted tumors lived longer when given anthocyanin from grape rinds.[1] Flavonoids administered in the diet of rats helped to reduce DNA damage from benzopyrene carcinogens.[2] Bioflavonoids are potent chelators, helping to eliminate toxic minerals from the system.[3] Bioflavonoids in general help to reduce allergic reactions, which create an imbalanced immune attack against cancer and infections. OPC traps lipid peroxides, hydroxyl radicals, delays the onset of lipid peroxidation, prevents iron-induced lipid peroxidation, inhibits the enzymes that can degrade connective tissue (hyaluronidase, elastase, collagenase) which then helps to prevent cancer cells from "knocking down the walls" of surrounding tissue for metastasis. Bioflavonoids may inhibit tumor promotion.[4] Bioflavonoids enhance the activity of T-lymphocytes.[5] Various flavonoids have produced striking reductions in cancer incidences in animals, sometimes up to almost total inhibition of tumorogenesis.[6]

Silymarin (milk thistle) 140 mg
Stimulates liver detoxification, may augment immune functions.

Silybum marianum, or milk thistle, is a stout annual plant that grows in dry rocky soils in parts of Europe and North America. Its seeds, fruit and leaves are widely prescribed medication in Europe for most diseases affecting the liver. Silymarin has been shown to help regenerate liver tissue, protect the liver against toxic chemicals, increase the production of glutathione (GSH) which is fundamental in the cell protecting itself against hydrogen peroxide produced.[7]

Since the liver is the primary detoxifying organ of the body and automatically becomes involved in the internal cancer battle, metastasis to the liver complicates cancer treatment. Among other functions, the liver also stores many vitamins and minerals, produces bile salts for fat digestion and absorption, and is generally one of the more versatile and essential organs in the body. For recovery from cancer to be possible, the liver must be healthy.

Echinacea (purpurea) 80 mg
Immune stimulant.

Echinacea species consist primarily of E. angustifolia, E. purpurea, and E. pallida. Native American herbalists used echinacea more than any other plant for medicinal purposes. There are over 350 scientific articles worldwide on the immune enhancing effects of echinacea, including the:
◊   activation of complement, which promotes chemotaxis of neutrophils, monocytes, and eosinophils; "gearing up" the immune cells
◊   solubilization of immune complexes
◊   neutralization of viruses.[8]

One of the components of echinacea, arabinogalactan, has shown promise as an anti-cancer agent in vitro.[9] In patients with inoperable metastatic esophageal and colorectal cancers, supplements of echinacea (as Echinacin) provided modest improvements in immune functions, slowed the growth of some tumors, and increased survival time.[10] Outpatients with advanced colorectal cancers were given echinacea as part of therapy with some patients experiencing stable disease, reduction in tumor markers, increases in survival time and no toxicity reported.[11]

Curcumin (curcuma longa) 50 mg
Potent antioxidant, protector of DNA.

Curry is an Indian spice that includes tumeric as one of the flavoring agents. The active component in tumeric appears to be a bright yellow pigment, curcumin (a.k.a.curcuma longa) which helps to enhance the immune system by protecting immune cells from their own poisons (pro-oxidants) used to kill cancer cells. Mustard is a good source of curcumin.

Curcumin appears to be a potent inhibitor of cancer.[12] In animal experiments, curcumin was shown to be directly toxic to tumor cells.[13] In a study with smokers, tumeric tablets were able to dramatically reduce the excretion of urinary mutagen levels (indicators of the possibility of cancer).[14] In patients with skin cancers (squamous cell carcinomas) who had failed therapy with chemo, radiation and surgery, supplements or ointment of tumeric were able to provide significant reduction in the smell, size, itching, pain, and exudate of the lesions.[15]

Ginkgo biloba (24% heteroside) 40 mg
Improves circulation, augments the production of healthy prostaglandin PGE-1, immune stimulant, and adaptogen (helps to regulate many cellular functions).

The ginkgo tree is one of the oldest living species on earth, having been around for over 200 million years. The ginkgo tree is an incredibly adaptable and tenacious plant. One ginkgo tree survived the near-ground zero nuclear blast in Hiroshima, Japan. Millions of these cone-shaped evergreen trees survive amidst air pollution, drought and poor soil throughout the world. A ginkgo tree may live as long as 1000 years. The leaves and berries contain a wide assortment of phytochemicals (collectively called "ginkgoflavonglycosides") that have been a pivotal medicine in China for 5000 years. There are now over 1,000 scientific studies published over the past 40 years demonstrating the medicinal value of ginkgo, with ginkgo extract becoming one of the more widely prescribed medications in Europe today. In 1989, over 100,000 physicians worldwide wrote over 10 million prescriptions for ginkgo.

There are several ways in which ginkgo may help the cancer patient:

◊ Vasodilator, expands the tiny capillaries that nourish 90% of the body's tissues, thus bringing oxygen and nutrients to the cells. In doing so, ginkgo improves depression[16] and general circulation to the organs.[17]

◊ Inhibits platelet aggregation, or the stickiness of cells. Stroke, heart attacks, and cancer metastasis are fueled by sticky cells which are generated by Platelet Activating Factor (PAF). Ginkgo inhibits PAF.[18] By modifying PAF, ginkgo helps to reduce inflammation and allergic responses.[19]

◊ Antioxidant of exceptional efficiency.[20] Slows down free radical destruction of healthy tissue, therefore protects immune cells in their semi-suicidal quest to kill cancer cells and also protects the favorable prostaglandin, PGE-1. This antioxidant activity also helps to stabilize membranes, where the lipid bi-layer is vulnerable to lipid peroxidation. This protection extends to the DNA, which is why Chernobyl workers were given ginkgo to protect them from further damage via radioactivity.

Astragalus (membranaceus) 167 mg
Adaptogen and immune stimulant.

Adaptogens are a small and elite group of herbal compounds, including garlic and ginseng, which coordinate and regulate a broad spectrum of biochemical processes, including prostaglandins, cell membranes, blood sugar levels, etc.. "Adaptogen" is the term coined in 1957 by the Russian pharmacologist I. Brekhman. Criteria for an adaptogen is that it must be:[21]
⇒ innocuous, cause minimal harm in reasonable quantities
⇒ non-specific in activity, that is, able to influence a wide range of physical, chemical and biochemical pathways in the body
⇒ a normalizer of functions; meaning that it will lower or raise a bodily measurement, depending on what needs to happen for improvement in overall health to occur, such as raising blood pressure in hypotensive individuals and lowering blood pressure in hypertensive individuals.[22]

Astragalus has also demonstrated anti-viral activity as it was able to shorten the duration and severity of the common cold in humans.[23] Researchers at M.D. Anderson Hospital in Houston found that astragalus was able to enhance the immune capacity using the cultured blood of 14 cancer patients[24] as well as augment the anti-tumor ability of Interferon-2.[25] In a study of 176 patients undergoing chemotherapy for cancers of the gastro-intestinal tract, astragalus and ginseng were able to prevent the normal immune depression and weight loss that occurs.[26] In a variety of human studies, astragalus has been shown to stimulate various parameters of the immune system, has anti-tumor activity, and inhibits the spreading (metastasis) of cancer.[27]

Panax ginseng (8%) 167 mg
Adaptogen, immune stimulant, anti-tumor activity, inhibits metastasis.[28]

Ginseng is one of the oldest, most widely used and scientifically studied of all the world's herbs. The original proponents of ginseng were Chinese physicians several thousand years ago, using it to treat nearly every conceivable ailment. Given the known "adaptogenic" qualities of ginseng, the enthusiasm of these ancient Chinese doctors may have been well placed. Ginseng is a plant species term (Panax) which is further subdivided into Panax quinquefolium (American ginseng), Panax japonicum (Japanese ginseng), Panax pseudoginseng (Himalayan ginseng) and Panax trifolium.[29] Eleutherococcus senticosus is a relative newcomer to this category, contains some ginseng-like compounds (triterpenoid saponins), but is not considered true ginseng. Panax ginseng C.A. Meyer is the Chinese or Korean ginseng used in ImmunoPower, best studied in the scientific literature and referred to in the following studies.

The wide disparity in outcome of clinical studies using ginseng probably stems from the lack of active ingredients in many substandard ginseng products sold today. Ginseng's therapeutic value comes from the 13 different triterpenoid saponins, collectively known as ginsenosides, which are found in various concentrations in various types of ginseng grown on various soils and experiencing various drying and storage techniques. While most ginseng is about 1-3% ginsenosides, the concentration in ImmunoPower is 8%. In one study published in 1979, of the 54 ginseng products analyzed, 60% were worthless and 25% had no ginseng at all![30] It is the regularly formed root from wild Panax ginseng that is the most highly prized. Nearly 60,000 people are employed in Korea for the raising and processing of ginseng.

Ginseng may help cancer patients for the following reasons:

◊ **Adaptogenic qualities**. Ginseng is nearly unsurpassed in the plant kingdom for its ability to bring about biochemical adjustments in whatever direction is necessary.

◊ **Central nervous system stimulant.**[31] In various animal and human studies, ginseng provides both calming and stimulating effects simultaneously. It allows people to better adapt to stressful situations, including cancer. It also provides for energizing effects and improvement of moods and alertness.

◊ **Blood glucose regulator**. While ginseng will lower blood glucose levels in the diabetic individual or the one fed a high sugar diet, it will not lower blood glucose in the healthy individual fed a normal diet.[32] Since cancer is a sugar feeder, keeping blood glucose levels in check is a crucial job of ginseng.

◊ **Immune-stimulating effects**. Ginseng has been shown to stimulate the reticuloendothelial system, which means getting more macrophages ("big eaters") to gobble up (phagocytosis) cancer cells and cell debris.[33] In animals, ginseng was shown to prevent viral infections.[34] Ginseng can dramatically bolster host defense mechanisms in animals and humans.

◊ **Liver cleansing, protection and stimulation**. Ginseng activates the macrophages in the liver, known as Kupffer cells, which are responsible for removing cellular debris from the body's most important detoxifying organ, the liver. Macrophages in the liver help to "take out the trash". Ginseng also helps to improve protein synthesis in the liver[35], reverse diet-induced fatty liver and protect the liver from chemically-induced damage.[36]

◊ **Anti-clotting and metastatic**. Cancer spreads by adhering to blood vessel walls. Hence reducing the stickiness, or platelet aggregation, of cells is a major plus. Ginseng reduces platelet aggregation.[37]

◊ **Anti-cancer properties**. Ginseng is a potent inhibitor of cancer in animals[38] and humans.[39] Ginseng has the unique, paradoxical and nearly miraculous ability to control cell growth, or hyperplasia. In healthy cells with adequate nourishment, ginseng encourages cell division. Yet under adverse conditions, ginseng helps to suppress abnormal cell division.[40] Ginseng helps to repair damaged DNA.[41]

In tumor bearing mice, 8 days of ginseng administration brought about a 75% reduction in average tumor size.[42] Oral administration of ginseng in tumor bearing mice inhibited the growth of liver cancer (solid ascites hepatoma), while inhibiting metastasis to the lungs.[43] Panax ginseng was able to enhance the uptake of mitomycin (an antibiotic and anti-cancer drug) into the cancer cells for increased tumor kill.[44] Ginseng was able to slow tumor growth and improve survival time in rats with chemically-induced liver cancer.[45]

SAFETY ISSUES
Ginseng and estrogen.

Of the 77 ingredients in ImmunoPower, 2 of them contain estrogen-like compounds: soy and ginseng, which merit a special discussion. There is some controversy in the scientific community regarding the use of estrogen-like compounds in the treatment of breast or ovarian cancer patients.

First, it is critical to set the records straight regarding the importance of estrogen. Estrogen is an essential hormone produced by women throughout their menstruating years as part of fertility. Estrogen has 260 different functions in the human body, including antioxidant, maintenance of bone structure, and protection against cardiovascular diseases. Estrogen does not cause breast or ovarian cancer, but it is a growth hormone and can accelerate the growth of anything, including hormone-dependent cancers.

There are 4 primary categories of estrogen-like compounds:

⇒ **Estrogen**, which actually refers to a family of hormones, including estradiol, estriol and estrone, manufactured in the female body for specific bodily functions.[46]

⇒ **Phytoestrogens**, which are estrogen-like compounds in plants, which have about 0.05% (1/2000) the strength of estrogen and have demonstrated beneficial effects both pre and post cancer diagnosis. These compounds compete with estrogen for binding to estrogen receptor sites.[47]

⇒ **Xenoestrogens**, which are estrogen-like compounds in herbicides, pesticides and other commercial chlorinated hydrocarbons. These have been shown to have disastrous consequences of antagonizing all of the negative aspects of estrogen.[48] Women with breast cancer have been found to have more chlorinated hydrocarbons, or xeno-estrogens, in their bloodstream. These xeno-estrogens are creating havoc in the wild, where male animals end up with dramatically deformed genitals and females have reduced fertility and increases in birth defects.

⇒ **Estrogen-receptors**, which are compounds that escort estrogen from the body, hopefully after it has performed its essential functions. The human body makes estrogen-receptors through the PGE-1 prostaglandin pathways when blood sugar levels are kept low and essential fatty acids (EPA, ALA, GLA, LA) are sufficient. Other compounds in ImmunoPower, sulforaphane and calcium D-glucarate, are included for the purposes of escorting estrogen from the body in a non-toxic manner.

Tamoxifen is an estrogen binder that can be of value in short term use to slow down breast cancer, but in long term use elevates the risk for heart attack[49] eye[50] and liver damage[51] and INCREASING the risk of endometrial cancer.[52]

Researchers, like Stephen Barnes, PhD at the University of Alabama, find that soy is able to inhibit the growth of hormone-dependent tumors, including breast and prostate. Soy and ginseng are Nature's "kinder, gentler" forms of Tamoxifen.

Adding all of this complex biochemistry together and trying to make the recommendations simple, there are several reasons why the 4 above-mentioned categories of estrogen-like compounds are not equal. Soy products and ginseng have been used both to prevent and reverse cancer. The macrobiotic diet, which uses soy as a pivotal source of protein, has not been shown to accelerate the course of breast or ovarian cancer. There are several soy-based products, including Haelan 851 and Dr. Ann Kennedy's Bowman Birk Inhibitor that help to slow various cancers, including breast and ovarian. While soy and ginseng products can reduce the symptoms of menopause by working as phytoestrogens, they do not increase the risk for breast or ovarian cancer nor do they accelerate the disease once present.

Green tea polyphenols 67 mg
Antioxidant, protector of DNA, immune stimulant.

America was founded upon a tea revolt. The American colonists decided that, rather than pay the English King's taxes on tea without representation in the British Parliament, the colonist would rather go into caffeine "cold turkey" by throwing the tea into Boston harbor. While the British have brought "high tea time" into its revered limelight, tea was first introduced to England in the 17th century via trade with China where it had been a favorite beverage for over 3,000 years. Of the 2.5 million tons of dried tea produced each year worldwide, most is grown and consumed in the Orient.

Tea comes from the plant Camellia sinensis, an evergreen shrub in which the young leaves can be either:
◊ lightly steamed to produce **green tea** or
◊ air dried and oxidized to produce **black tea.**

The potent polyphenols are maintained in green tea, since steaming denatures the enzymes that would normally convert the polyphenols to less beneficial ingredients. Green tea is healthier than black tea. While both forms of tea have caffeine, only 20% of tea produced annually comes as green tea.

One of the first scientific references to tea and cancer came from the watershed report from the World Health Organization in 1964, "Prevention of Cancer" in which these experts found a higher incidence of esophageal cancer among people in the Middle East who drink extremely hot tea on a regular basis.[53] This boiling tea burns the esophagus and creates a state of lifelong hyperproliferation, which invites cancer if nutrition intake is less than ideal. There is still some question as to whether black tea at normal drinking temperature constitutes a risk or a protection against cancer.[54] Green tea has such an extensive scientific foundation as a non-toxic and inexpensive anti-cancer agent, that the National Cancer Institutes of China and Japan are researching green tea with the same fervor that the American NCI researches chemotherapy drugs.

Green tea contains a variety of polyphenolic compounds, including catechin, epicatechin, and the reputed chief active ingredient, epigallocatechin gallate. One cup of green tea contains 300 to 400 mg of polyphenols and 50 to 100 mg of caffeine. Green tea works as an antioxidant, perhaps even more potent than vitamins C or E.[55] In animals, green tea was able to induce major improvements in antioxidant and detoxifying enzymes in the body.[56] In human studies, green tea users have about half the cancer incidence of non-tea drinkers.[57] In test tube studies, green tea shut down the tumor promoters involved in breast cancer.[58] Green tea inhibits the formation of cancer-causing agents in the stomach, including nitrosamines.[59]

The anti-cancer properties of green tea include:[60]
◊   Immune stimulant.
◊   Inhibits platelet adhesion, and possibly metastasis.
◊   Antioxidant which protects immune cells for a higher tumor kill rate while protecting the valuable prostaglandin PGE-1.
◊   Inhibits metastasis.
◊   Inhibits the breakdown of connective tissue via collagenase, which is the primary mechanism for the spreading of cancer cells.[61]

Cruciferous 400, sulforaphane 80 mg
Detoxifying agent, helps to neutralize the damaging effects of estrogen, may selectively slow the cancer process.

It was the cabbage family that was first highlighted in this new and exciting field of phytochemicals. Although the father of modern medicine, Hippocrates, taught us 2400 years ago "Let food be your medicine and medicine be your food", modern medicine has only recently begun to accept the importance of this ancient truth. For instance, researchers in the Cold War era of 1950 fed two different groups of animals either beets or cabbage and then exposed them to radiation. The animals fed cabbage had much less hemorrhaging and death from radiation. But since no one in those days could conceive of a radio-protective effect of a food, the scientists concluded that "something in beets makes radioactive exposure more lethal."[62]   Actually, "something" in cabbage makes radiation much less damaging to healthy tissue.

Cruciferous vegetables include cabbage, broccoli, brussel sprouts, cauliflower and others. Among the phytochemicals in cruciferous vegetables that have been researched, sulforaphane is one of the more 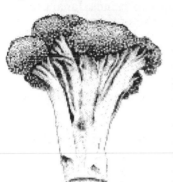 promising as a cancer fighter. It was Professor Lee Wattenburg of Minnesota who found that cabbage extract has the ability to prevent the initiation and promotion of cancer cells.[63] Of the various fractions in cruciferous plants, including indole-3-carbinol, isothiocyanates, glucosinolates, dithiolethiones and phenols; they are able to:[64]

◊   Prevent chemicals from being converted into cancer-causing compounds

◊   Induce liver detoxification systems, such as glutathione S-transferase and P-450, to help rid the body of poisons.

◊   Scavenge free radicals, thus working as an antioxidant.

◊   Prevent tumor promoters from reaching their cell targets, such as blocking the binding of estrogen to estrogen-dependent tumors.

Cat's claw, 3:1 concentrate 200 mg
   Immune stimulant, anti-inflammatory, protects DNA, antioxidant.

Cat's claw, or Uncaria tomentosa, is a relative newcomer to Western botanical medicine. It has been used therapeutically for centuries by Native South Americans in the higher elevations of the Peruvian Amazon rain forest. Cat's claw is a woody vine that grows to 100 feet by wrapping around nearby trees. The root and inner bark are used to prepare herbal concoctions that have demonstrated some effectiveness at cleansing the gastro-intestinal tract of parasites and re-establishing a favorable environment for healthy microflora bacteria.

Cat's claw may be able to:

◊   Inhibit free radicals.[65]

◊   Stimulate the immune system.[66]

◊   Cleanse and strengthen the intestinal tract.

◊   Inhibit auto-immune diseases, such as Crohn's

◊   Protect the DNA from damage.[67]

◊   Slow down cancer growth.[68]

Maitake D-fraction (33 mg)
   Adaptogen, immune stimulant.

Mushrooms, or fungi, have long been valued for their contributions as foods and medicines for humans. Penicillin was first discovered as bread mold, or fungi, and found to inhibit bacterial growth. Mushrooms usually grow as mold on rotten tree stumps or in manure. Of the various mushrooms that have been tested for their medicinal value, including lentinan, Shiitake, and PSK; Maitake (Grifola frondosa) has shown the most consistent anti-cancer effects from oral intake. The other mushrooms may have active ingredients that are effective when injected, but not when orally consumed.

Maitake literally means "dancing mushroom" since Japanese people who discovered these basketball-sized mushrooms growing on tree stumps would "dance with joy" at the prospects of the taste and health-giving properties. In the 1980s, Japanese firms began cultivating Maitake mushrooms on sawdust and intensely investigating the therapeutic value of this mushroom. An isolated fraction, D-fraction with active constituents of 1,6 and 1,3 beta-glucans, has been found to be the most potent and best absorbed from the diet.

Maitake may help cancer patients via:

◊ Immune stimulation, capable of doubling the activity of Natural Killer cells in animals. D-fraction was able to increase interleukin-1 production from macrophages and potentiate delayed type hypersensitivity response, which is indicative of tumor growth suppression.[69]

◊ Adaptogen that lowers hypertension[70], lowers excess blood sugar levels, protects the liver, and has anti-viral activity.[71]

◊ Inhibition of metastasis of cancer by 81% in one animal study.[72]

◊ Augmenting the anti-cancer activity of drugs like Mitomycin. In a comparison study between Maitake D-fraction and Mitomycin C, Maitake provided superior tumor growth inhibition of 80% vs. 45% for the drug. Yet when both were given together, but at half the dosage for each, tumor inhibition was 98%.

◊ Reducing toxic side effects from chemotherapy while augmenting tumor kill of the drug. There was a 90% drop in the incidence of appetite loss, vomiting, nausea, hair loss and leukopenia (deficiency of immune cells) in human cancer patients treated with Maitake D-fraction while undergoing chemotherapy.

L-glutathione (GSH) 100 mg
Stimulator of immune system, detoxification, regulator of cell division and prostaglandin metabolism.

Glutathione is one of the most widely distributed and important antioxidants in all of nature, yet there has been some confusion regarding its use in cancer patients and its absorption. So keep your thinking cap on as we review this nutrient.

Glutathione is a tripeptide, meaning a molecule formed from three amino acids: glutamine, cysteine and glycine. Some clinicians have chosen to use N-acetyl-cysteine, as a means of augmenting the production of glutathione in the body. Glutathione, also abbreviated GSH, is one of the most widely distributed antioxidants in plants and animals, and is the chief thiol (sulfur bearing) molecule in most cells. Glutathione plays a central role in the enzyme system glutathione peroxidase which is crucial for cell metabolism, cell regulation, detoxification, DNA synthesis and repair, immune function, prostaglandin metabolism and regulating cell proliferation through apoptosis (programmed cell death).[73] GSH is particularly helpful in protecting the liver from damage upon exposure to toxins.[74] GSH levels are decreased in most disease states, infertility, aging, toxic burden and other unfavorable health conditions.[75] Lower levels of blood GSH are associated with more illness, higher blood pressure, higher percent body fat, and reduced general health status.[76] Cancer patients have less GSH in their blood than healthy people.[77] So far, no controversy.

glutamine+cysteine+glycine=glutathione

Help cancer patients? Some oncologists have reasoned that GSH provides one of the main protective mechanisms for cancer cells to develop resistance to chemotherapy.[78] Thus, efforts have been made to develop drugs which deplete the cancer patient of GSH. However, supplements of glutathione in patients being treated for ovarian cancer with the drug cisplatin had an improvement in outcome and reduced kidney toxicity from the cisplatin.[79] In another study of 55 patients with stomach cancer, GSH prevented the neurotoxicity usually associated with cisplatin and did not reduce the anti-neoplastic activity of the drug.[80] In animals exposed to a potent carcinogen (DMBA), GSH provided significant reduction in the size and incidence of tumors.[81] Animals exposed to DMBA and given GSH, vitamin C, E, and betacarotene had substantial reduction in the number and size of cancers.[82]

In animals with chemically-induced (aflatoxin) liver cancer (an extremely poor prognostic cancer) 100% died within 20 months, while 81% of the animals with liver cancer who were treated with GSH were disease-free 4 months later.[83] Eight patients with advanced refractory (resistant to medical therapy) liver cancer were given 5 grams daily of oral GSH with most surviving longer than expected and one being cured.[84] Glutathione in the diet has been shown to protect the intestinal wall of animals from the insult of chemical carcinogens.[85] In cultured cancer cells, GSH was able to induce apoptosis (programmed cell death), which may be one of the ways that GSH can assist cancer patients.[86]

Can you absorb GSH in the gut? In one study, 7 healthy human subjects were given increasingly higher oral supplements of GSH up to 3 grams daily with blood levels showing no significant increase in glutathione, cysteine or glutamate.[87] However, many other studies with humans and animals[88] have found GSH well absorbed into the bloodstream. GSH may be converted into a different molecule for transport through the bloodstream. Best sources of GSH are dark green leafy vegetables, fresh fruit and lightly cooked fish, poultry and beef. Processing inevitably reduces the GSH levels of foods. On a logical basis, would Nature waste one of the more effective and pervasive antioxidants in plants and animals by making GSH unavailable for absorption? I don't think so.

ENDNOTES

[1] . Koide, T., et al., Cancer Biotherapy & Radiopharmaceuticals, vol.11, p.273, Aug.1996
[2] . LeBon, AM, et al., Chem.Biol.Interactions, vol.83, p.65, 1992
[3] . Havsteen, B, Biochem Pharmacol., vol.32, p.1141, 1983
[4] . Fujiki, H., et al., in Plant Flavonoids in Biology and Medicine, vol.1, p.429, Liss Publ., NY, 1986
[5] . Berg, P., et al., in Plant Flavonoids in Biology and Medicine, vol.2, p.157, Liss Publ., NY, 1988
[6] . Wattenberg, L., et al., Cancer Research, vol.30, p.1922, 1970
[7] . Werbach, M., et al., BOTANICAL INFLUENCES ON ILLNESS, p.30, Third Line Press, Tarzana, CA, 1994
[8] . Werbach, M., IBID, p.189
[9] . Luettig, B., et al., J. Natl.Cancer Inst., vol.81, p.669, 1989
[10] . Lersch, C., et al., Tumordiagen Ther., vol.13, p.115, 1992
[11] . Lersch, C., et al., Cancer Invest., vol.10, p.343, 1992
[12] . Nagabhushan, M., et al., J. Am.Coll. Nutr., vol.11, p.192, 1992
[13] . Kuttan, R., et al., Cancer Lett., vol.29, p.197, 1985
[14] . Polasa, K., Mutagen, vol.7, p.107, 1992
[15] . Kuttan, R., et al., Tumori, vol.73, p.29, 1987
[16] . Schubert, H., et al., Geriatr Forsch, vol.3, p.45, 1993
[17] . Kleijnen, J., et al., Br. J. Clin.Pharmacol. vol.34, p.352, 1992
[18] . Kleijnen, J., et al., Lancet, vol.340, p.1136, 1992
[19] . Koltai, M., et al., Drugs, vol.42, p.9, 1991
[20] . Pincemail, J., et al., Experientia, vol.45, p.708, 1989
[21] . Shibata, S., et al., Econ.Med.Plant Res., vol.1, p.217, 1985
[22] . Siegel, RK, JAMA, vol.243, p.32, 1980
[23] . Chang, HM, et al., Pharmacology and Applications of Chinese Materia Medica, vol. 2, World Scientific Publ., Teaneck, NJ, p.1041, 1987
[24] . Sun, Y, J. Biol Response Modifiers, vol.2, p.227, 1983
[25] . Chu, DT, et al., J. Clin.Lab.Immunol., vol.26, p.183, 1988
[26] . Li, NQ, et al., Chung Kuo Chung Hsi I Chieh Ho Tsa Chih, vol.12, p.588, 1992
[27] . Boik, J., CANCER AND NATURAL MEDICINE, p.177, Oregon Medical Press, Princeton, MN, 1995
[28] . Boik, J. CANCER AND NATURAL MEDICINE, p.180 Oregon Medical Press, Princeton, MN, 1995
[29] . Murray, MT, HEALING POWER OF HERBS, p.265, Prima Publ., Rocklin, CA 1995
[30] . Ziglar, W., Whole Foods, vol.2, p.48, 1979
[31] . Samira, MMH, et al., J.Int.Med.Res., vol.13, p.342, 1985
[32] . Ng, TB, et al., Gen.Pharmacol., vol.6, p.549, 1985; see also Yamato, M., et al., Proceedings of the 3rd Intl Ginseng Symp, p.115, 1980
[33] . Jie, YH, et al., Agents Actions, vol.15, p.386, 1984; see also Gupta, S., et al., Clin.Res., vol.28, p.504A, 1980
[34] . Singh, VK, et al., Planta Medica, vol.51, p.462, 1984
[35] . Oura, H., et al., Chem.Pharm.Bull., vol.20, p.980, 1972
[36] . Hikino, H., et al., Planta Medica, vol.52, p.62, 1985; see also Oh, JS, et al., Korean J.Pharmacol., vol.4, p.27, 1968
[37] . Yamamoto, M., et al., Am.J.Chin.Med., vol.11, p.84, 1983
[38] . Yun, TK, et al., Cancer Detect.Prev., vol.6, p.515, 1983
[39] . Yun, TK, et al., Int.J.Epidemiol., vol.19, p.871, 1990
[40] . Lee, KD, et al., Jpn.J.Pharmacol., vol.21, p.299, 1971; see also Fulder, SJ, Exp.Gerontol., vol.12, p.125, 1977
[41] . Rhee, YH, et al., Planta Medica, vol.57, p.125, 1991
[42] . Hau, DM, et al., Int. J. of Oriental Med., vol.15, p.10, 1990
[43] . Yang, G., et al., J. of Trad. Chin. Med., vol.8, p.135, 1988
[44] . Kubo, M., et al., Planta Med, vol.58, p.424, 1992
[45] . Li, X., et al., J. Tongji Med Univ., vol.11, p.73, 1991
[46] . Murray, RK, et al., HARPER'S BIOCHEMISTRY, 24th edition, p.550, Lange, Stamford, CT 1996
[47] . Boik, J., CANCER AND NATURAL MEDICINE, p.44, Oregon Medical Press, Princeton, MN 1995
[48] . Davis, DL, et al., Environmental Health Perspectives, vol.101, p.372, Oct.1993
[49] . Nakagawa, T., et al., Angiology, vol.45, p.333, May 1994
[50] . Pavlidis, NA, et al., Cancer, vol.69, p.2961, 1992
[51] . Catherino, WH, et al., Drug Safety, vol.8, p.381, 1993
[52] . Seoud, MAF, et al., Obstetrics & Gynecology, vol.82, p.165, Aug.1993

[53] . World Health Organization, PREVENTION OF CANCER, technical report 276, WHO, Geneva, 1964

[54] . LaVecchia, CL, et al., Nutr.Cancer, vol.17, p.27, 1992

[55] . Ho, C., et al., Prev.Med., vol.21, p.520, 1992

[56] . Khan, SG, et al., Cancer Res., vol.52, p.4050, 1992

[57] . Yang, CS, et al., J. Natl., Cancer Inst., vol.85, p.1038, 1993

[58] . Komori, A., et al., Jpn.J.Clin.Oncol., vol.23, p.186, 1993

[59] . Stich, HF, Prev.Med., vol.21, p.377, 1992

[60] . Boik, J., CANCER AND NATURAL MEDICINE, p.178, Oregon Medical Press, Princeton, MN 1995

[61] . Beretz, A, et al., Plant Flavonoids in Biology and Medicine II, p.187, Liss Publ., 1988

[62] . Lourau, G., et al., Experientia, vol.6, p.25, 1950

[63] . Wattenburg, LW, Cancer Res. (suppl), vol.52, p. 2085S, 1992

[64] . Kensler, TW, et al., p.154-196, in FOOD CHEMICALS AND CANCER PREVENTION, vol.1, American Chemical Society, Wash DC, 1994

[65] . McBrien, DC, et al., LIPID PEROXIDATION AND CANCER, Academy Press, NY 1982

[66] . Wagner, H., et al., Planta Medica, vol.12, p.34, 1985

[67] . Rizzi, R., et al., J. Ethnopharmacol., vol.38, p.63, 1993

[68] . DeOlivera, MM, et al., Anals Acad.Brasil Ciencias, vol.44, p.41, 1972

[69] . Hishida, I., et al., Chem.Pharm.Bull., vol.36, p.1819, 1988

[70] . Adachi, K., et al., Chem.Pharm.Bull., vol.36, p.1000, 1988

[71] . Nanba, H., J. Orthomolecular Med., vol.12, p.43, 1997

[72] . Nanba, H., Cancer Prevention, NYAS, p.243, Sept.1995

[73] . Bray, TM, et al., Biochem.Pharmacol., vol.47, p.2113, 1994; see also Shan, X, et al., Pharmacol.Ther., vol.47, p.61, 1990

[74] . DeLeve, LD, et al., Pharmac.Ther., vol.52, p.287, 1991

[75] . Bray, TM, et al., Biochem.Pharmacol., vol.47, p.2113, 1994

[76] . Julius, M., et al., J.Clin.Epidemiol., vol.47, p.1021, 1994

[77] . Beutler, E., et al., J.Lab.Clin.Ned., vol.105, p.581, 1985

[78] . Hercbergs, A., et al., Lancet, vol.339, p.1074, May 1992

[79] . DiRe, F., et al., Cancer Chemother.Pharmacol., vol.25, p.355, 1990

[80] . Cascinu, S., et al., J.Clin.Oncol., vol.13, p.26, 1995

[81] . Trickler, D., et al., Nutr.Cancer, vol.20, p.139, 1993

[82] . Shklar, G., et al., Nutr.Cancer, vol.20, p.145, 1993

[83] . Science, vol.212, p.541, May 1981

[84] . Hanek, DK, et al., Liver, vol.12, p.311, 1992

[85] . Lash, LH, et al., Proc.Natl.Acad.Sci., vol.83, p.4641, July 1986

[86] . Donnerstag, B., et al., Int.J.Oncol., vol.7, p.949, Oct.1995

[87] . Witschi, A., et al., Eur.J.Clin.Pharmacol., vol.43, p.667, 1992

[88] . Hagen, TM, et al., Am.J.Physiol., vol.259, p.G524, 1990

CHAPTER 4

✷

LIPIDS (Fats)

Not all fat is created equally. Fat-phobic Americans have lost sight of the fact that there are good, bad and ugly fats.

DIETARY FATS		
GOOD ☺	**BAD** ☺	**UGLY** ☹
flax, olive, canola, fish, primrose, borage, MCT, lecithin, rice bran, rapeseed, hemp	too much fat of any kind, especially in a deficiency state of vitamin E (protects against fat "rusting")	hydrogenated (lard), or oxidized (from fast food deep fryers), or not enough vit.E or too much sugar

Cod liver oil (1 cap) 1 gram, with 360 mg EPA & 240 mg DHA including naturally occurring Vitamin A 2500 iu & Vitamin D 270 iu
Augment immune system, improve production of favorable prostaglandin PGE-1, prevents metastasis of cancer cells by changing the stickiness of cells, improves cell membrane dynamics to augment nutrient absorption and toxin elimination.

When the Senate Diet Goals were released by a blue ribbon panel of nutrition experts in 1977, they included the recommendation to decrease fat intake from 40% of calories to 30%. Yet, experts then looked at the Greenland Eskimos, who get 60% of their calories from fat and practically no dietary fiber, yet mysteriously had little cancer or heart disease. Three factors saved these people from an otherwise disastrous diet:

1) genetic adaption, at least 40,000 years to adjust to this uniquely skewed diet

2) fish oil, which contains a very special and highly unsaturated fat, eicosapentaenoic acid, or EPA for short.

3) no sugar in the diet, which helps the body make PGE-1, a healthy prostaglandin

EPA is, essentially, Nature's anti-freeze. In the arctic regions of the world, the ocean temperature drops to below freezing, yet water-based life will explode at that temperature, like leaving out a water balloon on a sub-freezing night. So Nature provides the algae in the ocean with this special fat, EPA, that prevents freezing and bursting at low temperatures.

Smaller fish eat the algae, and bigger fish eat the smaller fish, until we have major concentrations of EPA in cold water fish, like cod, salmon, mackeral, tuna, and sardines. Much of the fat in seals and whales that were consumed by the Greenland Eskimos was rich in EPA, which provided these people with extraordinary protection against many diseases. EPA is so valuable against cancer that the National Library of Medicine has created a special report on the hundreds of scientific studies found in their data base on the therapeutic benefits of EPA.

EPA may help the cancer patient:

⇒**Changes membrane fluidity**. Cell membranes contain fats which are a direct reflection from our diet, including the unnatural hydrogenated fats found in Crisco and Pop Tarts. When we are talking about dietary fats, the old saying is literally true, "you are what you eat." Cell membranes that are fluid, flexible and allow the proper nutrients to pass into the cell will improve overall wellness, thus discouraging abnormal cell growths, like cancer. Cells that are flexible with EPA can squeeze down narrow capillaries to feed the distant tissue. Cells that are rigid with too much saturated or hydrogenated fat or having been "tanned" from too much sugar in the blood will not be able to move down narrow capillaries, like a car trying to get down a hotel hallway.

⇒**Increase prostaglandin E-1**, a.k.a. PGE-1, which favors reducing the stickiness of cells for less risk of metastasis.[1] PGE-1 also bolsters immune functions, dilates blood vessels, elevates production of estrogen receptors and other benefits for the cancer patient.

⇒**Slows tumor growth in animals**.[2] Slows tumor growth by altering protein synthesis and breakdown.[3]

⇒**Augments medical therapies**. EPA improves tumor kill in hyperthermia and chemotherapy by altering cancer cell membranes for increased vulnerability.[4] Increases the ability of adriamycin to kill cultured leukemia cells.[5] Tumors in EPA-fed animals are more responsive to Mitomycin C and doxorubicin (chemotherapy drugs).[6] EPA and GLA were selectively toxic to human tumor cell lines while also enhancing the cytotoxic effects of chemotherapy.[7]

⇒**Reduces initiation, promotion and progression of hormonally driven cancers**, such as breast, prostate and ovarian. An EPA-rich diet significantly lowered the levels of estradiol, a marker for breast cancer, in the 25 women studied who were at risk for breast cancer.[8] Modulates estrogen metabolism for reduced risk and spreading of breast cancer.[9]

Fish oil may be as effective as any cancer treatment

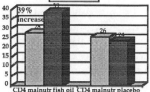

DOES FISH OIL SUPPLEMENTATION AS SOLE THERAPY IMPROVE OUTCOME IN PATIENTS WITH SOLID TUMORS?

"...consider alternative, less toxic treatment approaches..."

STUDY DESIGN:
64 cancer patients, refractory
No other TX for 4 mo Prior,
Solid tumors, randomized to
Placebo or fish oil 18 grams
MaxEPA (6 caps TID),
170 mg EPA +115 mgDHA
Per capsule, + 200 mg vit E,
Divided into well or malnourish,
Assessed at begin & day 40

"Omega 3 prolonged survival of all patients...resulted in significant (p<0.025) increase in survival for all patients compared with placebo" Gogos, et al., Cancer, vol.82, p.395, 1998 available. In a study examining end stage refractory cancer patients who have exhausted all chemo and radiation options, fish oil supplements provided a substantial improvement in length of life and immune functions compared to placebo.

A (preformed) 2500 iu
      Down regulates cancer at genetic level, immune stimulant, improves cell differentiation process, helps with cell to cell communication.

      Along with iron, vitamin A is one of the most common micronutrient deficiencies in the world. Around the world, an estimated 500,000 people each year go permanently blind because of clinical vitamin A deficiency. Vitamin A was the first micronutrient to be recognized for its role in preventing cancer. Vitamin A is one of the most multi-talented of all substances in human nutrition and plays a key role in preventing and reversing cancer. While vitamin A and beta-carotene are considered interchangeable, more recent evidence shows that these two nutrients have some overlapping functions and some distinctly different functions. A drug analog of vitamin A (all trans retinoic acid) has become a near cure all for acute promyelocytic leukemia, with one study showing a 96% cure rate.[10] Some companies use an emulsified vitamin A so that it stays in the blood stream longer, which may be important for extremely high doses of A (>100,000 iu/day) in cancer patients.
      All of the known functions of vitamin A relate either directly or indirectly to the cancer patient:
◊   **Cell division**. Billions of times each day, cells divide in the precarious process of cell division, a.k.a. proliferation or hyperplasia. Without vitamin A, this fragile process can easily turn into cancer, or neoplasia. Vitamin A is crucial for cancer prevention.[11] Vitamin A deficiency may be one of the primary insults leading to lung cancer.[12] There are probably binding sites on the human DNA for vitamin A. Researchers found that one of the most common cancers in Third World countries, cervical cancer, was linked to Human Papilloma Virus, which was then linked to shutting off the cancer-protective gene, called p53, which was then linked to a low intake of vitamin A. Essentially, vitamin A keeps the p53 active and protecting our DNA against cancer, even from viral attack.
◊   **Cell to cell communication**, a.k.a. gap junction. Cells communicate via a "telegraph" system of ions floating in and out of cell membrane pores. This intercellular communication helps to maintain cooperation and coordination of cell functions. Without vitamin A, the "telegraph" system becomes distorted and cancer can arise.
◊   **Maintenance of epithelial tissue**, or skin. The vast majority of cancers, including lung, breast, colon, and prostate, all arise from the epithelial tissue and are called carcinomas. Other categories of cancers include: leukemia (cancer of the bone marrow that produces red & white cells), lymphoma (cancer of the lymph cells and glands),

and sarcomas (cancers of the structural tissue).[13] When the body is deprived of vitamin A, skin (epithelial) cancer is more likely to result. Giving therapeutic doses of vitamin A has been shown to slow down and reverse some forms of cancer.

◊ **Immune stimulant**. Vitamin A deficiency brings changes in the mucosal membranes, changes in lymphocyte sub-populations, and altered T- and B-cell functions.[14] There are many studies linking vitamin A supplements to the curing of measles.[15] Vitamin A supplements brought a 19% reduction in respiratory infections in children.[16] Pregnant women with the lowest quartile of serum vitamin A had a 400% increase in the risk of transmitting their HIV virus to their unborn infant.[17]

◊ **Anti-cancer activity**. Vitamin A supplements as sole therapy in patients with unresectable (cannot be surgically removed) lung cancer measurably improved immune functions and tumor response.[18] Vitamin A, and not beta-carotene, improved lymphocyte levels and reduced complications after surgery in lung cancer patients.[19] In patients treated for bladder cancer, the incidence of recurrence was 180% higher in patients who consumed the lowest quartile of vitamin A in the diet.[20] High doses of vitamin A (200,000 iu/week) were able to reduce damaged and potentially cancerous mouth cells by 96%.[21] Vitamin A and its synthetic analogues have been shown to improve cancer treatment in oral leukoplakia, laryngeal papillomatosis, superficial bladder carcinoma, cervical dysplasia, bronchial metaplasia, and preleukemia.[22] Vitamin A supplements of 300,000 iu per day were provided in a placebo-controlled trial with 307 patients with stage I non-small-cell lung cancer. 37% of the treated group experienced a recurrence, while 48% of the non-treated group had a recurrence, thus bringing a 25% reduction in tumor recurrence when used as sole therapy.[23]

SAFETY ISSUES. While vitamins, in general, are much safer than drugs, it is important to discuss vitamin A toxicity, which is by far the most common cause of vitamin toxicity. Up to 1 million iu of vitamin A per day has been given for 5 years without side effects in European cancer clinics.[24] One study found that women taking as little as 10,000 iu/day during pregnancy had a slightly elevated risk for having a child with birth defects (teratogenicity).[25] Another study from the National Institutes of Health found no increase in birth defects in women taking 25,000 iu/day of vitamin A. An FDA biochemist, John Hathcock, PhD, states that toxicity with vitamin A at these low levels mainly involves people with confounding medical conditions, including compromised liver function.[26] Cancer clinics in Europe often administer up to 2.5 million iu/day of vitamin A in emulsified form for several months under medical supervision. While these doses are not recommended without medical supervision, it shows the relative safety of vitamin A in the general population. Giving at least 300,000 iu per day of retinol palmitate in 138 lung cancer patients for at least 12 months created self-terminating unremarkable symptoms in less than 10% of these patients and only caused interruption of treatment in 3% due to symptoms that were potentially related to vitamin A excess. Upset stomach (dyspepsia), headache, nosebleeds and mild hair loss were the most common and self-limiting symptoms.

Since meat eating populations would usually eat the liver of the animal first, which is the most concentrated source of pre-formed vitamin A, descendents of carnivorous people probably have a much greater tolerance and need for higher doses of A. By increasing the intake of vitamin E, many people will be able to avoid toxicity from high doses of vitamin A, since it is the lipid peroxide products from A that can cause damage to the liver. Vitamin E prevents lipid peroxidation.
PREGNANT WOMEN SHOULD NOT USE IMMUNOPOWER.

D (ergocalciferol) 270 iu
Helps to squelch cancer at genetic level, reducing the production of gene fragments (episomes) by working with calcium receptors.

As the fledgling science of nutrition grows in knowledge and analytical tools, we keep discovering more nutrients and more functions of the nutrients that we thought we already understood. Such is true for vitamin D, which actually is not a real vitamin in the sense of needing it in the diet.[27] We can manufacture vitamin D in the body by the action of sunlight on the skin converting cholesterol to D.

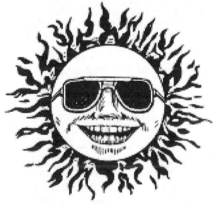

As a simple metaphor, think of most human cells containing a "switch" that can activate cancer, called the oncogene. Vitamin D puts a protective plate over that oncogene "switch" to prevent cancer from starting or spreading.

Nature always seems to provide. In areas of the world where sunshine is unpredictable at best, these people had traditional diets that were rich in fish liver, which is the most concentrated food source of vitamin D. Cloudy regions of the world have had notoriously higher rates of tuberculosis; cancers of the breast[28], ovaries[29], colon[30] and prostate; hypertension and osteoporosis[31]; multiple sclerosis, and other health problems.

If sunshine is the "medicine" in these diseases, then vitamin D and melatonin are the most likely by-products of sunlight exposure. Vitamin D has demonstrated the ability to enhance the immune system to fight off tuberculosis.[32] Our primitive ancestors consumed or produced about 5 times more vitamin D than we get because they ate whole foods, lots of fish and lived outside in the sun. Most Americans, and nearly all women receive far below the RDA (200-400 iu) for vitamin D.[33] One international unit (1 iu) of vitamin D-3 (a measurement of biological activity) is equal to 0.025 micrograms in weight.

Ergosterol is a plant steroid which is converted commercially to vitamin D-2 and used to fortify milk, a move that has virtually eliminated the deficiency syndrome of rickets in cloudy regions of the world. Vitamin D-3, cholecalciferol, is the natural vitamin produced in the skin by the action of sunlight. Ergosterol is the natural form of vitamin D that is concentrated in cod liver oil as the fish consumes various algae in the ocean. For centuries, cod liver oil has been the choice of doctors and mothers to prevent rickets from forming in young children. Once activated in the kidneys and liver, the steroid version of vitamin D-3 is: 1 alpha 25 dihydroxy cholecalciferol (1,25 D-3), which works with the hormones of parathyroid and calcitonin to regulate calcium metabolism, absorption, transport and more.

So, how does all of this information relate to the cancer process? Probably by regulating calcium transport into and out of the cell, which has been shown to be crucial in the cell differentiation process.[34]

◊ In animals fed a high fat diet, which normally would produce a higher incidence of colon cancer, supplements of calcium and vitamin D blocked this carcinogenic effect of the diet.[35]

◊ Vitamin D inhibits the growth of breast cancer in culture, and also seems to subdue human breast cancer.[36]

◊ Cells from human prostate cancer were put into a "...permanent nonproliferative state.", or shut down the cancer process, by the addition of vitamin D.[37]

◊ Human cancer cells have been shown to have receptor sites, or stereo specific "parking spaces" for vitamin D.[38]

Vitamin D prevents the formation of gene fragments, episomes, that may be the beginning of the cancer process. Bone cells that generate new blood and immune cells (hematopoietic cells) have receptors for 1,25 D-3 and activated macrophages from the immune system can synthesize 1,25 D-3.[39] Vitamin D induces differentiation to suppress cell growth in numerous tumor lines tested.[40] In tumor-bearing mice, vitamin D-3 supplements inhibited the immune suppression from the tumor secretion (granulocyte/macrophage colony stimulating factor, GM-CSF), while also reducing tumor growth and metastasis.[41] Due to the success of vitamin D at down-regulating various forms of cancer, many drug companies are researching patentable vitamin D analogs to treat cancer. But nothing works like Mother Nature's original.

SAFETY ISSUES. Nature has checkpoints in place to control the possibility of vitamin D toxicity in the body. People who are native to sunny climates have darker skin which is full of melanin to reduce the production of vitamin D in the skin while also protecting against the damaging effects of ultraviolet light. Dark skinned people are also more vulnerable to rickets (vitamin D deficiency) when moving to cloudy climates. Also, African-American men have a much higher incidence of prostate cancer, perhaps due to variations in vitamin D metabolism.

In order for dietary intake of vitamin D to become toxic, there needs to be activation of vitamin D in the kidney and liver, which are other safeguards in the body. Nonetheless, young children are potentially vulnerable to vitamin D toxicity, which may begin as low as 1800 iu/day for extended periods of time.[42] Symptoms of toxicity include hypercalcemia, hypercalciuria, anorexia, nausea, vomiting, thirst, polyuria, muscular weakness, joint pains, and disorientation.[43] At full dosage, ImmunoPower contains 810 iu/day, which is well within the safety range, even for the few people who consume large amounts of vitamin D in the diet.

Evening primrose oil (2 caps) 1000 mg (90 mg GLA)
Improves production of PGE-1, selectively toxic to tumor cells.

Our ancestors consumed a diet of range fed animals who grazed on wild grain, nuts and seeds. In these foods is a wide assortment of valuable fatty acids, including gamma linolenic acid (GLA), which is richly concentrated in the evening primrose and borage plants. Intake of GLA in modern Americans has dropped off substantially with the consumption of corn-fed beef, which is rich in linoleic acid that generates the tumor-promoting eicosanoid of arachidonic acid. The reason why range-fed lean buffalo was good for Native Americans, yet corn-fed high fat beef is not so good for modern Americans is primarily the quality and quantity of fats in these two animals. A ratio of approximately 4:1 of EPA to GLA is very favorable for host defense mechanisms to fight off cancer.

We are able to make less GLA internally as we age, are exposed to stress and toxins, become compromised by disease, and eat hydrogenated fats--which describes millions of Americans. GLA in the diet helps to drive PGE-1, mentioned above, while also being selectively toxic to tumor cells.[44] GLA was selectively toxic to cultured human breast cancer cells.[45] In 21 human cancer patients with refractory (failed medical treatment) and untreatable malignancies, GLA was able to provide measurable benefits, including weight gain and reduction in tumor mass based on radiological evidence.[46] When healthy and cancer cells are cultured with EPA and GLA, the healthy cells begin to outgrow the cancerous cells.[47]

Shark oil (1 capsule) 1 gram
Improves the production of white (immune) and red (erythrocyte) cells from the bone marrow. Protects against the damaging effects of radiation therapy. 200 mg alkylglycerols.

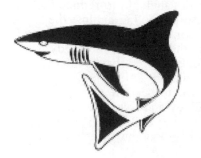

While it may be true that "sharks don't get cancer", it is more than cartilage that works in the shark's favor. Shark liver oil is rich in a compound called "alkoxyglycerols" or "alkylglycerols". The highest concentration of alkoxyglycerols in Nature are found in mother's milk, bone marrow and shark liver oil, which is an indication of the importance of this fatty compound. Bone marrow seems to derive the greatest benefit from alkoxyglycerol administration by nourishing the "cradle of all blood cells". Bone marrow is responsible for manufacturing red blood cells (hemopoiesis, or hematopoiesis) and white blood cells for the immune system.

Shark oil may help cancer patients:

⇒**Reversing anemia**. Many cancer patients become anemic, or deficient in red blood cells, which leads to weakness and increased risk for infections. Shark liver oil encourages normal production of red blood cells; which is a much better strategy than giving high dose iron supplements. See the section on "iron" in chapter 6 on minerals. I have found significant improvement in red blood cell (hemoglobin) and white blood cell (lymphocyte) counts in patients taking shark liver oil capsules.

⇒**Protecting healthy tissue** from radiation damage. In cancer patients given shark oil capsules before, during and after radiation therapy; there was a 67% reduction in radiation induced injuries.[48] Prior administration of shark oil capsules to radiation provided a 47% reduction in both severe (such as fistulas) and less harmful injuries from radiation therapy for cervical/uterine cancer.[49]

⇒**May slow cancer growth**. Shark oil (as Alkyrol, used in ImmunoPower) was able to reduce cancer mortality in a human clinical trial.[50] Patients with uterine cancer who were given alkylglycerols throughout their cancer treatment had regression of tumor growth.[51]

Conjugated linoleic acid, or CLA (1 capsule) 1 gram
    Improves cellular communication to prevent and reverse cancer, stabilizes blood glucose, antioxidant and immune regulator.

Recently, I had to find a cable to connect my computer to my monitor. This was no easy task. In describing my needs to the salesperson, we got into a spirited discussion of how many pins in how many rows for each end of the cable. "Close" is not good enough in either computer cables or fatty acid requirements in the human body. Americans often consume fats that are unhealthy, like hydrogenated fats, and are deficient in valuable fats, like CLA. A tiny difference in molecular structure, just like computer cables, can make a huge difference in whether this fat will help or hinder your cellular machinery.

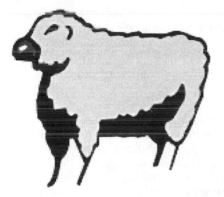

        CLA is a collection of unique "18 pin" fatty acids found primarily in the meat and milk of grazing animals, like beef and dairy. CLA is one of the more exciting recent developments in anticarcinogenic fats. There is 300-400% more CLA in spring and summer milk and most Australian dairy products due to the availability of fresh green pasture land, which augments CLA content in the milk and fat of grazing animals.[52]

CLA is just another example of my first axiom of nutrition: "Nature knows best." Scientific studies in the past have come up with some conflicting results regarding diet and cancer. While most studies find that a high fat diet increases the risk for cancer, one recent study found that milk fat may protect women against breast cancer.[53] While most nutritionists argue that beef, in general, increases the risk for cancer, one prospective epidemiological study found that people consuming meat along with green or yellow vegetables on a daily basis had up to a 75% reduction in colon cancer incidence compared to those who consumed either meat or vegetables alone.[54]

CLA makes a good argument for humans consuming an omnivorous diet, since there is far more CLA, carnitine, EPA, taurine, and lipoic acid in animal foods than plants foods. Dr. Weston Price was a dentist and, in my humble opinion, one of the more important nutritionists in history. He toured the world in the 1930s with his nurse-wife visiting numerous cultures and found many different diets. But he never found a group of people who were complete vegans...all of our ancestors ate some animal food. Maybe CLA is one of the nutrients that we need from a healthy mixed diet.

CLA is a unique fat, derived from linoleic acid, which is one of the two essential fatty acids in human nutrition, along with alpha-linolenic acid. CLA has unsaturated bonds in either the 9 & 11 position or the 10 & 12 carbon position. It comes in both "cis" (looks like a horseshoe) and "trans" (looks like a lightning bolt) isomers. Bacteria in the gut of ruminants, like cows, sheep, deer and buffalo, can produce CLA. Yet there is more CLA in grilled beef than raw beef, so the cooking process also enhances CLA content.[55] Of all the nutrition factors studied, CLA is one of the more impressive at arresting cancer cells in animal and test tube studies.[56]

CLA may be able to help the cancer patient through:

➤ Cellular communication. Healthy cells know when to grow and when to stop growing and when to die. Cancer cells lose this crucial "knowledge". There is evidence that CLA assists in "signal transduction" pathways that tell cancer cells to commit suicide (apoptosis).

➤ Protection from toxins. CLA provided major cancer protection against toxins (like DMBA) in animal studies.[57] CLA may protect us from cancer by encouraging detoxification pathways.[58]

➤ Antioxidant. There is a large and growing list of non-essential dietary antioxidants, including CLA, ellagic acid, curcumin, quercetin, and epicatechin (all found in ImmunoPower), which have shown remarkable abilities to slow down the oxidative damage, or the "rusting" that occurs constantly in all human beings.[59] Antioxidants can provide immune cells with a protective shield as they dowse the cancer cells with potent free radicals. Antioxidants can protect the healthy tissue of the patient while the chemotherapy and radiation become more selective at destroying tumor tissue that does not absorb antioxidants as effectively as do healthy cells. However, other researchers found that if CLA is an antioxidant, then it does not protect cells in the usual antioxidant fashion, as shown by protection of cell membranes in culture.[60]

➤ Inhibitor of the cancer cascade. Cancer results from a series of deterioration steps in the cells. Cancer results after the stages of initiation, promotion, and progression have occurred. Hyperplasia (rapid cell growth), can worsen into metaplasia (above normal cell growth), can further deteriorate into dysplasia (abnormal cell growth), which can become neoplasia (new form of cell growth, or cancer). There are numerous pre-cancerous conditions, including fibrocystic breast disease, diverticulosis (colon), oral leukoplakia (mouth), cervical dysplasia (cervix), and benign prostatic hypertrophy (prostate), which all bear more attention from both patient and physician. CLA seems to prevent this cancer cascade or avalanche from occurring. CLA also reverses cancer in animals even when they possess a genetic predisposition for cancer.[61]

➤ Neutralizing the potential damage from other fats. Animals fed varying levels of fat (10-20% by weight, similar to American diet) in the diet and different types of fat (corn oil vs lard) were protected against breast cancer when fed only 1% of the diet as CLA.[62]

➤ Generating unknown but valuable fatty acid by-products from the liver. In animal studies, CLA in the diet generated a unique collection of fats in the liver and outside of the liver.[63] Maybe CLA also provides the raw ingredient for the liver to make something very valuable in the body.

➤ Shuts down abnormal cell growth. CLA in test tube studies (in vitro) has shown a remarkable ability as a cytotoxic (kills cancer cells) and cytostatic (stops or slows cancer growth) agent in a wide variety of human cancers, including melanoma, colorectal, prostate, ovarian, glioblastoma (brain), mesothelioma, leukemia, and breast.[64]

➤ Some studies have found that CLA enhances immune functions[65] while another study showed no effect on the immune system while feeding the animals a diet that was 50% sucrose.[66] As I have stated repeatedly, a high sugar diet will encourage cancer growth beyond the inhibitory effect of any single anticancer nutrient, including CLA. A high sugar diet is a much more powerful "vector" than micronutrients.

➤ Improve glucose and insulin levels. CLA manages to also make cells more sensitive to insulin, thus lowering insulin requirements and blood glucose levels. These researchers from Penn State and Purdue boldly state: "CLA may prove to be an important therapy for the prevention and treatment of non-insulin dependent diabetes mellitus."[67] Controlling blood glucose can provide the cancer patient with major assistance in slowing cancer growth.

➤ Timing is crucial. Studies with animals show that when CLA is fed to animals from post-weaning through puberty, it can prevent breast cancer from occurring even when a potent carcinogen is injected in the animals. However, if animals are deprived of CLA until the breast cancer occurs, then CLA must be fed to the animal for the remainder of its life in order to prevent a recurrence of cancer.[68] Apparently, CLA in young animals helps to insure proper maturation of the mammary glands and to prevent the initiation and promotion phases of cancer.

Basically, CLA is one of the more promising, non-toxic, inexpensive, anti-cancer, anti-heart disease, anti-diabetes nutrients to come along in the history of nutrition science.

ENDNOTES

[1] . Gorlin, R., Archives Intern. Med., vol.148, p.2043, Sept.1988
[2] . Karmali, RA, J. Nat. Cancer Inst., vol.73, p.457, 1984; see also Gabor, H., et al., J.Nat.Cancer Inst. vol.76, p.1223, 1986
[3] . Wan, JM, et al., Fed. Amer Soc Exper Biol., vol.A350, p.21, 1988
[4] . Burns, CP, et al., Nutrition Reviews, vol.48, p.233, June 1990
[5] . Guffy, MM, et al., Cancer Research, vol.44, p.1863, 1984
[6] . Cannizzo, F., et al., Cancer Research, vol.49, p.3961, 1981
[7] . Begin, ME, et al., J.Nat.Cancer Inst., vol.77, p.1053, 1986
[8] . Karmali, RA, J.Internal Med. suppl, vol.225, p.197, 1989
[9] . Osborne, MP, et al., Cancer Investigation, vol.6, p.629, 1988
[10] . Huang, ME, Am.J.Hematol., vol.28, p.124, 1988
[11] . Watson, R., et al., Nutr.Res., vol.5, p.663, 1985
[12] . Zhang, XM, et al., Virchows Archiv.B Cell.Pathol., vol.61, p.375, 1992
[13] . Friedberg, EC, CANCER QUESTIONS, p.32, Freeman & Co, NY, 1992
[14] . Semba, RD, Clin. Infect.Dis., vol.19, p.489, 1994
[15] . Rumore, MM, Clin.Pharm., vol.12, p.506, 1993
[16] . Pinnock, CB, et al., Aust.Paediatr.J., vol.22, p.95, 1986
[17] . Nutrition Reviews, vol.52, p.281, 1994
[18] . Micksche, M., et al., Onkologie, vol.1, p.57, 1978
[19] . Vagner, VP, et al., Klin.Med., vol.69, p.55, 1991
[20] . Michalek, AM, et al., Nutrition and Cancer, vol.9, p.143, 1987
[21] . Stich, HF, Am.J.Clin.Nutr., vol.53, p.298S, 1991
[22] . Lippman, SM, et al., J.Am.Coll.Nutr., vol.7, p.269, 1988
[23] . Pastorino, U., et al., J. Clin.Oncol., vol.11, p.1216, 1993
[24] . Hruban, Z, Am.J.Pathol., vol.76, p.451, 1974
[25] . Rothman, KJ, et al., N.Engl.J.Med., vol.333, p.1369, 1995
[26] . Hathcock, JN, et al., Am.J.Clin.Nutr., vol.52, p.183, 1990
[27] . Norman, AW, in PRESENT KNOWLEDGE IN NUTRITION, p.120, Ziegler, EE (eds), ILSI, Washington 1996
[28] . Gorham, ED, et al., Intern.J.Epidemiol. vol.20, p.1145, Dec.1991
[29] . Lefkowitz, ES, et al., Intern.J.Epidemiol., vol.23, p.1133, Dec.1994
[30] . Garland, CF, et al., Lancet, p.1176, Nov.18, 1989
[31] . Barger-Lux, MJ, J. Nutr., vol.124, p.1406S, Aug.1994
[32] . Crowle, AJ, et al., Infection and Immunity, vol.55, p.2945, Dec.1987
[33] . Newmark, HL, Adv.Exp.Med.Biol., vol.364, p.109, 1994
[34] . Lancet, p.1122, May 16, 1987
[35] . Pence, B., et al., Proc Amer.Assoc. Cancer, vol.28, p.154, 1987
[36] . Colston, KW, et al., Lancet, p.188, Jan.28, 1989
[37] . Peehl, DM, et al., J. Endocrinol. Invest., vol.17, p.3,, 1994
[38] . Eisman, JA, et al., Modulation and Mediation of Cancer by Vitamins, p.282, Karger, Basel, 1983
[39] . Kizaki, M., et al., Vitamins and Cancer Prevention, p.91, Wiley-Liss, NY, 1991
[40] . DeLuca, HF, Nutrients and Cancer Prevention, p.271, Humana Press, NY, 1990
[41] . Rita, M., et al., Cancer Immunol. Immunother., vol.41, p.37, 1995
[42] . Food and Nutrition Board, National Research Council, Recommended Dietary Allowances, National Academy Press, p.97, Washington, DC, 1989
[43] . Buist, RA, Intern.Clin.Nutr.Rev., vol.4, p.159, 1984
[44] . Begin, ME, et al., Prostaglandins, Leukotriennes, and Medicine, vol.19, p.177, Aug.1985; see also Begin, ME, Anticancer Research, vol.6, p291, 1986

[45]. Takeda, S., et al., Anticancer Research, vol.12, p.329, 1992
[46]. Vander Merwe, CF, et al., British J.Clin.Practice, vol.41, p.907, 1987
[47]. Begin, ME, et al., Prostaglandins, Leukotrienes & Medicine, vol.19, p.177, 1985
[48]. Brohult, A., et al., Acta.Obstet.Gynecol.Scand., vol.56, p.441, 1977
[49]. Brohult, A., et al., Acta.Obstet. Gynecol.Scand., vol.58, p.203, 1979
[50]. Brohult, A., et al., Acta. Chem.Scand., vol.24, p.730, 1970
[51]. Brohult, A., et al., Acta Obstet.Gynecol.Scand., vol.65, p.779, 1986; see also
Acta.Obstet.Gynecol.Scand., vol.57, p.79, 1978
[52]. Riel, RR, J.Dairy Sci., vol.46, p.102, 1963
[53]. Knekt, P., et al., Br.J.Cancer, vol.73, p.687, 1996
[54]. Hirayama, T., in DIET AND HUMAN CARCINOGENESIS, Joosens, JV , p.191, Elsevier, NY
[55]. Sebedio, JL, et al., Biochimica et Biophysica Acta, vol.1345, p.5, 1997
[56]. Ip, C., et al., Nutrition & Cancer, vol.27, no.2, p.131, 1997
[57]. Ip, C., et al., Cancer Research, vol.54, p.1212, 1994
[58]. Liew,C., et al., Carcinogenesis, vol.16, no.12, p.3037, 1995
[59]. Decker, EA, Nutrition Reviews, vol.53, no.3, p.49, Mar.1995
[60]. van den Berg,JJM, et al., Lipids, vol.30, no.7, p.599, 1995
[61]. Ip, C., et al., Carcinogenesis, vol.18, no.4, p.755, 1997
[62]. Ip, C., et al., Carcinogenesis, vol.17, no.5, p.1045, 1996
[63]. Belury, MA, et al., Lipids, vol.32, no.2, p.199, 1997
[64]. Shultz, TD, et al., Cancer Letters, vol.63, p.125, 1992; see also Visonneau, S., et al.,
J.Fed.Amer.Society Experimental Biology, vol.10, p.A182, 1996
[65]. Cook, ME, et al., Poultry Science, vol.72, p.1301, 1993; see also Miller, CC, et al.,
Biochem.Biophys.Res.Commun., vol.198, p.1107, 1994
[66]. Wong, MW, et al., Anticancer Research, vol.17, p.987, 1997
[67]. Houseknecht, KL, et al., Biochem. Biophys.Res.Commun., vol.244, p.678, 1998
[68]. Ip, C., et al., Nutrition & Cancer, vol.24, p.241, 1995

CHAPTER 5
✷
VITAMINS

Betacarotene 15 mg (=25,000 iu)
Immune stimulant, helps with cell to cell communication.

It is easy to appreciate the beauty of carotenoids on a crisp fall day with the autumn foliage at its peak. Carotenoids are usually pigmented substances produced by plants to assist in photosynthesis and protect the plant from the damaging effects of the sun's radiation. Of the 800 or so carotenoids that have been isolated, the most famous are beta-carotene, alpha-carotene, lutein, zeaxanthin, lycopene, and beta-cryptoxanthin. Most carotenoids are pigmented molecules that are red, yellow or orange in color. A few carotenoids, such as phytoene and phytofluene, are colorless.

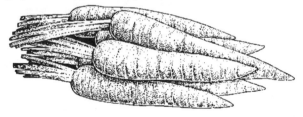

Over 200 epidemiological studies[1] show that a diet rich in fruit and vegetables will lower the risk for a variety of cancers. Of the 15% of annual lung cancer patients who are not smokers, which totals over 22,000 deaths per year, fruits and vegetables can provide major protection against lung cancer.[2]

Beta-carotene and other carotenoids have been thoroughly reviewed regarding their role in cancer and found: "...carotenoids exert an important influence in modulating the actions of carcinogens."[3] Beta-carotene has been shown to play a major role in the "telegraph" communication between cells that prevents or reverses abnormal growths. This "gap junction communication" is one of many reasons why beta-carotene protects us from cancer.[4] Beta-carotene selectively inhibited the growth of human squamous cancer cells in culture.[5] Beta-carotene and canthaxanthin provided significant protection in animals against the cancer-causing effects of radiation.[6]

Carotenoids may partially compensate for the "sins" of our unhealthy lifestyles. In one study, researchers from the National Cancer Institute and Harvard tracked over 47,000 healthy individuals and found that lycopenes, even from pizza sauce, were protective against prostate cancer.[7] Other studies have found that beta-carotene supplements can reverse the pre-cancerous condition (oral leukoplakia) brought about by chewing betel nut,[8] which is a Third World version of chewing tobacco.

Beta-carotene affects the cancer process in a variety of ways:

◊ alters the adenylate cyclase activity in melanoma cells in culture, which affects cell differentiation, and thus whether a cell will turn cancerous or not[9]

◊ potent anti-oxidant,[10] which spares immune cells in the microscopic "war on cancer" and protects the healthy prostaglandins

◊ provides a certain level of tumor immunity in mice innoculated with cancer cells[11]

◊ protects the DNA against the damaging effects of carcinogens[12]

◊ according to studies by Food and Drug Administration researchers, beta-carotene protects against the cancer causing effects of a choline deficient diet in animals

◊ once cancer has been initiated, either chemically or physically, beta-carotene inhibits the next step in the cancer process of neoplastic transformation[13]

◊ there is a synergistic benefit of using vitamin A with carotenoids in patients who have been first treated with chemo, radiation and surgery for common malignancies[14]

◊ beta-carotene and vitamin A together provided a significant improvement in outcome in animals treated with radiation for induced cancers[15]

◊ carotenoids (from Spirulina and Dunaliella algae) plus vitamin E and canthaxanthin were injected in animal tumors, with the result being complete regression as mediated by an increase in Tumor Necrosis Factor (TNF) in macrophages in the tumor region[16]

◊ in 20 patients with mouth cancer who were given high doses of radiation and chemo, beta-carotene provided significant protection against mouth sores (oral mucositis) induced by medical therapy, although there was no significant difference in survival rates[17]

◊ in animals, beta-carotene provided cancer protection against a carcinogenic virus, which would normally damage the DNA[18]

Beta-carotene in ImmunoPower is provided by Betatene, a special mixed carotenoid extract from Dunaliella algae, which has been shown in scientific studies to potently inhibit the development of breast tumors in animals.[19] Betatene consists of a rich mixture of various carotenoids, primarily naturally occurring betacarotene, along with smaller amounts of lycopene (also found separately in ImmunoPower), alpha-carotene, zeaxanthin, cryptoxanthin and lutein.

BETA CAROTENE CAUSES LUNG CANCER?

SAFETY ISSUES. There is virtually no toxicity to beta-carotene at any dosage, other than the mild pigmentation (carotenemia) that occurs in the skin region.[20] With our primitive analytical tools, scientists isolated out the most likely champion of the carotenoids, beta-carotene, and conducted several human intervention trials funded by the National Cancer Institute to examine if beta-carotene would reduce the incidence of lung cancer in heavy smokers. It didn't.[21] And in two studies, the beta-carotene supplemented groups had slightly elevated incidences of lung cancer. The press loved this huge controversy and made sure that everyone knew about it. Unfortunately, only a small portion of the story was told.

Issues not covered by the press included:

-Those individuals who had the highest SERUM beta-carotene at the start of these two studies had a lower incidence of lung cancer. Beta-carotene ABSORBED does indeed reduce the risk of suicidal lifestyles, like smoking

- Prominent researchers in nutrition and cancer have published papers showing that antioxidants, like beta-carotene, can become pro-oxidants in the wrong biochemical environment, such as the combat zone of free radicals generated by heavy tobacco use.[22] Nowhere in Nature do we find a food with just beta-carotene. All foods contain a rich and dazzling array of anti-oxidants.

-After 35 years of heavy smoking, the damage is done. The damaging effects of tobacco cannot be neutralized by one "magic bullet" pill of synthetic beta-carotene with coal tar based food dyes added to insure a homogenous color in the beta-carotene capsules.

-It is the synergism of multiple carotenoids that protects people. If beta-carotene truly provoked lung cancer then what about the 200 studies showing that a diet rich in fruit and vegetables (best sources of beta-carotene) significantly lowers the incidence of cancer.

-At the International Conference on Nutrition and Cancer, sponsored by the University of California at Irvine, held in July of 1997, there were several watershed presentations showing that one nutrient alone may be ineffective or counterproductive for cancer patients while a host of compatible nutrients in the proper ratio can be extremely effective at slowing or reversing cancer.

E (2/3 succinate, 1/3 natural) 400 iu
Natural E (mixed tocopherols) stimulates immune functions and works as an antioxidant. E succinate may be selectively toxic to tumor cells.

More than a few physicians have assumed that, since vitamin E is an antioxidant and chemo and radiation work by generating prooxidants to kills cancer cells, therefore vitamin E will reduce the efficacy of medical therapy in cancer patients. Nothing could be further from the truth. Vitamin E is a valuable ally for both the cancer patient and the oncologist.

My college professors in the 1970s would facetiously chuckle at the "health nuts" who popped vitamin E capsules, claiming that "vitamin E was in search of a disease." In one study, healthy students were deprived of vitamin E in the diet for up to 2 years with no blatant vitamin deficiency syndrome, such as is found with vitamin C and scurvy, or vitamin D and rickets. Deficiencies of vitamin E cause an increase in lipid peroxidation (prooxidants) that decrease energy production (due to mitochondrial membrane damage), increase mutation of DNA, alter the normal transport mechanisms in the cell membrane.[23] Hemolytic anemia (premature bursting of red blood cells) has been found in infants who are fed a diet high in polyunsaturated fats (which generate lipid peroxides) and iron (which is a prooxidant). Malabsorption syndromes, such as biliary cirrhosis (blockage of the liver duct to the gallbladder), can generate blatant vitamin E deficiency in humans.[24]

Actually, clinical deficiencies of vitamin E probably take decades to turn into full blown cataracts, Alzheimer's, heart disease, arthritis or cancer. While 1 milligram of vitamin E (alpha tocopheryl acetate) equals 1 international unit, other versions (racemates) of E are not as potent, and hence have less iu per mg.

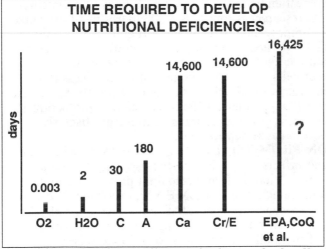

TIME REQUIRED TO DEVELOP NUTRITIONAL DEFICIENCIES

Most substances in life are either fat soluble (can be dissolved in alcohol) or water soluble, with a few magical substances, like lecithin, able to work in either universe. Vitamin E is the most critical of all fat soluble antioxidants. Imagine that little "fires", or prooxidants, break out all over the human body all of the time. The primary "fire extinguisher" that can put out fires in the fat soluble portion of the body, including the vulnerable cell membrane--is vitamin E.[25] Because of this fundamental role in cell biology, vitamin E helps to:

◊ protect the beneficial prostaglandins
◊ stimulates immune function
◊ protects healthy cells against toxins and radiation while making cancer cells more vulnerable to medical therapy
◊ a special form of vitamin E (succinate) is selectively toxic to cancer cells.

Vitamin E actually refers to a family of 8 related compounds, the tocopherols and tocotrienols. ImmunoPower also contains tocotrienols. More on that subject later. Tocopherols got their name from "pherein", meaning to carry, and "tocos", meaning birth, because vitamin E from wheat germ was found to be essential for fertility. True natural vitamin E is a mixture of alpha, beta, delta and gamma tocopherols plus some tocotrienols, which are more concentrated in rice bran and palm oil. ImmunoPower contains 1/3 mixed natural tocopherols and 2/3 vitamin E succinate because the two compounds each have a unique way of attacking cancer. Vitamin E may help the cancer patient in numerous ways:

NUTRITIONAL SYNERGISM. Zinc deficiency in animals further compounds a vitamin E deficiency, meaning that zinc must be present to properly utilize vitamin E.[26] Also, vitamin E protects the body against the potentially damaging effects of iron and fish oil. Human volunteers given high doses of fish oil experienced an immune abnormality (mitogenic responsiveness of peripheral blood mononuclear cells to concanavalin A) which was reversed with supplements of vitamin E.[27]

IMMUNE REGULATOR. Vitamin E plays a powerful role as an immune regulator.[28] When 32 healthy elderly adults were given supplements of 800 iu daily of vitamin E there were measurable improvements in immune functions.[29] Following 28 days of supplements of vitamins E, C and A; researchers found that 30 elderly institutionalized patients had substantial improvements in immune functions (absolute T-cells, T4 subsets, T4:T8 ratio and lymphocyte proliferation).[30] E seems to work by protecting immune factors from immediate destruction in their suicidal plunge at cancer cells. E also works by bolstering the activity of the thymus and spleen organs to stimulate lymphocyte proliferation. In burned animals, vitamin E supplements offered substantial protection in the intestinal mucosa to prevent bacterial translocation (gut bacteria migrating into the blood to cause septicemia).[31]

PROTECTION FROM TOXINS. Vitamin E protected animals from the cancer-causing effects of alcohol on the esophagus[32] and a carcinogen on the colon.[33] Vitamin E and selenium protected animals against the potent carcinogenic effects of DMBA from tobacco.[34] Vitamin E protected the damaged liver of rats from developing fatty liver and collagen content.[35] Vitamin E protects us against the greatest toxin and essential nutrient of them all--oxygen, as shown in exercised animals.[36] By sparing fats in the blood from becoming lipid peroxides, vitamin E supplements were very effective at preventing heart disease.[37] Vitamin E prevents the formation of one of the more common carcinogenic agents in humans; nitrosamines, which are formed by the combination of nitrates in the diet and amino acids in the stomach. Vitamin E prevents the damage to the skin from ultraviolet radiation.[38] According to researchers from Bulgaria, vitamin E protects us against the harmful effects of too much iron-generating free radicals and damage to our detoxification system, cytochrome P-450. Much of the damage caused by iron in the human body is due to: 1) wrong form of iron, we need chelated iron, not iron salts as we get in fortified white flour, 2) not enough antioxidants to prevent this oxidizing metal from "rusting" in the cell and creating harm.

REVERSE PRE-CANCEROUS CONDITION. Vitamin E supplements (200-400 mg/d for 3 months) reversed fibrocystic breast disease (a major risk for breast cancer) in 22 out of 26 women.[39] Other women have found reversal of fibrocystic breast disease through elimination of caffeine, chocolate, and colas which contain methylxanthines.

PROSTAGLANDINS. We can generate very healthy prostaglandins if we have the right dietary precursors in our blood, which comes from:
⇒ enough fish oil (EPA) or flax oil (ALA) and borage oil (GLA)
⇒ healthy levels of blood sugar (60-100 mg%)
⇒ optimal amounts of vitamin E.[40]

Because of this beneficial impact on prostaglandins, vitamin E helps to inhibit platelet adhesion[41], which helps to slow down the spreading of cancer. And yet, as shown below, vitamin E does not influence blood clotting, or prothrombin time, which is good news for people worried about proper clotting during and after surgery.

SLOWS AND REVERSES CANCER. In human studies, low intake of vitamin E increases the risk for cancer of various body sites.[42] Patients with head and neck cancers are more likely to have a recurrence if they have low blood levels of vitamins E, A and betacarotene.[43] Vitamin E injected into animal mouth tumors was able to significantly reduce or completely eliminate tumors.[44] In patients with colorectal cancer, vitamin E, C, and A supplements were able to reduce the growth of abnormal cells in the colon, indicating a possible slowing of the cancer process.[45] In human epidemiology studies, people with the highest intake of E (still very low compared to ideal intake) had a 40% reduction in the risk for colon cancer.[46] In animals, vitamin E supplements prevent lung tumors from developing.[47]

VITAMIN E SUCCINATE AND CANCER. For some unknown reason, when vitamin E is esterified (combined) with succinic acid, a new molecule is formed with surprising ability to selectively shut down cancer growth, but not harm healthy tissue, [48] slowing the growth of brain (glioma and neuroblastoma) and melanoma cells in culture.[49] E succinate is able to reduce the genetic expression of c-myc oncogenes in cultured cancer cells.[50] E succinate inhibits virally-induced tumors in culture.[51] E succinate has been studied as a potent regulator of cell proliferation.[52]

IMPROVES MEDICAL THERAPY OF CANCER. Vitamin E helps generally toxic medical therapies to distinguish between healthy and cancerous cells. The best proposed mechanism for this action is the anaerobic state of many tumors. Vitamin E apparently is not well absorbed, or needed, by tumors, since they are anaerobic (without oxygen). An antioxidant is of little interest to an oxygen independent cell. Because of this function of vitamin E, chemotherapy and radiation can be made much more selectively toxic to the cancer cells, while protecting the patient from host damage.

It has long been known that a vitamin E deficiency, common in cancer patients, will accentuate the cardiotoxic effects of adriamycin.[53] The worse the vitamin E deficiency in animals, the greater the heart damage from adriamycin.[54] Patients undergoing chemo, radiation and bone marrow transplant for cancer treatment had markedly depressed levels of serum antioxidants, including vitamin E.[55] Given the fact that both chemo and radiation can induce cancer, which reduces the chances for survival, it is noteworthy that vitamin E protects animals against a potent carcinogen, DMBA.[56] Vitamin E supplements prevented the glucose-raising effects of a chemo drug, doxorubicin.[57] Since cancer is a sugar-feeder, preventing this glucose-raising effect may be another valuable contribution from vitamin E in patients receiving chemo. Meanwhile, vitamin E improves the tumor kill rate of doxorubicin.[58] Vitamin E modifies the carcinogenic effect of daunomycin (chemo drug) in animals.[59]

Human prostate cancer cells were killed at a higher rate when adriamycin (chemo drug) was combined with vitamin E at concentrations that can easily be obtained from supplementation.[60] Vitamin E supplements (1600 iu/day) taken one week prior to adriamycin therapy protected 69% of patients from hair loss, which is nearly universal in adriamycin-treated patients.[61] Vitamin E helped to repair kidney damage caused by adriamycin in animals.[62] Vitamin E and selenium supplements in animals helped to reduce the heart toxicity from adriamycin.[63] Selenium and vitamin E supplements were given to 41 women undergoing cytotoxic therapy for ovarian and cervical cancers, with a resulting drop in the toxicity-related rise in creatine kinase.[64] Vitamin E, A and prenylamine reduced the toxicity of adriamycin on the heart of animals studied.[65]

In animals with implanted tumors, those pretreated with vitamin E had a much greater tumor kill from radiation therapy.[66] Radiation therapists know that the ability to kill cancer with radiation diminishes as the tumor becomes more anaerobic or hypoxic. Vitamin E seems to sensitize tumors, making them more vulnerable to radiation therapy. In cultured human cancer cells, vitamin E increased the damaging effects of radiation on tumor cells.[67] Brain cancer cells were easier to kill once pretreated with vitamin E succinate.[68] Tumor kill in animals receiving radiation therapy was greatly increased by pretreatment with vitamin E.[69] Vitamin E supplements reduced the breakage of red blood cells in animals given radiation therapy.[70] Vitamin E supplements improved the wound recovery in animals given preoperative radiation.[71]

Vitamin E combined with vitamin K, leucovorin (anti-metabolite cancer drug) and 5FU (fluorouracil) significantly enhanced the cell growth inhibition curves for 5FU.[72] One of the more troublesome side effects of chemotherapy is peripheral neuropathy, or a tingling numbness in the extremities. Low vitamin E status is likely to blame for peripheral neuropathy.[73]

Mouth sores (oral mucositis) are a common problem arising from the use of many chemotherapy drugs. These mouth sores are so painful that cancer patients stop eating, which creates malnutrition, which really deteriorates the general health picture. Vitamin E topically applied healed 67% of cancer patients in a double blind trial at M.D. Anderson Hospital in Houston.[74] To use this therapy, puncture the end of a soft gelatin vitamin E capsule and spread the vitamin E oil over the mouth sore. Do this several times each day.

Can't get enough in food

Vitamin E supplements have even been endorsed by the National Cancer Institute[75], American Heart Association and the United States Department of Agriculture, because in order to consume 400 international units of vitamin E, you would have to eat either:
-2 quarts of corn oil, or
-5 pounds of wheat germ, or
-8 cups of almonds, or
-28 cups of peanuts

SAFETY ISSUES. Taking many times the RDA of vitamin E had some researchers worried about toxicity, so they fed 900 iu (90 times the RDA) daily to healthy college students for 12 weeks with no changes in liver, kidney, thyroid, **blood clotting** or immunoglobulin levels.[76] These results are valuable because vitamin E inhibits the platelet aggregation that can cause stroke, heart disease or cancer metastasis; yet does not alter blood clotting activity. Therefore, pre-surgical patients do not need to reduce vitamin E intake for fear of not clotting during and after surgery. According to a review of the world's literature on vitamin E toxicity, there are virtually no side effects at dosages under 3200 iu/day.[77]

K (menadione) 100 mcg
Selectively toxic to tumor cells, forms anti-cancer compound with C

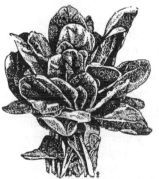

When vitamin K was first researched in 1929, it was labelled the "Klotting" factor by the Dutch scientist Henrik Dam. Since then, much has been learned about this fascinating molecule. There are three primary variations of vitamin K, all with certain levels of activity in the body.
⇒ K-1, or phylloquinone, is produced in higher plants such as spinach, broccoli, brussel sprouts and kale.
⇒ K-2, or menaquinone, is produced by bacterial fermentation, which means that we manufacture varying amounts of vitamin K in a healthy human gut; also fermented foods like cheeses and soy foods carry some K.
⇒ K-3, or menadione, is the synthetically derived version of vitamin K, called Synkavite in drug form.

Although mother's milk will quickly begin generating vitamin K in the infant's gut, physicians have developed a standard hospital protocol of giving injections of Synkavite to all newborns. About 1/3 of all patients with chronic gastrointestinal problems have clinical vitamin K deficiency.[78]

There are several handsome lessons to be learned as we review vitamin K in ImmunoPower:

◊ **Metavitamin functions**. Many nutrients develop unique functions when given at anything beyond survival doses. Niacin, vitamin A, vitamin C, fish oil and others all reflect the fact that low dose of a nutrient will give you basic survival functions, while higher doses give us "above-vitamin" or meta-vitamin functions. In this case, vitamin K is basically a clotting factor that helps to activate prothrombin so that we do not bleed to death when cutting open the skin envelope.[79] In higher doses, vitamin K becomes a potent anti-cancer agent which is non-toxic to healthy cells.[80]

◊ **Synergism yields two main benefits**: Increase in healing capacity while lowering the dosage requirements. Researchers found that combining vitamins C and K-3 against cultured human breast cancer cells allowed for inhibition of the cancer growth at doses 90-98% less than what was required if only one of these vitamins was used.[81]

◊ **Look beyond the obvious**. Coumadin (a.k.a. dicumarol, warfarin) is an anti-coagulant drug that holds promise in cancer treatment by shuting down cancer cell metabolism and helping to slow metastasis. Vitamin K has a primary function of inducing coagulation. The obvious deduction is that vitamin K (a coagulant) would neutralize the benefits of coumadin (anti-coagulant). In real life, Vitamin K-3 does not neutralize the effects of coumadin[82] but actually improves the anti-cancer effects of coumadin.[83] The reason that K-1 reverses the effects of coumadin and K-3 does not lies in the slight difference in chemical structure in which K-3 cannot participate in the gamma carboxylation of prothrombin.

◊ **Similar is not the same as identical in chemical structures**. Oftentimes, drug companies find a substance that has therapeutic action, such as vitamin A or indole-3-carbinol from broccoli, and will try to create a slightly different molecule so that it can be patented. These slight differences nearly always translate into high toxicity from these newly-formed molecules. For instance, the difference between a man and woman rests primarily on the difference between the hormones testosterone and estrogen, which are nearly identical molecules except for one OH group. Over 40 years ago, Professor J.S.Mitchell of England showed that patients receiving K-3 had measurable shrinkage of tumors. Later, the drug doxorubicin was introduced as an anti-cancer drug. K-3, doxorubicin and coumadin all share related chemical structures as "naphthoquinone" molecules. Yet, of all these compounds, K-3 has been shown by Chlebowski and colleagues at the University of California Los Angeles to have 70 times (7000%!!!) more anti-cancer activity than coumadin and 25 times more cancer killing capacity than vitamin K-1.

Vitamin K-3 works against cancer both by directly antagonizing cell replication in cancer cells[84] and by inhibiting metastasis. K-3 also works as a potentiator of radiation therapy. In one study, patients with mouth cancer who were pre-treated with injections of K-3 prior to radiation therapy doubled their odds (20% vs. 39%) for 5 year survival and disease free status.[85] Animals with implanted tumors had greatly improved anti-cancer effects from all chemotherapy drugs tested when vitamins K and C were given in combination.[86] In cultured leukemia cells, vitamins K and E added to the chemotherapy drugs of 5FU (fluorouracil) and leucovorin provided a 300% improvement in growth inhibition when compared to 5FU by itself.[87] Animals given methotrexate and K-3 had improvements in cancer reversal with no increase in toxicity to the host tissue.[88] In one case study, a patient with recurrent and drug refractory bone cancer metastasized to the lungs, was put on a regimen of hydrazine sulfate and vitamin K-3 injections, with a resulting weight gain and complete regression of her cancer.[89] In 13 cancer patients, some with demonstrated drug resistant tumors, menadiol (vitamin K analog, a.k.a. K-4) was given at up to 3200 mg per meter squared per week along with various chemo drugs with no increase in host toxicity but some improvements in tumor responses.[90]

SAFETY ISSUES. There is no known toxicity associated with the plant-derived version, K-1.[91] The toxicity of menadione (K-3) is very low, with animals having no adverse side effects after being fed 1000 times the daily requirement.[92] The typical dietary intake of K-1 in America is somewhere between 100-500 micrograms daily, with little understanding of the role played by the production of K-2 in the healthy human gut.

A special note on coumadin. Many cancer patients on coumadin are directed by their physician to avoid foods high in vitamin K-1, including kale, spinach, broccoli and other anti-cancer greens. The doctor will take blood samples and conduct a Pro test (prothrombin test, time required for the blood to clot) and prescribe coumadin based on this test. It is much more essential to have a PREDICTABLE amount of vitamin K-1 in the diet than to avoid it, which will allow for the safest and most effective use of anti-coagulant drugs.

C 2500 mg; 1000 mg as ascorbic acid & 1500 mg as sodium ascorbate
Immune stimulant, antioxidant, envelops & shuts down cancer.

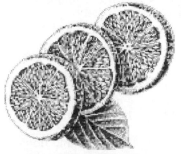

If vitamin A was the mother of all anti-cancer vitamins, then vitamin C is the grandmother of all. The problem started millions of years ago when primates lost the liver enzyme necessary to convert sugar into vitamin C.[93] Of the millions of animals, reptiles, amphibians, insects and other things that walk, crawl, fly and swim--humans are among the few creatures on earth that do not make our own vitamin C. Our primitive ancestors were able to consume 300-500 milligrams daily of vitamin C, which definitely prevents scurvy. Throughout the golden ages of world exploration by ship, thousands of people died--sometimes up to half of the crew--due to scurvy. Highly perishable fresh fruits and vegetables are the richest sources of vitamin C and were unavailable on ship voyages longer than a few weeks. Around 1750, the English physician, James Lind, found that limes could prevent and reverse scurvy (does that make limes a prescription drug?).

"Time lags" are a known phenomenon that separate a discovery from the actual implementation of a breakthrough. It was another 50 years after Dr. Lind's research before limes were required to be carried aboard ships, thus costing the world thousands of unnecessary deaths in this delay. Are we doing the same thing by delaying aggressive nutrition support for millions of cancer patients?

Vitamin C is one of the more versatile vitamins in human nutrition. Its functions include:
⇒ potent protector against free radicals
⇒ maintenance of tough connective tissue (collagen and elastin) which is the "glue" that keeps our body together
⇒ production of adrenaline for energy
⇒ production of serotonin for thought and calmness
⇒ stimulates various immune components to protect against infections and cancer
⇒ converts cholesterol into bile for its elimination in the bowels
⇒ maintains fat stores in the adipose tissue to prevent heart disease
⇒ important for bone formation
⇒ critical in many detoxification pathways to better tolerate pollutants
⇒ reduces allergic reactions by preventing histamine release
⇒ helps insulin to better control blood sugar levels.

And remember, these are just the normal everyday functions in healthy people. In sick people, vitamin C develops additional therapeutic roles.

HOW MUCH???

Part of the controversy surrounding vitamin C is the extreme range of dosages that can be consumed in humans or produced in animals:
⇒ 10 milligrams daily will prevent blatant scurvy in most healthy adults
⇒ 60 mg is the Recommended Dietary Allowance
⇒ 200-300 mg would be consumed by people who are following the NCI suggestion of 5 servings of fruit and vegetables daily
⇒ 300 mg of supplemental vitamin C was shown to increase quantity of life by 6 years in men
⇒ 1000 mg is required in many hospitalized patients just to maintain adequate serum ascorbate levels
⇒ 10,000 to 20,000 mg is often taken by many people using C to curtail some illness, like cancer, AIDS, viral infections, and injury recovery
⇒ 100,000 mg/day has been given IV, or intravenously with no side effects
⇒ 20,000 mg is produced daily by many animals, like goats and dogs, on a per weight basis using a 154 pound reference man; internal production goes up further when the animal is exposed to stress, infections, or toxins

Although Linus Pauling, PhD was not the first scientist to suggest that vitamin C might help cancer patients, he was definitely the most vocal and decorated of the lot. With 2 unshared Nobel prizes and 3 Presidential citations, you would think that the scientific community would be more open to Dr. Pauling's comments. Though Pauling was considered to be one of the 2 greatest scientists of the 20th century, along with Albert Einstein, the 1970s found Pauling to be an academic nomad for his innovative views on vitamin C.

However, as time marched on, data continued to gather to support Pauling's viewpoint. By 1982, the National Academy of Sciences was willing to admit that vitamin C might prevent cancer.[94] And by 1990, the National Institutes of Health hosted a conference on "Vitamin C and Cancer", which showed that Pauling was truly on to something.[95] While Pauling's strident critics claimed that he was trying to cure cancer with vitamin C, in fact Pauling only suggested high doses of C in concert with medical therapies would augment cancer outcome, as he wrote:

> "The optimum treatment of the cancer patient requires a concerted multi-disciplinary approach employing the full resources of surgery, radiotherapy, chemotherapy, immunotherapy and supportive care. The last named has received the least attention, although it might well possess great potential for therapeutic advance."[96]
> Linus Pauling, PhD,1974

Pauling later went on to explain the reasons that vitamin C may improve outcome in cancer treatment, including the increased need for C in cancer patients, ability of C to prevent cancer breaking down connective tissue for metastasis, ability of C to help "wall off" or encapsulate the tumor, role of C in immune attack on cancer, and the role of C in hormonal balance.[97] One of the highlights of my career has been having Dr. Pauling eat supper at my house in 1992 while he was spry and alert at 91 years of age.

Vitamin C can help cancer patients in several critical categories:

1) Prevention. Cancer patients have already demonstrated a genetic vulnerability to cancer and toxins. Cancer patients will likely be exposed to even more potent carcinogens in medical therapy. Therefore, the need to prevent secondary and iatrogenic tumors is great. In a study encompassing 16 groups in 7 countries covering 25 years, higher vitamin C intake was strongly related to lowering cancer incidence.[98] Another study examined the cancer protective effect of vitamin C and found that 33 of 46 epidemiological studies showed it helped, while none showed any increase in cancer with higher vitamin C intake.[99] Vitamin C protects humans against a whole assortment of toxic chemicals[100] while accelerating wound recovery[101] and stabilizing iron compounds (ferritin) in the blood.[102] C reduced the incidence and severity of kidney tumors in animals exposed to the hormones estradiol or diethylstilbestrol.[103]

Through a wide variety of mechanisms, vitamin C is a potent inhibitor of cancer.[104]

  2) Augmenting medical therapy. C may be able to enhance the toxicity of chemo and radiation against the cancer cells while protecting the patient from possible harm. C was able to enhance the effectiveness of a drug (misonidazole) that improves outcome in radiation treatment of cancer.[105] C improved the tumor-stopping abilities of a wide range of medical therapies against brain cancer (neuroblastoma) cells in culture.[106] Animals given the chemo drugs vincristine (from the periwinkle plant) and vinblastine were given supplements of vitamin C with an increase in the excretion of these very toxic drugs.[107] Animals given adriamycin (a common chemotherapy drug) along with vitamin C had a significant prolongation of life and reduction in the expected heart damage (cardiotoxicity) from this drug.[108] Given the widespread use of adriamycin and its known lethal toxicity on the heart[109], it should be standard procedure to give high doses of antioxidants prior to administration of adriamycin.

  Animals with implanted tumors were injected with high doses of C one hour prior to whole body radiation therapy, all scaled to mimic the effects in a human cancer patient. Vitamin C did not affect the tumor killing capacity of the radiation, but did provide substantial protection to the animals.[110] 50 previously untreated cancer patients were randomly divided into 2 groups, with #1 receiving radiation therapy only and #2 receiving radiation plus 5 grams daily of C. After 1 month, 87% of the vitamin C group had achieved a complete response (disappearance of all tumors) compared to 55% in the control group.[111]

  3) Slowing or reversing cancer. High doses of C are preferentially toxic to tumor cells while not harming healthy tissue. One of the explanations for why C kills cancer but not healthy cells lies in the fact that C generates large amounts of hydrogen peroxide, H_2O_2, a potent free radical, which is neutralized in healthy cells by catalase.[112] Cancer cells do not have catalase to protect them. Animals exposed to a carcinogen and then vitamin C had their basal cell cancers examined under electron microscope. The cancer cells exposed to C showed a disintegration of cell structure, cell membrane disruption, increased collagen synthesis and general reduction in the number and size of tumors.[113] The researcher concluded: "...vitamin C exerts its antineoplastic effects by increasing cytolytic and autophagic activity, cell membrane disruption, and increased collagen synthesis, and thus, inhibits cancer cell metabolism and proliferation."

  C may be the ultimate selective toxin against cancer that researchers have been searching for.[114] Vitamin C was toxic to melanoma cells but not healthy cells in culture.[115] When researchers took leukemia cells from 28 patients and cultured them with vitamin C, 25% of the cultures were inhibited by at least 79%.[116] In animals with implanted tumors, vitamin C and B-12 together provided for significant tumor regression and 50% survival of the treated group, while all of the animals not receiving C and B-12 died by the 19th day.[117] C and B-12 seemed to form a cobalt-ascorbate compound that selectively shut down tumor growth. When vitamin C and K were combined to cancer cells in culture, the dosage required to slow and kill cancer cells dropped to only 2% compared to the dosage required by either of these vitamins alone.[118] Vitamin C or essential fatty acids were able to inhibit the growth of melanoma in culture, yet when combined their anti-cancer activity was much stronger.[119]

In both case studies and clinical trials in the scientific literature, C helps many cancer patients and hurts no one. Show me a drug that has the same risk to benefit to cost ratio. In one case report, a 70 year old man had been treated for kidney cancer, and then experienced a metastatic recurrence. He refused further medical therapy and started on 30 grams daily of intravenous vitamin C. Six weeks later, his chest X-rays showed that he was disease free.[120] A 42 year old man with reticulum cell sarcoma was treated on two different occasions with high dose intravenous vitamin C as sole therapy and each time resulted in a complete remission with 17 years of followup.[121]

Pauling and Cameron found that 10,000 mg (10 grams) daily of vitamin C brought a 22% survival rate in end-stage untreatable cancer patients after 1 year on C, compared to a 0.4% survival in patients without C.[122] Charles Moertel, MD of the Mayo Clinic allegedly followed the Pauling protocol and found no benefit with vitamin C.[123] Actually, even though Moertel did not follow Pauling's protocol, none of the untreatable, drug refractory colon cancer patients in Moertel's study died while on vitamin C for 3 months.

Finnish oncologists used high doses of nutrients (including 2-5 grams of C) along with chemo and radiation for lung cancer patients. Normally, lung cancer is a "poor prognostic" malignancy with a 1% expected survival at 30 months under normal treatment. In this study, however, 8 of 18 patients (44%) who were given vitamin C and other nutrients were still alive 6 years after diagnosis.[124]

Oncologists at West Virginia Medical School randomized 65 patients with transitional cell carcinoma of the bladder into either the "one-per-day" vitamin supplement providing the RDA, or into a group which received the RDA supplement plus 40,000 iu of vitamin A, 100 mg of B-6, 2000 mg of vitamin C, 400 iu of vitamin E, and 90 mg of zinc. After 10 months, tumor recurrence was 80% in the control group (RDA supplement) and 40% in the experimental "megavitamin" group. Five year projected tumor recurrence was 91% for controls and 41% for "megavitamin" patients. Essentially, high dose nutrients, including vitamin C, cut tumor recurrence in half.[125]

In a non-randomized clinical trial, Drs. Hoffer and Pauling instructed patients to follow a reasonable cancer diet (unprocessed food low in fat, dairy, and sugar), coupled with therapeutic doses of vitamins (including 12 grams of C) and minerals.[126] All 129 patients in this study received concomitant oncology care. The control group of 31 patients who did not receive nutrition support lived an average of less than 6 months. The group of 98 cancer patients who received the diet and supplement program were categorized into 3 groups:

-Poor responders (n=19) or 20% of treated group. Average lifespan of 10 months, or a 75% improvement over the control group.

-Good responders (n=47), who had various cancers, including leukemia, lung, liver, and pancreas; had an average lifespan of 72 months (6 years).

-Good female responders (n=32), with involvement of reproductive areas (breast, cervix, ovary, uterus); had an average lifespan of over 10 years, which is a 2100% improvement in lifespan over untreated patients!! Many were still alive at the end of the study.

4) Higher need. There is an elevated need for this nutrient during disease recovery. In one study, 15 patients with melanoma and colon cancer who were receiving immunotherapy (interleukin 2 and lymphokine-activated killer cells) showed blood levels of vitamin C indicative of scurvy.[127] In 20 adult hospitalized patients on Total Parenteral Nutrition (TPN), the mean daily vitamin C needs were 975 mg, which is over 16 times the RDA, with the range being 350-2250 mg.[128] Of the 139 lung cancer patients studied, most tested deficient or scorbutic (clinical vitamin C deficiency).[129] Another study of cancer patients found that 46% tested scorbutic while 76% were below acceptable levels for serum ascorbate.[130]

SAFETY ISSUES. Vitamin C is extremely safe, even in high doses. In one review of the literature regarding safety of vitamin C, 8 different double blind placebo controlled trials giving up to 10,000 mg daily of C for years produced no side effects.[131] In some sensitive individuals, doses of as little as 1000 mg produce gastro-intestinal upset, including diarrhea. Allegations that vitamin C mega-doses would produce oxalate kidney stones or cause B-12 deficiency have never been seen in millions of humans taking mega-doses of C for years. Up to 100,000 mg of C has been safely administered IV. As doses of oral C increase, the percentage that is absorbed goes down. Some experts claim that 10-20 grams of C per day is the upper threshold of what humans can tolerate and efficiently absorb. In a full dosage of 3 scoops daily of powdered ImmunoPower, the user will get 7500 mg, of which 3000 mg is as provided as ascorbic acid and the remaining 4500 mg as sodium ascorbate. There is some evidence that ascorbic acid is quickly absorbed, more likely to cause GI upset and quickly excreted; all of which has certain value. Meanwhile, mineral bound ascorbate (such as sodium ascorbate found in ImmunoPower) provides a more prolonged and sustained blood level of serum ascorbate.

B-1 (thiamine mononitrate) 10 mg
Improves aerobic metabolism.

Everytime humans process our food into something less than whole we learn a valuable, if not painful, lesson. When the British first learned to mill wheat and remove the outer bran and inner germ, they called the remaining cadaver of a food substance "the Queen's white flour". Bringing this technology around the world, the Dutch showed the South Pacific people of Java how to refine their rice, leaving only white rice behind and disposing of the bran and germ. Many of these people developed a condition of weakness and inability to function, called beri-beri, or literally translated: "I cannot. I cannot." Thiamin was one of the first vitamins to be studied and isolated in the early 20th century.

The importance of thiamin lies in its critical role in energy metabolism and the need for energy in every cell of the body. Thiamin becomes incorporated into a critical enzyme (thiamin pyrophosphate) for production of ATP energy. Low intake of thiamin was associated with an increase in the risk for prostate cancer.[132] Although thiamin is added back to enriched white flour, it is not added back to pastry flour (as in doughnuts) and is often deficient in the elderly[133] and those who regularly consume alcohol.[134] Best food sources of thiamin include brewers yeast, peas, wheat germ, peanuts, whole grains, beans, liver.

B-2 (riboflavin) 10 mg
    Improves aerobic metabolism.

Again, like thiamin above, riboflavin is mainly concerned with generating ATP energy from foodstuffs through the enzyme FAD (flavin adenine dinucleotide). However, riboflavin is also essential for the generation of a critical protective enzyme, glutathione peroxidase, which mops up free radicals. With optimal amounts of riboflavin in the body, there is less damage to cell membranes, DNA and immune factors. Low intake of riboflavin is associated with an increased risk for cancer of prostate and esophagus. Although riboflavin is added back to enriched white flour, many elderly[135] and poor people are low in riboflavin intake.[136] Alcohol interferes with the absorption and metabolism of riboflavin. Best food sources of riboflavin include brewer's yeast, kidney, liver, broccoli, wheat germ, milk and almonds.

B-3 (hexanicotinate) 500 mg
    Improves aerobic metabolism & tumor killing capacity of medical therapy, also may work like an enzyme to dissolve protective coating surrounding tumor.

Like the energy vitamins mentioned above, niacin generates ATP energy via the enzyme NAD (nicotinamide adenine dinucleotide) and also has other duties that impact the cancer patient. Niacin supplements in animals were able to reduce the cardiotoxicity of adriamycin while not interfering with its tumor killing capacity.[137] Niacin combined with aspirin in 106 bladder cancer patients receiving surgery and radiation therapy provided for a substantial improvement in 5 year survival (72% vs. 27%) over the control group.[138]

Tumors can hide from radiation therapy as hypoxic (low oxygen) lumps. Niacin seems to make radiation therapy more effective at killing these hypoxic cancer cells.[139] Loading radiation patients with 500 mg to 6000 mg of niacin has been shown to be safe and one of the most effective agents known to eliminate acute hypoxia in solid malignancies.[140] There is also intriguing evidence that high doses of niacin can act like enzymes, which means:

⇒ changing the coating of the tumor to make it more vulnerable to the immune system and medical intervention.

⇒ breaking up inefficient clumps of immune cells, or circulating immune complexes

⇒ altering Tumor Necrosis Factor (TNF) that can lead to depression, weight loss and pain.

B-5 (D-calcium pantothenate) 20 mg
    Improves stress response.

Pantothenic acid is named for "pantos", which is Greek for "found everywhere". Indeed, all plants and animals require or make pantothenic acid as part of a crucial energy enzyme, acetyl Coenzyme A, which is vital for generating ATP energy and a chemical for stress response. Injections of pantothenic acid improved wound healing in rabbits.[141] Based on the fact that the average American diet provides about 6 mg of pantothenic acid daily, the recommended intake (no formal RDA) is 4-7 mg. Deficiencies of pantothenic acid will generate symptoms of paresthesia (burning, prickling, tingling of extremities), headache, fatigue, insomnia, and GI distress. Pantothenic acid works closely with carnitine and CoQ (both in ImmunoPower) to maximize the efficiency of burning dietary fats. Supplements of pantothenic acid can help in the stress response, proper balancing of adrenal hormones, energy production and manufacturing of red blood cells. Best food sources of pantothenic acid are royal bee jelly, liver, kidney, egg yolk, and broccoli.

B-6 total of 50 mg
3.3 mg Pyridoxal 5 pyrophosphate & 46.6 mg pyridoxine HCl
Improves immune functions, may reduce toxicity from radiation therapy.

B-6 occurs in 3 natural forms: pyridoxine, pyridoxal, and pyridoxamine. B-6 works chiefly in an enzyme, pyridoxal-5-phosphate, which shifts amine groups from molecule to molecule. At least 100 different enzyme systems in humans involving protein metabolism, catabolism, anabolism or enzyme production all require B-6. B-6 is essential for:

⇒ regulating proper blood glucose levels

⇒ production of niacin from tryptophan

⇒ lipid metabolism and carnitine synthesis

⇒ making nucleic acids (RNA and DNA)

⇒ immune cell production

⇒ regulation of hormones.

Among its many functions, B-6 is required for producing thymidine, without which cells are more likely to develop cancerous mutations.[142] In a group of 12 non-medicated newly diagnosed cancer patients who had been smokers, all showed indications (based on coenzyme stimulation) of B-6 deficiency.[143] A low intake of B-6 increases tumor susceptibility and tumor size.[144]

In huge surveys conducted by the United States Department of Agriculture, 80% of Americans did not consume the RDA of 2 mg daily of B-6. There are many aspects of the typical American lifestyle that will exacerbate a marginal deficiency of B-6: many drugs, common food dyes, alcohol, and a high protein intake. Deficiency symptoms will reflect the functions of B-6, which means that almost anything can go wrong.

In one study, 25 mg (1250% of RDA) provided measurable improvements in immune functions in healthy adults. B-6 supplements (50-500 mg) have been shown to cure up to 97% of Carpal Tunnel Syndrome, a painful condition of the wrist and hands. B-6 is very helpful in: ⇒preventing and reversing neuropathy, or a tingling numbness in the hands and feet, which is common in chemo patients.
⇒preventing the "tanning" of blood proteins, a.k.a. glycosylation or glycation, that occurs when too much sugar is regularly found in the bloodstream.[145] Above-normal intake of B-6 offers many possible benefits to the cancer patient, including:
◊   Immune stimulation.[146]
◊   Blood sugar control
◊   Protection from radiation damage.
◊   Inhibits growth in melanoma.

Early studies in animals indicated that depriving them of B-6 might slow down tumor growth and increase survival time.[147] More recent studies find the opposite to be true. Animals supplemented with B-6 and then injected with a deadly strain of cancer, melanoma, showed an enhanced resistance to the disease.[148] B-6 inhibits melanoma in vivo.[149] B-6 supplements of 25 mg/day in 33 bladder cancer patients provided for marked reduction in tumor recurrence compared to the control group.[150] More recently, oncologists randomized 65 patients with transitional cell carcinoma of the bladder into either the "one-per-day" vitamin supplement providing the RDA, or into a group which received the RDA supplement plus 40,000 iu of vitamin A, 100 mg of B-6, 2000 mg of vitamin C, 400 iu of vitamin E, and 90 mg of zinc. High dose nutrients, including B-6, cut tumor recurrence in half.[151] B-6 supplements of 300 mg/day throughout 8 weeks of radiation therapy in patients with endometrial cancer provided a 15% improvement in survival at 5 years.[152]

SAFETY ISSUES. Less than 500 mg/day appears to be safe for most adults.[153] P-5-P appears to be the more readily available and active form of B-6, yet most people can convert pyridoxine into active P-5-P. ImmunoPower contains both forms of B-6.

> **B-12 (cyanocobalamin) 1 mg**
> Assists in proper cell growth, i.e. making of new immune factors and proper division of other cells. Combines with vitamin C to create selective anti-cancer compound.

In 1926, Minot and Murphy were awarded the Nobel prize for showing that feeding large quantities of liver could cure the dreaded disease, pernicious anemia, or B-12 deficiency. As people mature beyond age 40, the likelihood of developing pernicious anemia goes up substantially as the gut loses its efficiency at binding with this gigantic molecule and escorting it across the intestinal mucosa. The RDA of 2 micrograms (mcg) can easily be obtained in a typical "meat and potatoes" diet in America, since the best sources are liver, meat, fish, chicken, clams and egg yolk. However, absorbing the nutrient is another challenge. When this "intrinsic factor" in the gut is missing, large amounts in the diet can somewhat overwhelm the mucosal barrier in the gut and allow some absorption into the bloodstream, which is what happened when liver was used to cure pernicious anemia.

Since B-12 is a methyl donor, it is involved in all new cell growth, which makes it rather important in processes like red blood cell and immune cell formation, energy metabolism, and nerve function. There is a huge body of data now pointing to B-12 and folacin as primary nutrients that can interrupt the production of homocysteine, which is a major risk factor in heart disease.

For the cancer patient, B-12 supplements may bolster host defense mechanisms, plus it can combine with vitamin C to form a unique cobalt ascorbate complex that is selectively toxic to tumor cells. [154]

> **Folic acid 200 mcg**
> Assists in proper cell growth, immune stimulant, helps to check abnormal DNA production.

Folic acid (a.k.a. folate, folacin) presents a unique challenge in cancer treatment. On one side of the fence stand the oncologists who use have used the chemotherapy drug methotrexate for decades as an antagonist to the B vitamin, folic acid, to slow cancer growth, with leucovorin (folinic acid) as the rescue agent to summon the patient back from near death, or "the vital frontier". On the other side stand nutritionists who understand the pivotal role that folic acid plays in HEALTHY cell growth. The efficacy of methotrexate, now being used to treat some cases of rheumatoid arthritis, is not affected by patients taking supplements of folic acid. [155]

Without optimal amounts of folic acid in the cell, growth is erratic and prone to errors, such as birth defects and cancer. Low folate status during pregnancy will generate common birth defects, including spinal bifida. Humans with low B-12 and folate status present a clinical picture that looks like leukemia. [156] The importance of folate in new cell growth is highlighted in the fact that it is the only nutrient whose requirement doubles during pregnancy.

Folic acid may be the most common vitamin deficiency in the world, since more people are chosing animal foods (poor source of folic acid) over plant foods.[157] The name, folic acid, comes from the Latin term "folium", meaning foliage, since dark green leafy vegetables are a rich source of folic acid. Other good sources of folic acid include brewer's yeast, legumes, asparagus, oranges, cabbage, root vegetables and whole grains. Since folic acid is essential for all new cell growth, disturbances in folic acid metabolism are far reaching, including heart disease (due to more homocysteine in the blood), birth defects, immune suppression, cancer, premature senility and a long list of other conditions. Without adequate folate in the diet, cell growth is like a drunk driver heading down the highway--more likely to do some harm than not.

Since folic acid and B-12 work together in methyl donor reactions, a deficiency of one can be masked by an excess of the other. Hence, the FDA has stipulated that non-prescription supplements cannot contain more than 800 micrograms of folic acid. Experts have estimated that up to 20% of all senility in older adults is merely a long term deficiency of folic acid and vitamin B-12. The RDA of folate is 200 mcg for adults and 400 mcg for pregnant women, although the Center for Disease Control has recommended that 800 mcg of folic acid would prevent most cases of spinal bifida. Without adequate folic acid in the body, there is a buildup of homocysteine in the blood, which probably generates 10% or more of the 1 million cases of heart disease each year in the U.S..

Cancer is not an "on-off" switch. There are varying shades of gray in between the black and white of normal cells and full blown metastatic malignancies. In cervical cancer, there is a rating system where a stage I dysplasia shows abnormal cell growth, while stage IV is life-threatening cancer. In one study, 40% of women with stage I and II cervical dysplasia showed clear signs of folic acid deficiency.[158] In a double blind placebo controlled trial, 10 milligrams daily of folate (50 times the RDA) reversed cervical dysplasia in the majority of women tested.[159] Low folate intake increases the risk for colorectal cancer.[160] Human cells in a culture of low folate show immune suppression (impaired delayed hypersensitivity).[161] Folate deficiency is common throughout the world and America, especially among the elderly and adolescent females.[162] Alcohol and many drugs interfere with the absorption and metabolism of folate. Average intake of folate in the U.S. is about 240 mcg, which is one half to one fourth of what a good diet will contribute.

> **Biotin 50 mcg**
> Improves energy metabolism for glucose and fats, involved in pH
> maintenance through carbon dioxide binding, helps regulate cell growth.

Biotin is a B vitamin that is incorporated into 4 different
carboxylase enzymes, which makes it essential for processing fats, sugar
and various amino acids. Biotin is also involved in the production of
glucokinase, an enzyme in the liver that is essential for burning glucose.
Biotin supplements have been helpful at improving glucose tolerance in
insulin-dependent diabetics (Type 1, using 16 milligrams/day) and non-
insulin dependent diabetics (Type 2, using 9 mg/day).[163] Biotin
supplements have been able to improve peripheral neuropathy (tingling
numbness) in diabetics. Peripheral neuropathy is common in patients
after extensive chemotherapy.

ENDNOTES

[1] . Block, G., et al., Nutr.Cancer, vol.18, p.1, 1992
[2] . Mayne, ST, et al., J. Nat.Cancer Inst., vol.86, p.33, 1994
[3] . Krinsky, NI, Amer.J.Clin.Nutr., vol.53, p.238S, 1991
[4] . Zhang, L., et al., Carcinogenesis, vol.12, p.2109, 1991
[5] . Schwartz, JL, Biochem.Biophys Res.Comm., vol.169, p.941, 1990
[6] . Mathews-Roth, MM, et al., Photochem Photobiol., vol.42, p.35, 1985
[7] . Giovannucci, E., et al., J.Nat.Cancer Inst., vol.87, p.1767, 1995
[8] . Garewal, HS, et al., Archives Otolaryngol Head Neck Surg., vol.121, p.141, Feb.1995
[9] . Hazuka, MB, et al., J. Amer.Coll.Nutrition, vol.9, p.143, 1990
[10] . Burton, GW, J.Nutrition, vol.119, p.109, 1989
[11] . Tomita, Y., et al., J.Nat.Cancer Inst., vol.78, p.679, 1987
[12] . Santamaria, L., et al., Modulation and Mediation of Cancer by Vitamins, p.81, Karger, Basel, 1983
[13] . Bertram, JS, et al., Nutrients and Cancer Prevention, Prasad, KN (eds), p.99, Humana , 1990
[14] . Santamaria, L., et al., Nutrients and Cancer Prevention, p.299, Prasad, KN (eds), Humana, 1990
[15] . Seifter, E., et al., J.Nat.Cancer Inst., vol.71, p.409, 1983
[16] . Shklar, G., et al., Eur.J.Cancer Clin.Oncol., vol.24, p.839, 1988
[17] . Mills, EED, British J.Cancer, vol.57, p.416, 1988
[18] . Seifter, E., et al., J.Nat.Cancer Inst., vol.68, p.835, 1982
[19] . Nagasawa, H., et al., Anticancer Res., vol.9, p.71, 1989
[20] . Meyers, DG, et al., Archives Internal Med., vol.156, p.925, 1996
[21] .New England Journal of Medicine, vol.330, p.1029, 1994
[22] . Schwartz, JL, Journal of Nutrition, vol.126, 4 suppl, p.1221S, 1996
[23] . Sokol, RJ, in PRESENT KNOWLEDGE IN NUTRITION, p, 132, Ziegler, EE (eds), ILSI, Wash DC, 1996
[24] . Munoz, SJ, et al., Hepatology, vol.9, p.525, 1989
[25] . Niki, E. et al., Amer.J.Clin.Nutr., vol.53, p.201S, 1991
[26] . Bunk, MJ, et al., Proc.Soc.Exp.Biol.Med., voo.190, p.379, 1989
[27] . Kramer, TR, et al., Am.J.Clin.Nutr., vol.54, p.896, 1991
[28] . Nutrition Reviews, vol.45, p.27, Jan.1987
[29] . Meydani, SN, et al., Am.J.Clin.Nutr., vol.52, p.557, 1990
[30] . Penn, ND, et al., Age Ageing, vol.20, p.169, 1991
[31] . Kuroiwa, K, et al., J.Parenteral Enteral Nutr., vol.15, p.22, 1991
[32] . Odeleye, OE, et al., Nutr.Cancer, vol.17, p.223, 1992
[33] . Cook, MG, et al., Cancer Research, vol.40, p.1329, 1980
[34] . Horvath, PM, et al., Anticancer Research, vol.43, p.5335, Nov.1983
[35] . Sclafani, L, et al., J.Parenteral Enteral Nutr., vol.10, p.184, 1986
[36] . Packer, L., Med.Biol., vol.62, p.105, 1984
[37] . Rimm, EB, et al., New Engl J.Med., vol.328, p.1450, 1993
[38] . Record, IR, et al., Nutr.Cancer, vol.16, p.219, 1991
[39] . J.Amer Med.Assoc, vol.244, p.1077, 1980
[40] . Panganamala, RV, et al., Annals NY Acad Sci, vol.393, p.376, 1982

[41] . Jandak, J., et al., Blood, vol.73, p.141, Jan.1989
[42] . Knekt, P., et al., Am.J.Clin.Nutr., vol.53, p.283S, 1991
[43] . deVries, N., et al., Eur.Arch.Otorhinolaryngol, vol.247, p.368, 1990
[44] . Shklar, G., et al., J.Nat.Cancer Inst., vol.78, p.987, 1987
[45] . Paganelli, GM, et al., J.Nat.Cancer Inst., vol.84, p.47, 1992
[46] . Longnecker, MP, et al., J.Nat.Cancer Inst., vol.84, p.430, 1992
[47] . Yano., T., et al., Cancer Letters, vol.87, p.205, 1994
[48] . Prasad, KN, et al., J. Amer.Coll.Nutr., vol.11, p.487, 1992
[49] . Rama, BN, et al., Proc.Soc.Exper.Biol. Med., vol.174, p.302, 1983
[50] . Cohrs, RJ, et al., Int.J.Devl.Neuroscience., vol.9, p.187, 1991
[51] . Kline, K., et al., Nutr.Cancer, vol.14, p.27, 1990
[52] . Prasad, KN, et al., NUTRIENTS AND CANCER PREVENTION, Prasad, KN (eds), p.39, Humana Press, 1990
[53] . Singal, PK, et al., Mol.Cell.Biochem., vol.84, p.163, 1988
[54] . Singal, PK, et al., Molecular Cellular Biochem., vol.84, p.163, 1988
[55] . Clemens, MR, et al., Am.J.Clin.Nutr., vol.51, p.216, 1990
[56] . Shklar, G., et al., J.Oral Pathol.Med., vol.19, p.60, 1990
[57] . Geetha, A., et al., J.Biosci., vol.14, p.243, 1989
[58] . Geetha, A., et al., Current Science, vol.64, p.318, Mar.1993
[59] . Wang, YM, et al., Molecular Inter Nutr.Cancer, p.369, , Arnott, MS, (eds), Raven Press, NY, 1982
[60] . Ripoll, EAP, et al., J.Urol., vol.136, p.529, 1986
[61] . Wood, L, N.Engl.J.Med., vol.312, p.1060, 1985
[62] . Washio, M., et al., Nephron, vol.68, p.347, 1994
[63] . VanVleet, JF, et al., Cancer Treat.Rep., vol.64, p.315, 1980
[64] . Sundstrom, H., et al., Carcinogenesis, vol.10, p.273, 1989
[65] . Milei, J., et al., Am.Heart J., vol.111, p.95, 1986
[66] . Kagerud, A., et al., vol.20, p.1, 1981
[67] . Prasad, KN, et al., Proc.Soc.Exper.Biol.Med., vol.161, p.570, 1979
[68] . Sarria, A., et al., Proc.Soc.Exper.Biol.Med., vol.175, p.88, 1984
[69] . Kagerud, A., et al., Anticancer Research, vol.1, p.35, 1981
[70] . Hoffer, A., et al., Radiation Research, vol.61, p.439, 1975
[71] . Taren, DL, et al., J.Vit.Nutr.Res., vol.57, p.133, 1987
[72] . Waxman, S., et al., Eur.J.Cancer Clin.Oncol., vol.18, p.685, 1982
[73] . Traber, MG, et al., N.Engl.J.Med., vol.317, p.262, 1987
[74] . Wadleigh, RG, et al., Amer.J.Med,vol.92, p.481, May 1992
[75] . J.Nat.Cancer Inst., vol.84, p.997, July 1992
[76] . Kitagawa, M., et al., J. Nutr.Sci. Vitaminology, vol.35, p.133, 1989
[77] . Hathcock, JN, NY Acad Sciences, vol.587, p.257, 1990
[78] . Nutrition Reviews, vol.44, p.10, Jan.1986
[79] . Suttie, JW, in PRESENT KNOWLEDGE IN NUTRITION, p.137, Ziegler, EE (eds), ILSI, Washington, 1996
[80] . Chlebowski, RT, et al., Cancer Treatment Reviews, vol.12, p.49, 1985
[81] . Noto, V., et al., Cancer, vol.63, p.901, 1989
[82] . Dam,H., et al., in Harris, RS (eds), VITAMINS AND HORMONES, p.329, vol.18, Academic Press, NY, 1960
[83] . Chlebowski, RT, et al., Proc.Am.Assoc.Cancer Res., vol.24, p.653, 1983
[84] . Nutter, LM, et al., Biochem.Pharmacol., vol.41, p.1283, 1991
[85] . Krishanamurthi, S., et al., Radiology, vol.99, p.409, 1971
[86] . Taper, HS, et al., Int.J.Cancer, vol.40, p.575, 1987
[87] . Waxman, S., et al., Eur.J.Cancer Clin.Oncol., vol.18, p.685, 1982
[88] . Gold, J., Cancer Treatment Reports, vol.70, p.1433, Dec.1986
[89] . Gold, J., Proc.Amer Assoc Cancer Researchers, vol.28, p.230, Mar.1987
[90] . Nagourney, R., et al., Proc.Amer.Assoc.Clin.Oncol., vol.6, p.35, Mar.1987
[91] . National Research Council, VITAMIN TOLERANCE OF ANIMALS, National Academy Press, Washington, DC 1987
[92] . Suttie, IBID
[93] . Levine, M., et al., in PRESENT KNOWLEDGE IN NUTRITION, p.146, ILSI, Washington, 1996
[94] . National Academy of Sciences, DIET NUTRITION AND CANCER, National Academy Press, Washington, 1982
[95] . Block, G., Annals Intern.Med., vol.114, p.909, 1991
[96] . Cameron, E, and Pauling, L., Chem.Biol.Interactions, vol.9, p.272, 1974
[97] . Cameron, E., Pauling, L., Cancer Research, vol. 39, p.663, Mar.1979
[98] . Ocke, MC, et al., Int.J.Cancer, vol.61, p.480, 1995
[99] . Block, G., Am.J.Clin.Nutr., vol.53, p.270S, 1991
[100] . Tannenbaum, SR, et al., Am.J.Clin.Nutr., vol.53, p.247S, 1991

[101]. Ringsdorf, WM, et al., Oral Surg, p.231, Mar.1982
[102]. Nutrition Reviews, vol.45, p.217, July 1987
[103]. Liehr, JG, Am.J.Clin.Nutr., vol.54, p.1256S, 1991
[104]. Bright-See, E., Modulation and Meditation of Cancer by Vitamins, p.95, Karger, Basel., 1983
[105]. Josephy, PD, et al., Nature, vol.271, p.370, Jan.1978
[106]. Prasad, KN, et al., Proc.Natl.Acad.Sci., vol.76, p.829, Feb.1979
[107]. Sethi, VS, et al., in Modulation and Mediation of Cancer by Vitamins, p.270, Karger, Basel, 1983
[108]. Fujita, K., et al., Cancer Research, vol.42, p.309, Jan.1982
[109]. Minow, RA, et al., Cancer Chemother.Rep., vol.3, p.195, 1975
[110]. Okunieff, P., Am.J.Clin.Nutr., vol.54, p.1281S, 1991
[111]. Hanck, AB, Prog.Clin.Biol.Res., vol.259, p.307, 1988
[112]. Koch, CJ, et al., J.Cell.Physiol., vol.94, p.299, 1978
[113]. Lupulescu, A., Exp.Toxic.Pathol. vol.44, p.3, 1992
[114]. Riordan, NH, et al., Medical Hypotheses, vol.44, p.207, 1995
[115]. Bram, S., et al., Nature, vol.284, p.629, Apr.1980
[116]. Park, CH, et al., Cancer Research, vol.40, p.1062, Apr.1980
[117]. Poydock, ME, Am.J.Clin.Nutr., vol.54, p.1261S, 1991
[118]. Noto, V., et al., Cancer, vol.63, p.901, 1989
[119]. Gardiner, N, et al., Pros.Leuk., vol.34, p.119, 1988
[120]. Riordan, HD, et al., J. Orthomolecular Med., vol.5, p.5, 1990
[121]. Campbell, Al, Oncology, vol.48, p.495, 1991
[122]. Cameron, E., Pauling, L., Proc.Natl.Acad.Sci., vol.75, p.4538, Sept.1978
[123]. Moertel, CG, et al., N.Engl.J.Med., vol.312, p.137, 1985
[124]. Jaakkola, K., et al., Anticancer Res 12,599-606, 1992
[125]. Lamm, DL, et al., J Urol, 151:21-26, 1994
[126]. Hoffer, A, Pauling, L, J Orthomolecular Med, 5:3:143-154, 1990
[127]. Marcus, SL, et al., Am.J.Clin.Nutr., vol.54, p.1292S., 1991
[128]. Abrahamian, V., et al., Ascorbic acid requirements in hospital patients, JPEN, 7, 5, 465-8, 1983
[129]. Anthony, HM, et al., Vitamin C status of lung cancer patients, Brit J Ca, 46, 354-9, 1982
[130]. Cheraskin, E., Scurvy in cancer patients?, J Altern Med, 18-23, Feb.1986
[131]. Bendich, A., in BEYOND DEFICIENCIES, NY Acad.Sci., vol.669, p.300, 1992
[132]. Kaul, L., et al., Nutr.Cancer, vol.9, p.123, 1987
[133]. Bowman, BB, et al., Am.J.Clin.Nutr., vol.35, p.1142, 1982
[134]. Rindi, G., in PRESENT KNOWLEDGE IN NUTRITION, p.163, ILSI, Washington, 1996
[135]. Elsborg, L., Int.J.Vitamin Res., vol.53, p.321, 1983
[136]. Lopez, R., et al., Am.J.Clin.Nutr., vol.33, p.1283, 1980
[137]. Schmitt-Graff, A., et al, Pathol.Res.Pract., vol.181, p.168, 1986
[138]. Popov, Al, Med.Radiol. Mosk., vol.32, p.42, 1987
[139]. Kjellen, E., et al., Radiother.Oncol., vol.22, p.81, 1991
[140]. Horsman, MR, Radiotherapy Oncology, vol.22, p.79, 1991
[141]. Aprahamian, M., et al., Am.J.Clin.Nutr., vol.41, p.578, 1985
[142]. Prior, F., Med.Hypotheses, vol.16, p.421, 1985
[143]. Chrisley, BM, et al., Nutr.Res., vol.6, p.1023, 1986
[144]. Ha, C., et al., J.Nutr., vol.114, p.938, 1984
[145]. Solomon, LR, et al., Diabetes, vol.38, p.881, 1989
[146]. Gridley, DS, et al., Nutrition Research, vol.8, p.201, 1988
[147]. Tryfiates, GP, et al., Anticancer Research, vol.1, p.263, 1981
[148]. DiSorbo, DM, et al., Nutrition and Cancer, vol.5, p.10, 1983
[149]. DiSorbo, DM, et al., Nutrition and Cancer, vol.7, p.43, 1985
[150]. Byar, D., et al., Urolog7, vol.10, p.556, Dec.1977
[151]. Lamm, DL, et al., J Urol, 151:21-26, 1994
[152]. Ladner, HA, et al., Nutrition, Growth, & Cancer, p.273, Alan Liss, Inc., 1988
[153]. Cohen, M., et al., Toxicology Letters, vol.34, p.129, 1986
[154]. Poydock, ME, Am.J.Clin.Nutr., vol.54, p.1261S, 1991
[155]. Leeb, BF, et al., Clin.Exper.Rheumat., vol.13, p.459, 1995
[156]. Dokal, IS, et all, Br.Med.J., vol.300, p.1263, 1990
[157]. Bailey, LB, FOLATE IN HEALTH AND DISEASE, Marcel Dekker, NY 1995
[158]. Fekete, PS, et al., Acta. Cytologica, vol.31, p.697, 1987
[159]. Butterworth, CE, et al., Am.J.Clin.Nutr., vol.35, p.73, 1982
[160]. Freudenheim, J., Int.J.Epidemiol., vol.20, p.368, 1991
[161]. Levy, JA, BASIC AND CLINICAL IMMUNOLOGY, p.297, Lange, Los Altos, 1982
[162]. Werbach, M., NUTRITIONAL INFLUENCES ON ILLNESS, p.625, Third Line , Tarzana, 1996
[163]. Koutsikos, D., et al., Biomed.Pharmacother., vol.44, p.511, 1990

CHAPTER 6

★

MINERALS

Calcium (aspartate) 150 mg
Electrolyte balance and cellular communication.

Calcium is the most abundant mineral in the human body. While 99% of the body's calcium is bound up in the bones, the remaining 1% that is circulating is crucial for nerve and muscle function as well as regulating cell metabolism. There are calcium receptor sites on most cell membranes which help to control the flow of nutrients into and out of the cell as well as cell proliferation.

More than 5% of hospitalized cancer patients have elevated levels of calcium in the blood (hypercalcemia).[1] This is not because the patient is eating too much calcium, but caused by either:

⇒ a parathyroid hormone substance secreted by the tumor
⇒ or that tumors cause the release of bone stores
⇒ or that elevated calcium levels are caused by cell membranes not being able to maintain cell integrity. The calcium may get jettisoned when the cell is full of illness.

Best food sources of calcium include dairy products, dark green leafy vegetables (like kale and spinach) and cooked bones (like in canned salmon). Even though dairy products are a rich source of calcium, there are a number of health problems that can be associated with milk, cheese and butter intake:

While the RDA of calcium is 800-1200 milligrams daily, most Americans fall well short of this mark. Best supplemental sources of calcium are soluble forms of aspartate, citrate, lactate, orotate, etc. Calcium works with magnesium, sodium, potassium and some ultra-trace minerals to regulate the "battery of life", or cell membrane potential that is crucial. Calcium also works with magnesium, phosphorus, protein, zinc, vitamin C, B-6, boron and other nutrients to maintain proper mineralization of the skeleton, while dumping just the right amount of calcium into the bloodstream to keep the heart pumping merrily. Calcium metabolism is truly a delicate balancing act.

A low calcium intake increases the risk for colon cancer.[2] This effect may be due to calcium binding to bile acids in the colon to prevent carcinogenic by-products from forming, or due to the role calcium may play in regulating new cell growth. In human cancer patients, supplemental calcium increased the efficacy of radiation therapy to the bones and vulva.[3] Half of the patients with colon polyps (pre-cancerous growth) who were given supplements of calcium (1250 mg as carbonate) had a significant decrease in cell proliferation. Calcium seems to tame the beast of hyperproliferative growth, like pre-cancerous growths.[4] Patients at high risk for developing colon cancer all showed a decrease in colon cell proliferation with calcium supplements.[5]

Magnesium (aspartate) 150 mg
Essential for energy metabolism. Low intake can spontaneously induce lymphoma.

Magnesium is essential in at least 300 different enzyme reactions in the human body, including the pervasive conversion of ATP for energy. In animals, magnesium deficiency can spontaneously generate bone tumors and lymphomas.[6] Numerous studies show that a diet low in magnesium will increase the risk for various forms of cancer. Magnesium not only works with other electrolytes to maintain the sodium-potassium pump, but also has a central role in regulating DNA synthesis and the cell cycle.

The RDA for magnesium has been lowered from 400 milligrams daily to 350 mg, not because the evidence warranted this change but because few Americans came even close to consuming the RDA. The average American intake is 143-266 mg/day; which explains why low magnesium intake has been linked to an increase in the incidence of hypertension, heart disease, migraines, fatigue, immune suppression, fibromyalgia, glaucoma, and much more. Best food sources of magnesium are kelp, whole grains, nuts, and molasses. Magnesium aspartate is the best absorbed form of magnesium supplements.

Symptoms of magnesium deficiency include depression, excess sweating, fatigue, frequent infections and high blood pressure; which all are common in cancer patients. Many drugs, including diuretics, and alcohol cause a loss of magnesium from the system.

Potassium (citrate) 333 mg
Essential ingredient for "electrolyte soup" that dictates healthy cell membrane.

Potassium is the primary cation (positively charged ion) inside the human cell. Potassium is found primarily in plant foods, with the richest sources being avocado, banana, tomato and potato. Meats and fish can provide a significant amount of potassium to the diet. Many studies show that a diet high in sodium (or salt) and low in potassium (found in plant food) increases the risk for heart disease and cancer, among other diseases.[7] Potassium is crucial for nerve and muscle function and the conversion of glucose into glycogen for storage. The first symptom of potassium deficiency is usually weakness and fatigue.

The FDA has set an upper limit of 99 mg allowed of potassium in tablet form due to the concerns that people with poorly functioning kidneys (less than 1% of the population) might suffer potassium overload. Meanwhile, 90% of the population do not get optimal amounts of potassium in the diet, especially in the right ratio with the other crucial electrolytes of sodium, calcium and magnesium. The range of potassium intake that is recommended by the RDA board is 1.9 to 5.6 grams daily. Up to 3 grams daily can be lost in perspiration and through the use of diuretics, like anti-hypertensive medication, alcohol and coffee. While many American health authorities have crusaded against the use of salt (sodium) at the table, actually a deficiency of potassium, magnesium and calcium are much more likely to be at fault in hypertension, heart disease and various forms of cancer.

Zinc (chelate) 10 mg
Potent immune stimulant, essential in over 200 enzyme reactions in the body, including immune cell production and cell replication.

Zinc is the most multi-talented mineral in the body, participating in everything from sexual development, to immunity, to maintenance of nerve tissue, to the zinc-dependent antioxidant enzyme SOD (superoxide dismutase). Apoptosis, or programmed cell death, which is missing in cancer cells, may be regulated by zinc.[8] The average American consumes about 10 milligrams of zinc daily, which is well shy of the 15 mg RDA. Best food sources of zinc include shell fish, organ meats, meat, fish, pumpkin seeds, ginger root, nuts and seeds.

Zinc is a crucial mineral for optimal immune functioning. Low zinc status will lower T cell counts, reduce thymic hormone levels and reduce reactions to pathogens and cancer. Reduced zinc levels and cancer are both common in the elderly. Zinc supplements of only 20 mg/day improved immune functions via jump starting the thymus gland in institutionalized elderly subjects.[9] Loss of appetite is one of the first symptoms of zinc deficiency. Zinc supplements usually restore appetite, which is a common problem in cancer patients. A low intake of zinc increases the risk for cancers of the esophagus[10] lung[11] and prostate.[12] Cadium from tobacco and pollution will readily replace zinc in the prostate and may lead to benign prostatic hypertrophy (enlarged prostate) and prostate cancer.[13]

SAFETY ISSUES. Supplements of zinc should be in the 20-60 mg/day range, since doses of 150 mg/day have been shown to trigger copper deficiency and depress the cardio-protective HDL-cholesterol.

> **Iron (chelate) 3.3 mg**
> Essential for red blood cell synthesis (hematopoeisis) to properly oxygenate tissues, essential for energy metabolism and immune cell production.

Iron has the narrowest "window of efficacy" of all nutrients and is the best nutritional example of "too much or too little will create a health problem". Iron is one of the most commonly deficient nutrients in America and around the world.[14] Yet consuming iron salts through enriched white flour without eating enough antioxidants can bring about a troublesome biochemical environment where the iron can create free radicals, damage the DNA and cause heart disease or cancer.[15] Iron can be hoarded by infecting bacteria and cancer cells to further invade healthy tissue. I have seen many cancer patients who developed anemia while the cancer was winning the fight, yet had a sudden rise in serum ferritin iron stores when the cancer cells are being destroyed and releasing their iron content. Iron deficiency can lead to suppressed immune function.[16] Therefore, iron supplements must be provided:
⇒ in conservative doses, as in ImmunoPower
⇒ in the most bioavailable form, as the chelated version used in ImmunoPower
⇒ in conjunction with multiple antioxidants (such as provided in ImmunoPower) to protect against the potential free radical damage from iron.

Iron is involved in:
◊ hemoglobin production for transporting oxygen to the cells
◊ myoglobin in the muscles
◊ oxidative burst as immune cells kill cancer cells
◊ one of the ways to induce cancer death through chemo drugs
◊ cytochromes for energy metabolism
◊ other iron containing enzymes like NADH.

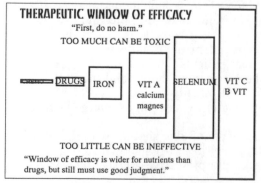

THERAPEUTIC WINDOW OF EFFICACY
"First, do no harm."
TOO MUCH CAN BE TOXIC
DRUGS IRON VIT A calcium magnes SELENIUM VIT C B VIT
TOO LITTLE CAN BE INEFFECTIVE
"Window of efficacy is wider for nutrients than drugs, but still must use good judgment."

Symptoms of deficiency include anemia, lethargy, behavioral problems, poor body temperature regulation, reduced immunity and others. Since the RDA for iron is 10-15 mg and most Americans do not consume this amount, the right form (chelated) of iron supplements may be extremely valuable for people who also get adequate antioxidants at the same time to prevent the metabolic wrecking ball effect from iron as a free radical.

SAFETY ISSUES. Many cancer patients are found to be anemic, which can precipitate the "knee jerk" response for recommending high doses of iron supplements, such as ferrous sulphate. This is a very bad idea. As mentioned above, iron supplements should be taken in conservative doses and in chelated versions, such as the heme form found in the blood. Any other strategy of supplementing iron can be counterproductive for the cancer patient.

Copper (chelate) 1 mg
    Involved in several important enzyme reactions, including cytochromes for energy and superoxide dismutase for free radical protection.

Copper is important for the construction of tough connective tissues, which is how the body tries to envelop a tumor. Copper is crucial for energy metabolism via cytochrome c. Copper supplements have slowed tumor growth in animals.[17] Copper, via ceruloplasmin, helps to prevent the oxidation of fatty acids that can destroy DNA and cell membranes. The RDA of copper is 1.5-3 mg/day. Best sources of copper in the diet include organ meats, shellfish and legumes.

Iodine (potassium iodide) 50 mcg
    Assists the thyroid gland in regulating basal metabolism, which is often low in cancer patients. Is a selective toxin for disease-causing microorganisms in the gut.

Iodine is primarily involved in the thyroid hormone, thyroxin, which regulates basal metabolism throughout the body. Additionally, iodine seems to modify the effects of estrogen on breast tissue, thus reducing fibrocystic breast disease, which doubles the risk for developing breast cancer.[18] Low thyroid output is a fundamental insult in many women with breast cancer.[19]

    Seafood, especially kelp, provides the best sources of iodine. The fortification of salt with iodine (iodized salt) has been a classic example of public health measures that significantly reduced the incidence of goiter, or iodine deficiency expressed as clinical hypothyroidism. Yet, for various reasons, subclinical hypothyroidism is still rampant in the U.S. Iodine is also a selective toxin for microorganisms in the gut, helping to kill parasites and intestinal infections.

    NOTE. If basal temperature is below 97.8 F, then medical assistance may be needed in the form of prescription thyroxin supplements to bolster basal metabolism.

Manganese (chelate) 1.67 mg
Essential mineral cofactor in various enzyme reactions, including an important antioxidant system of SOD (superoxide dismutase).

Manganese deficient animals develop low insulin output, problems with the connective tissue and processing of fats. Recommended intake is 2-5 milligrams daily for adults, with over half the female population consuming less than adequate amounts of manganese.[20] Best food sources of manganese are whole grains, nuts and fruits grown on manganese rich (properly fertilized) soil. There are at least 3 different minerals, including manganese, copper, and zinc, that play a role in variations of the critical antioxidant enzyme system SOD.

Chromium (GTF niacinate) 200 mcg
Essential mineral for proper energy metabolism, especially related to controlling blood sugar levels and preventing lean tissue wasting.

Chromium is at the center of the Glucose Tolerance Factor (GTF) which works with insulin to allow glucose into body cells. Without adequate GTF in the body, insulin levels are raised, which can be disastrous. Glucose-dependent tissues, like the brain, lens of the eye, kidney and lungs suffer the most when blood sugar levels are abnormal. Without proper burning of glucose in the cells, the body resorts to the backup energy substrates of protein (which causes lean tissue wasting, a.k.a. cachexia) and fat (which elevates levels of fats in the blood for increased risk of heart disease). GTF is also critical for immune functions and may even play a role in regulating cell growth.[21] Deficiencies of chromium in humans typically lead to impaired glucose metabolism, elevated blood fats, and peripheral neuropathy (tingling numbness in extremities).

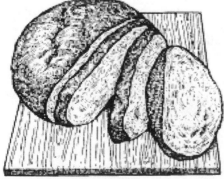

An estimated 90% of the American population do not consume the minimum recommended intake of 50 micrograms daily. Researchers at the United States Department of Agriculture have estimated that up to 25% of heart disease in America could be prevented merely by consuming adequate quantities of chromium. Human subjects who took 400 micrograms daily of chromium supplements lost more fat and gained more lean tissue than those who took 200 mcg.[22] Another study found that 600 mcg of chromium provided signficant drops in fasting blood glucose in diabetics.[23] Several studies have shown that chromium supplements lower fasting blood glucose levels in normal healthy individuals.[24] Remember, a crucial strategy in fighting cancer is to starve the cancer of its favorite fuel, which is sugar.

Chromium is concentrated in whole grains and beans grown on chromium-rich soil, which is rare since chromium is not typically used in fertilizer. Brewer's yeast, liver, black pepper and molasses are decent sources of chromium. Chromium is stripped out of most food refining processes, including the milling of wheat to white flour and cane sugar to refined white sugar. 86% of Americans consume white bread rather than whole grain bread. The average American consumes 132 pounds per year of refined sugar, which increases the need for chromium while increasing the EXCRETION of chromium. The most bioavailable forms of chromium supplements are GTF, chromium picolinate and chromium polynicotinate; with the least bioavailable being the chromium salts like chromium chloride.

Selenium (selenomethionine) 200 mcg
    Immune stimulant, detoxifying agent via glutathione peroxidase, may selectively control the growth of abnormal tissue.

Selenium presents a fascinating story for the cancer patient. Until the 1960s, selenium was considered a toxic mineral by the FDA. In 1982, I developed a line of vitamin supplements made in the U.S. and shipped to Australia but were rejected at their customs office because these supplements contained selenium, which was still considered toxic by the Australian FDA. An abundance of information beginning to appear in the 1960s showed that selenium may be one of our greatest allies in the war on cancer. Selenium is found is widely varying amounts in the diet, due to huge differences of selenium found in the soil. In places like South Dakota and Montana, there is so much selenium in the soil, that animals grazing on the grass can develop selenium toxicity, or "blind staggers", which involves nerve and behavior problems. Some historians claim that General Custer's horses bolted on him in the Battle of Little Bighorn because the horses were suffering from selenium toxicity. In Finland, where the selenium-deficient soil leads to a high incidence of cancer and heart disease, wheat flour is enriched with selenium just like we add iron to our white flour.

Wheat germ, seafood and Brazil nuts are the best sources of selenium. The RDA is 70 micrograms while the average intake is just over 100 micrograms. When lining up maps showing selenium content in the soil with cancer incidence, there is a strong link between low selenium intake and higher cancer risk.[25] In a recent prospective double blind human intervention study, supplements providing 200 mcg of selenium were able to reduce the incidence of various cancers by up to 60%.[26] Selenium is a potent immune stimulator.[27]

Selenium-deficient animals have more heart damage from the chemo drug, adriamycin.[28] Supplements of selenium and vitamin E in humans did not reduce the efficacy of the chemo drugs against ovarian and cervical cancer.[29]   Animals with implanted tumors were then treated with selenium and cis-platin (chemo drug) and showed a reduced toxicity to the drug with no change in anti-cancer activity.[30] Selenium supplements helped repair DNA damage from a carcinogen in animals.[31] Selenium was selectively toxic to human leukemia cells in culture.[32]

Selenomethionine is the preferred form of selenium supplements. Garlic grown on selenium enriched soil develops a unique anti-cancer activity, which is how the Kyolic garlic used in ImmunoPower is cultured.

SAFETY ISSUES. Selenium toxicity may begin as low as 1000 mcg/day in some people, but toxicity is more common at about 65,000 micrograms (65 mg) for the average healthy adult.[33]

Molybdenum (chelate)   167 mcg
Essential mineral that functions as a cofactor in various enzyme reactions, including detoxification pathways.

M olybdenum functions as a mineral cofactor in hydroxylation enzyme reactions, such as uric acid and sulfite processing.   When sulfites build up in the human system, cysteine metabolism is affected, which is crucial for detoxification. Most diets supply only around 50-100 micrograms daily of molybdenum and do not meet the safe and adequate levels of 75-250 mcg recommended by the Food and Nutrition Board. There is no RDA for molybdenum. Large scale farming does not add molybdenum to the soil as part of broad spectrum fertilization, which further compounds the problems of common molybdenum deficiencies. It is found in vegetables which are grown on molybdenum-rich soil. Beans and organ meats are the best sources of molybdenum. This is an extremely non-toxic mineral, with animal studies showing that an intake of 100-5000 milligrams per kilogram of diet is necessary to produce toxicity symptoms.[34]

Vanadium (vanadyl sulfate) 33 mcg
Crucial mineral for controlling blood glucose, which is very important to control prostaglandin metabolism and cancer growth.

V anadium is not added back to the soil in agri-business, and hence may be missing from the American diet, which typically contains 10-60 micrograms daily of vanadium.[35] When non-insulin dependent diabetics were supplemented with 100 milligrams daily (100,000 micrograms) of vanadyl sulfate, blood glucose levels dropped by 14%.[36] Vanadium in the form of vanadyl sulfate has shown promise in helping to control rises in blood glucose in human diabetics.[37] Toxicity may begin at 13 milligrams (13,000 micrograms) of vanadium daily.   Best food sources of vanadium include mushrooms, shellfish, dill, parsley and black pepper.

Nickel (sulfate) 3.3 mcg
Essential mineral that participates in hydrolysis, reduction & oxidation, gene expression, stabilizing certain structures.

Nickel is probably missing in the American diet. While a diet rich in nuts, beans, peas and whole grains could provide up to 900 micrograms per day, the typical American diet provides less than 100 micrograms. Based on sketchy knowledge of this ultra-trace mineral, experts have guessed at 25-35 micrograms daily as a requirement for adults.

Tin (chloride) 3.3 mcg
Essential mineral in human nutrition. May be missing in diet.

ENDNOTES

[1] . Heath, DA, Br., Med.J., vol.298, p.1468, 1989
[2] . Sorenson, AW, et al., Nutr.Cancer, vol.11, p.135, 1988
[3] . Iakovkeva, SS, Arkh.Patol., vol.42, p.93, 1980
[4] . Wargovich, MJ, J.Am.Coll.Nutr., vol.7, p.295, 1988
[5] . Buset, M., et al., Cancer Res., vol.46, p.5426, 1986
[6] . Seelig, MS, in ADJUVANT NUTRITION IN CANCER TREATMENT, p.284, Quillin, P (eds), Cancer Treatment Research Foundation, Arlington Heights, IL 1994
[7] . Jansson, B., Cancer Detect.Prevent., vol.14, p.563, 1991
[8] . Cousins, RJ, in PRESENT KNOWLEDGE IN NUTRITION, p.293, ILSI, Washington, 1996
[9] . Boukaiba, N, et al., Am.J.Clin.Nutr., vol.57, p.566, 1993
[10] . Barch, DH, J.Am.Coll.Nutr., vol.8, p.99, 1989
[11] . Allen, JI, et al., Am.J.Med., vol.79, p.209, 1985
[12] . Whelen, P., et al., Br.J.Urol., vol.55, p.525, 1983
[13] . Feustel, A., et al., Urol.Res., vol.12, p.253, 1984
[14] . Yip, R., et al., in PRESENT KNOWLEDGE IN NUTRITION, p.277, ILSI, Washington, 1996
[15] . Beard, J., in IRON DEFICIENCY ANEMIA, p.99, National Academy Press, 1993
[16] . Dallman, PR, Am.J.Clin.Nutr., vol.46, p.329, 1987
[17] . Sorenson, RJ, in TRACE SUBSTANCES IN ENVIRONMENTAL HEALTH XVI, U.Missouri 1982
[18] . Ghent, WR, et al., Can.J.Surg., vol.36,p.453, 1993
[19] . Callebout, E., in THE DEFINITIVE GUIDE TO CANCER, Diamond, J. (eds), p.116, Future Medicine, Tiburon, 1997
[20] . Keen, CL, et al., in PRESENT KNOWLEDGE IN NUTRITION, p.339, ILSI, Washington, 1996
[21] . Stoecker, BJ, in PRESENT KNOWLEDGE IN NUTRITION, p.347, ILSI, Washington, 1996
[22] . Evans, GW, et al., J.Inorganic Biochem., vol.49, p.177, 1993
[23] . Mossop, RT, Central African J.Med., vol.29, p.80, 1983
[24] . Anderson, RA, et al., Metabolism, vol.32, p.894, 1983
[25] . Schrauzer, GN, in VITAMINS, NUTRITION, AND CANCER, p.240, Karger, Basel, 1984
[26] . Clark, LC, et al., J.Amer.Med.Assoc., vol.276, p.1957, 1996
[27] . Kiremidjian-Schumacher, L., et al., Environmental Res., vol.42, p.277, 1987
[28] . Coudray, C., et al., Basic Res.Cardiol., vol.87, p.173, 1992
[29] . Sundstrom, H., et al., Carcinogenesis, vol.10, p.273, 1989
[30] . Ohkawa, K., et al., Br.J.Cancer, vol.58, p.38, 1988
[31] . Lawson, T., et al.,Chem.Biol.Interactions, vol.45, p.95, 1983
[32] . Milner, JA, et al., Cancer Research, vol.41, p.1652, 1981
[33] . Hathcock, JN, in MICRONUTRIENTS AND IMMUNE FUNCTIONS, vol.587, p.257, NY Acad.Sci., 1990
[34] . Nielsen, FH, in PRESENT KNOWLEDGE IN NUTRITION, p.359, ILSI, Washington, 1996
[35] . Harland, BF, et al., J.Am.Diet.Assoc., vol.94, p.891, 1994
[06] . Cohen, N., et al., J.Clin.Invest., vol.95, p.2501, 1995
[37] . Brichard, SM, et al., Trends Pharmacol.Sci., vol.16, p.265, 1995

CHAPTER 7

⭐

ACCESSORY FACTORS

WHAT ARE "ACCESSORY FACTORS"?

While there are around 50 nutrients that are considered essential in the diet of humans, there are literally thousands of other "accessory factors" found in various foods. There is increasing evidence that we may need these substances in our diet in order to maintain optimal health. These accessory factors may someday be considered "conditionally essential" nutrients, which means that during some phases of life (i.e. very young, older, sick), these nutrients would become essential in the diet. Cancer patients often have a compromised system which is unable to manufacture optimal amounts of these nutrients in the body. A poorly chosen diet, which is common in cancer patients, further compounds the possibility that these accessory factors will be deficient in the cancer patient. The difference between "surviving" and "thriving to beat cancer" may rest in the intake of these accessory factors

Aloe powder 167 mg
Immune stimulant, aids in cellular communication.

For 5000 years, many cultures and herbalists around the world have been using aloe vera as a primary medicinal plant. King Solomon used it as his favorite laxative. Hippocrates, the father of modern medicine 2400 years ago, used at least 14 different medicine formulas containing aloe. Alexander the Great conquered an island in order to have aloe for his soldiers. As I write this section, I am looking at one of many aloe plants that we keep in our house. Aloe thrives on neglect. All the plant needl is decent soil and a little water and sun, then you get to harvest one of Nature's most versatile and impressive healers. Fresh aloe gel applied topically may be the greatest skin creme on the planet earth. The yellow bitter part of the plant leaf is a proven laxative that has brought relief to many of my patients. And whole leaf extracts have the ability to gear up the immune system, reduce swelling, improve healing, kill bacteria and viruses, and improve communication between cells (intercellular) and within the cell (intracellular).

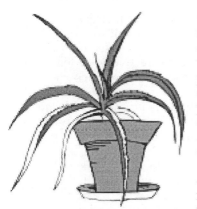

Of the 300 species of aloe, it is aloe vera that has received the most attention. Aloe certainly typifies the complexity of understanding the healing properties of plants. There are over 200 biologically active ingredients in aloe vera, including prostaglandins, essential fatty acids (including GLA), vitamins, minerals, anthraquinones, and polysaccharides (longer chains of sugar-like molecules).[1]

In the movie, MEDICINE MAN, a doctor (Sean Connery) discovered a cure for cancer from a plant in the Amazon forest, which was rapidly being levelled by bulldozers and fire. But now he cannot reproduce his original concoction from the same plant. To ruin the suspense and tell you the ending, the active ingredient in his original cancer cure was from the spider feces that was found in the sugar used to dilute the herbal concoction. Moral of the story: We are still neophytes when it comes to understanding just what is the active ingredient (s) in medicinal plants. Which is why using low heat processing of the whole leaf aloe is crucial for preserving the active ingredient, as is done in ImmunoPower.

While once discussing the merits of aloe with a noted researcher on the subject, I commented: "It seems like aloe cures almost everything[2], as if it were an essential nutrient that we are not getting in our diet!!" He grinned and commented: "You may be right. For most of the millions of years of human history, our ancestors ate food that was not refrigerated, hence our food supply had all sorts of mold (yeast) growing on it. I think that we have an essential need for the unique collection of sugar-like molecules (mannans) that come from the cell wall of yeast and the aloe plant."

Indeed, there are receptor sites on immune cells (macrophages) for D-mannose (one of the sugars in aloe) just like a key fitting a keyhole.[3] Aloe seems to act like a mild vaccination in the human body, by bringing a substance that appears to be a bacterial cell wall into the bloodstream, which then whips the immune system into a state of red alert preparedness.

Aloe may help the cancer patient in many ways.

◊ **Antibacterial & antifungal**. Aloe vera applied topically to burn regions of animals was superior to the common antibacterial medication used, silver sulfadiazine.[4]

◊ **Antiviral activity**. Feline leukemia is a form of cancer contracted by cats and caused by a virus. This disease is invariably fatal, with 70% of cats dying within 8 weeks of early symptoms. Most cats are euthanized as soon as the diagnosis is made. In one study, acemannan from aloe was injected weekly for 6 weeks into the cats, with a followup 6 week waiting period. After this 12 week study, 71% of the cats were alive and in good health.[5] Acemannan has also demonstrated a potent ability to fight the flu virus, measles and the HIV virus while also reducing the dosage required of the drug AZT.[6]

◊ **Anti-inflammatory**. Drugs, like cortisone, that are effective at reducing inflammation also shut down wound recovery. Aloe has the ability to reduce swelling while also enhancing wound recovery.

◊ **Immune stimulant**. Aloe has been shown to increase the activity of the immune system.[7] Aloe seems to provide neutrophils with more "bullets", or toxic substances to kill cancer and invading organisms.[8] Aloe (acemannan) increases the production of nitric oxide, a potent anti-cancer "napalm" used by immune cells.[9]

◊ **Anti-cancer activity**. Various fractions of aloe (mannans and glucans) have been found to have potent anti-neoplastic activity.[10]

◊ **Radio-protective**. Some forms of mannan are bone marrow stimulants and can protect mice against cobalt-60 radiation.[11] In my experience with cancer patients, those who took aloe before and during radiation therapy had minimal damage of healthy tissue while still getting an impressive anti-cancer effect from the radiation. Generalized radiation to the pelvic region for prostate or colon cancer can be particularly nasty in harming the bladder and gastro-intestinal tract. I remember one cancer patient who used aloe throughout 40 rounds of pelvic radiation and suffered no burns and only mild GI distress.

◊ **Cell communication**. Many forms of carbohydrates, called glycoproteins, may play a key role in promoting healthy communication within the cell and between cells. Aloe may contribute an important carbohydrate (mannan) which becomes part of this crucial "telegraph system" which prevents or slows down cancer.[12] Given the 8 monosaccharides used in the body and the 18 configurations used to arrange these molecules, the possible "words" in this complex "telegraph" system works out to 18 to the 8th power, or over 11 billion "messages". No doubt, more important breakthroughs will come out of this new and exciting field of cell communication.

　　SAFETY ISSUES. While aloe can be a valuable laxative, too much aloe can cause diarrhea. In 1983, the Food and Drug Administration Advisory Panel for over-the-counter drugs reviewed over a hundred reports on aloe and found that no adverse events had been reported, concluding "clearly, the substance is safe."

Dimethylglycine 16.7 mg
　　Once called "vitamin" B-15. Immune stimulant and energizer.

　　Dimethylglycine, or DMG, has a relatively short but colorful track record in nutrition science. Ernst Krebs, MD discovered pangamic acid (also called "vitamin" B-15) in the pits of apricots along with laetrile ("vitamin" B-17) in 1951. Neither DMG nor pangamic acid are considered essential vitamins, though whole grains, brewer's yeast, pumpkin seeds and beef blood are rich sources of pangamic acid. DMG combines with gluconic acid in the body to form pangamic acid[13], which was the subject of considerable attention and research in Russia and Europe, thus initially branding pangamic acid as a non-essential substance with only foreign research documentation to support it. Pangamic acid has been used to enhance athletic performance and to reverse the aging process in European clinics. DMG may work by:

⇒ becoming part of pangamic acid in the body
⇒ being broken down into glycine, which may help to generate more glutathione peroxidase (see glutathione above).

DMG has been shown to increase immune functions (antibody titer) by 300-500% in vaccinated animals.[14] In a double blind study with healthy human subjects, 120 mg daily of DMG along with 180 mg of calcium gluconate provided a 400% increase in antibody response to pneumococcal vaccine.[15] The 10 subjects with illness showed similar improvements in immune response, adding that mitogen response to lymphocytes in the patients with diabetes and sickle cell anemia was increased by 300%. DMG may improve aerobic energy metabolism, detoxify the body and liver, inhibit allergic responses, reduce blood pressure, and stimulate the nervous and endocrine systems.

Bovine cartilage 3 gm
Immune stimulant, anti-mitotic agent (shuts down cell division in abnormal cells), anti-angiogenesis (shuts down production of blood vessels from tumors), adaptogen.

Of the many ingredients in ImmunoPower, bovine tracheal cartilage (BTC) is one of the more crucial and expensive ($180/month alone) of all nutrition factors to help the cancer patient, so we will spend more than a little time discussing this ingredient. Imagine these headlines: "Major drug company finds new treatment for cancer, arthritis, shingles, and many other infectious disorders". The story would be featured on TV and newspapers around the world. The stock value of that company would skyrocket. But what if that same substance was a humble little unpatentable food extract? Would the enthusiasm be as great? Bovine cartilage may be in that category.

Good luck never hurt anyone's career. In 1954 John Prudden, MD (Harvard), PhD (Columbia) noticed an article from the reknowned Columbia-Presbyterian researchers, Drs. Meyer, Regan, and Lattes, on how topical cartilage could neutralize the disastrous effect that cortisone had on inhibiting wound recovery. This tip on the therapeutic value of cartilage had come from a mysterious "Dr. Martin" from Montreal, who has never since been located.

The next lucky event for Prudden came when a 70 year old woman came to him with advanced breast cancer that was literally eating away her chest cavity, stage IV fungating breast cancer. Prudden tried the topical bovine cartilage along with injecting bovine cartilage solutions into obvious tumor areas with the hopes that it might help to heal these awful ulcerated wounds. Surprisingly, the woman returned to Dr.

Prudden with the wounds healed AND the cancer gone. It has been said that "chance favors the prepared mind".

Over the course of 40 years, Prudden has been involved in $7 million of research to better understand BTC. Prudden received a patent on cartilage in 1962 for its anti-inflammatory properties when topically applied to arthritic regions of the body. Prudden is an affable man and dog lover who saved one of his dogs from mastocytoma (a terminal cancer) using BTC.

Prudden found that the "wind pipe" of cows was considered offal or waste products of the butchering process. Given the world's hunger for beef, this seemed to be a bountiful supply of inexpensive raw material. Prudden developed the complex process for removing the fat from the cartilage, then drying and powdering. He named his original product Catrix, short for Cicatrix, which means "healed wound".

While some people might think that eating shark cartilage is just rewards for a predatory animal, actually many environmental groups are concerned about endangering the shark population, which sits atop the ocean's precarious food chain. Sharks have a pivotal role in population control and "pruning" the sick and unfit creatures of the oceans. You are much more likely to be struck by lightning than bitten by a shark while swimming in the ocean.

Cartilage resembles fetal mesenchyme, which is the source for developing muscle, bones, tendons, ligaments, skin, fat, and bone marrow. It probably is this unique origin which gives rise to the many therapeutic benefits of cartilage. Initially, there was some interest in using only young (less than 6 month old) cows for BTC. Prudden feels that this is an unnecessary effort and an unproven theory.

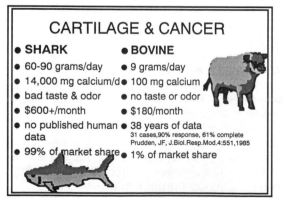

CARTILAGE & CANCER

● SHARK	● BOVINE
● 60-90 grams/day	● 9 grams/day
● 14,000 mg calcium/d	● 100 mg calcium
● bad taste & odor	● no taste or odor
● $600+/month	● $180/month
● no published human data	● 38 years of data 31 cases,90% response, 61% complete Prudden, JF, J.Biol.Resp.Mod.4:551,1985
● 99% of market share	● 1% of market share

SHARK VERSUS BOVINE. In the 1970s, I. William Lane, PhD, served as a consultant to the Shah of Iran on harvesting sharks from the Persian Gulf. In the 1980s, Dr. Lane was taught how to process cartilage by Prudden. In December of 1991, Lane received a use patent on anti-angiogenesis therapy using shark cartilage. In 1993, the "60 Minutes" TV show popularized Lane's book, SHARKS DON'T GET CANCER[16], and made shark cartilage a leading contender among alternative cancer therapies. Although the National Cancer Institute initially showed interest in helping Lane, they backed out on endorsing or researching shark cartilage.

Advantages of bovine cartilage over shark cartilage:

◊ Efficacy. The original research involving cartilage in human intervention trials all used bovine. In published peer reviewed literature, and after 22 years clinical use by Prudden, and 40 years of safety studies costing over $7 million, bovine cartilage is by far the safest and most effective of the cartilage products:

◊ More potent. Ten times more shark cartilage (1000% more) in weight must be used in order to get a clinical response in cancer patients.

◊ No taste or odor. Compared to shark cartilage, which induces nausea & diarrhea in many users, bovine cartilage is relatively free from taste and odor.

◊ More economical. Bovine cartilage saves 75% in cost over shark cartilage.

◊ Calcium content. Hypercalcemia is common in cancer patients. 22% of shark cartilage is calcium, which provides 14 grams of calcium (14,000 mg, or 14 times the RDA) compared to 1% calcium concentration in bovine cartilage. The 9 gram/day of bovine cartilage in ImmunoPower contains 90 mg of calcium.

◊ Additional components. Among the other substances in cartilage that may have therapeutic benefit, including chondroitan sulfate and glycosaminoglycans, shark cartilage contains less than 10% while bovine cartilage contains greater than 20% by weight.

◊ Reduce toxic side effects in chemo & radiation. Bovine may improve outcome in herpes zoster (shingles) and AIDS.

Active ingredient(s)?? Finding the active ingredient may not be easy with cartilage, which is a complex collection of protein, carbohydrate, fats, minerals, and accessory factors. Some companies boast that their cartilage product is higher in the protein factors that inhibit the making of blood vessels (anti-angiogenesis) from tumors.

Prudden thinks that some mucopolysaccharide, or starch-like molecule, is responsible for all the therapeutic magic of BTC. This theory makes sense, given the therapeutic mucopolysaccharides that have been isolated from Maitake mushroom and aloe vera gel.

Anti-angiogenesis? Lane's theory that shark cartilage may shut down the making of blood vessels from tumors (anti-angiogenesis) has some foundation. In 1976 Dr. Robert Langer of MIT and Dr. Judah Folkman of Harvard published work showing that something in cartilage can shut down angiogenesis in cultured tumors.[17] Later studies by this same group showed that rabbits with corneal cancers had measurable benefits from cartilage topically applied in slowing the growth of tumors.[18] In 1983, Langer and colleague Anne Lee found that something in shark cartilage could slow the growth of tumors through anti-angiogenesis.[19]

Langer pursued this line of research, finding that tumors could not grow larger than 1-2 centimeters (1/2 to 1 inch) without vascularization to support further growth.[20] Dr. Patricia D'Amore of Harvard endorsed the concept that if you shut down angiogenesis then you shut down tumor growth.[21] Folkman's team then found that when a cell switches from normal growth (hyperplasia) to rapid and uncontrolled tumor growth (neoplasia), then the angiogenesis process gears up dramatically.[22] Other Harvard researchers found that something in cartilage definitely shuts down angiogenesis, which is essential for tumor growth.[23] Japanese researchers reported on this anti-angiogenic agent found in shark cartilage.[24] More Harvard researchers reported on the strong link between angiogenesis and tumor progression.[25] Folkman further explained the importance of anti-angiogenesis in cancer, yet added that perhaps genetic regulation is more important than some dietary protein.[26]

In discussions with pathologists and Dr. Prudden, there seems to be a difference between the blood vessels that extend "cork screw-like" from a tumor and the blood vessels that extend "tree root-like" from healthy tissue. If there is an anti-angiogenesis factor in cartilage, then it cannot inhibit the making of normal healthy blood vessels. How does a baby shark grow into a large adult shark if shark cartilage shuts down the making of ALL blood vessels?

"Sharks don't get cancer" while cows do get cancer. Yet, the shark's skeleton is entirely cartilage, or roughly 20% of its weight; while cartilage is found in much smaller quantities in a cow's body.

Alan Gaby, MD, President of the American Holistic Medical Association stated in the April 1994 Townsend Letter: "I have not met any physicians who are excited about their results with shark cartilage."

Prudden believes that BTC is effective because it is a biodirector, or "normalizer". There are parallels of these "homeostatic regulators" in the botanical medicine field called adaptogens, like ginseng or astragalus, which will raise your blood pressure if it is too low or lower it if it is too high. Think about the enigma of cartilage:

⇒ topically applied, it **accelerates** healthy growth for wounds but **slows** abnormal cancer growth
⇒ taken internally, it **increases** various immune factors, including B-cells (from the bone), macrophages (literally: "big eaters"), and cytotoxic T-cells (important in the "war on cancer"); YET it also **slows** down auto-immune attacks involved in allergies, arthritis, and lupus
⇒ taken internally, it slows the wasting disease, cachexia, caused by cancer and AIDS
⇒ taken internally, it **slows** the division in abnormal cells (anti-mitotic), but **allows** healthy cells to divide
⇒ taken internally, it **reduces** inflammation, such as in arthritis

Prudden pioneered the use of BTC for its
•wound healing properties, which culminated in textbook acceptance[27]
•anti-inflammatory agent in arthritis[28]
•anti-cancer activity.[29]

Prudden's peer-reviewed article showed a 90% response rate in 31 human cancer patients followed for 15 years. Of the 31 total patients, 35%, or 11 of these terminal patients were **cured** using 9 grams daily of oral bovine tracheal cartilage as sole therapy, while 55% or 17 showed some benefit then relapsed, and 10% or 3 showed no improvement. Prudden has used BTC in over 1000 cancer patients, with good followup on 100 patients. His latest research paper has been submitted for peer review before being published in a journal.

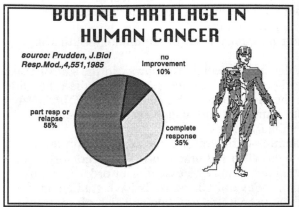

BOVINE CARTILAGE IN HUMAN CANCER

source: Prudden, J.Biol Resp.Mod.,4,551,1985

no Improvement 10%

part resp or relapse 55%

complete response 35%

Dr. Brian Duric has found equally impressive results using BTC to halt cancer growth in vitro.[30] Prudden's other research shows that BTC probably works by turbo-charging the immune system.[31] For his noteworthy persistence and brilliance in spearheading BTC research, Prudden received the coveted "Linus Pauling Scientist of the Year" award at the Third International Symposium on Adjuvant Nutrition in Cancer Treatment in Tampa in September of 1995.

Of all the impressive healing agents in Nature's "pharmacy", none is more safe, cost-effective, versatile, and promising than BTC.

Nucleic acids (nucleotides from brewer's yeast): DNA 500 mg and RNA 500 mg
Immune stimulants, help to regulate genetic expression and discourage the excessive production of Tumor Necrosis Factor, which can lead to tissue wasting.

At the very core of our cells are the "blueprints" of DNA that allow that cell to make another exact copy. RNA has various forms that basically are the "servants" of DNA, clamping on the DNA to read the base pair sequence, then going out into the cell to construct proteins, enzymes or whatever the cell needs based on the DNA blueprints. Obviously, this is a very crucial pathway for human health. When DNA goes awry, cancer can result. Somehow the DNA in the healthy host tissue can become corrupted and start creating cells that lack normal regulation properties, have no plan and reproduce without any restraint.

We make our own DNA and RNA (also called nucleic acids) in our cells from amino acids in the purine and pyrimidine pathways. We also eat some DNA/RNA in metabolically active foods including brewer's yeast, liver, seeds (especially the germ), organ meats, and bee pollen. The debate has never been over the value of DNA/RNA, but rather "can we absorb these nutrients into the bloodstream intact?" To answer that question, we need to step back and look at other examples of:

* fatty acids that are dissected with bile salts and enzymes in the GI tract and then reassembled in the bloodstream
* the known passage of large proteins through the intestinal wall to cause food allergies in the bloodstream

* the use of glandular therapy (such as natural dessicated thyroid) to treat the target gland with a large protein molecule that should be destroyed in the acid bath of the gut.
* how infants receive their immunity from the immunoglobulins in mother's millk.

Either these molecules have special "windows" in the gut or these molecules are torn apart in the gut and then reassembled on the other side of the intestinal mucosa in the bloodstream. Supplements of RNA/DNA have shown benefits in both immunity and wound recovery when taken orally in both human and animal studies.

Animals fed a nucleotide-deficient diet had impaired immune functions which were corrected when fed uracil (a DNA precursor).[32] In protein depletion, RNA supplements may be essential in order to return immune functions to normal.[33] Several human trials have studied an enteral formula, Impact, which uses RNA, arginine and fish oil to provide substantial improvement in immune factors.[34] RNA seems to improve wound recovery after surgery.[35] RNA supplements provide a boost to memory in the elderly.[36] RNA supplements were able to help regenerate the damaged livers of rats.[37] Early indications were that RNA may be able to help cancer patients.[38] Of course, a patentable drug (Poly A/Poly U) was developed to continue these studies, with very encouraging results.[39] RNA supplements seem to encourage Natural Killer cells to attack cancer and bacteria.[40]

In personal discussions with Arsinur Bircaglu, MD, an oncologist from Turkey, she showed very intriguing human clinical data that large amounts of RNA and DNA taken orally could shut down the tissue wasting process (cachexia) that is so common in cancer and AIDS. Precursors to make more nucleic acids seems to dampen down the cytokines (Tumor Necrosis Factor) that trigger the downward spiral of cancer cachexia.

FOS, fructo-oligosaccharides 1 gm
Stimulates growth of probiotic organisms in gut, with the far-reaching effects of favorable bacterial growth, reduced production of carcinogens in the gut, maintenance of gut integrity and immune functions.

In order to better appreciate the importance of FOS for cancer patients, we need to rewind the video cassette recorder to Louis Pasteur's deathbed confession in 1895: "I have been wrong. The germ is nothing. The terrain is everything."

Among carbohydrate molecules, there are:
⇒ short length molecules (mono and disaccharides)
⇒ medium length molecules (oligosaccharides)
⇒ long chain molecules (polysaccharides).

Oligosaccharides made from the monosaccharide fructose are the subject of this discussion, because they have been very potent at stimulating the growth of "friendly" bacteria. Oligosaccharides are poorly digested by human digestive juices, but easily digested by many forms of bacteria in the gut. Some oligosaccharides, such as stachyose and raffinose from beans and certain nuts, can feed bacteria that cause intestinal gas. FOS feeds the bacteria that fortify your gut wall and immune system, and should actually help to control gas. Best food sources of FOS are onions and whole grains.

In an extensive review of the scientific literature, FOS supplements have been shown to:

◊ encourage the growth of bifidobacteria
◊ reduce detrimental bacteria and their toxic metabolites
◊ prevent and reverse diarrhea or constipation caused by pathogenic bacteria
◊ protect liver functions
◊ reduce blood pressure
◊ induce the production of essential nutrients.[41]
◊ encourage the growth of "friendly" bacteria which have shown considerable anti-cancer activity in animal studies.[42]

For more information on the importance of healthy bacteria in the colon, please see the section that discusses "probiotics".

Tocotrienols 20 mg
    Antioxidant, immune stimulant, regulates fatty acid metabolism.

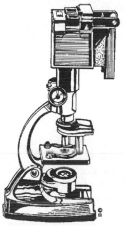

I hiked up to the top of Mount San Gorgonio in southern California in 1984. The view was spectacular. However, when I pulled out my binoculars, I could see much more detail. And when I borrowed a pair of high powered binoculars from a friend, the details of the surrounding landscape became even more defined and clear. The same thing is happening in the field of nutrition. As our analytical equipment becomes more sophisticated, our ability to see subsets of molecules that work together becomes more impressive. The star nutrient of today may become a supporting actress tomorrow. Such may be the case for vitamin E (tocopherols) and its kissing cousin, tocotrienols.

While some nutritionists campaign against the use of palm oil, since it has a higher content of saturated fats than soy or corn oil, the data actually shows that palm oil may LOWER the risk for heart disease, since it is rich in tocotrienols which are potent antioxidants that protect the blood vessel walls.[43] Palm oil is the second largest volume of vegetable oil produced in the world.

Tocotrienols are very similar in structure to tocopherols, which is vitamin E. Palm oil and rice bran are the richest sources of tocotrienols. Tocotrienols have only 30% the vitamin E activity when compared to D-alpha-tocopherol, the "gold standard" of vitamin E.[44] Yet tocotrienols

have demonstrated a greater anti-cancer activity than vitamin E.[45]
Tocotrienols were able to delay onset of cancer in animals, while mixed
carotenes from palm oil were able to regress these same cancers.[46] In
vitro and in vivo, dietary palm oil (richest source of tocotrienols) was able
to exhibit a "dose dependent" anti-tumor activity against several
carcinogenic compounds.[47] Just as some researchers now feel that
bioflavonoids are more important in human nutrition than the vitamin C
that was discovered first, there are some very bright scientists who feel that
the primary role of vitamin E is to help manufacture and protect
tocotrienols, which may have the ultimate antioxidant and immune-
stimulating activity in the human body.

Medium chain triglycerides (MCT) 1 gm
Slows down lean tissue wasting, enhances thermogenesis (making
of heat) and augments burning of fat, a fuel source which cancer cells
cannot use.

Fatty acids can have a length of anywhere from 2 carbons to 24
carbons. The long chain fats (or triglycerides, called LCT) include most
dietary fats of soy oil and beef fat. LCT is difficult to absorb and
requires special bile acids and absorption pathways in the lymphatic
ducts.[48] Medium chain triglycerides (MCT) are much easier to absorb
and are quickly burned in the human system. MCTs are primarily found
in coconut oil and smaller amounts in other nuts. Almost like adding
kindling (MCT) to a group of logs (LCT), medium chain triglycerides
actually promote the burning of the body's fat stores, which helps to
encourage thermogenesis (making of heat) in humans.[49] Cancer cells can
be selectively destroyed by elevating the body temperature.
MCT has been shown to be a useful tool:
◊ in the control of obesity
◊ lowering serum cholesterol
◊ as a concentrated and readily available source of energy
◊ helps to prevent immune suppression in critically ill people[50]
◊ maintains body (visceral) protein stores during wound recovery.[51]
MCT is extremely safe, provides quick energy for the person,
does not feed the cancer, protects protein reserves in the body and helps
to slowly melt away unwanted fat stores in the adipose tissue.

Lecithin, phosphatidylcholine 1500 mg
Helps to detoxify the liver, regulates cell growth, contributes
choline for many other functions in the body, becomes part of healthy
cell membranes for proper nutrient intake and toxin removal.

Lecithin is an incredible substance with great potential to help the
cancer patient. Most substances in life are either fat soluble, such as
butter, or water soluble, such as vitamin C. Lecithin is on a very short list
of substances that can dissolve both fat and water soluble substances at the
same time, also known as an emulsifier. Lecithin is used widely in the

food industry to prevent separation of ingredients in cookies, etc. Richest sources of lecithin are soybeans and egg yolks. For a little experiment, next time you finish with blending some eggs for scrambling, add water to the container and use an electric blender to see the "soap bubbles" rise from the leftover lecithin-rich egg yolks.

Lecithin is a molecule that is similar in structure to triglycerides found in soy oil and beef, except that one of the fatty acids has been replaced by phosphatidylcholine. This simple exchange gives lecithin unique properties, including the:

⇒ lowering of serum cholesterol and reduction of platelet aggregation in humans[52]
⇒ reversing the skin disease psoriasis[53]
⇒ improving the course of Alzheimer's disease[54]
⇒ reducing the tremors in tardive dyskinesia.[55]

Lecithin seems to work in the cell membrane to enhance "cell membrane dynamics", works in the nervous tissue (sphingomyelin), and contributes a key B-vitamin, choline. Choline works with folate, methione and B-12 as methyl donors, which are responsible for all new cell growth.

Choline is one of the few nutrients tested in which merely a deficiency (without any other compounding factor, like toxins or aging) is enough to spontaneously generate liver cancer in animals.[56] In animal and human studies, choline deficiency leads to fatty liver and compromised liver functions.[57] Lecithin is a major protective nutrient for the liver, helping to regenerate healthy liver tissue and excrete toxins. Protecting the liver, with substances like lecithin and milk thistle, is crucial for cancer patients.

Genistein (from soy) 6 mg
Helps to selectively slow down cancer growth.

When scientists reviewed the world's cancer incidences, they found some strange disparities. Japanese men had 1/5 the incidence of prostate cancer and Japanese women had 1/5 the incidence of breast cancer when compared to Americans. The reasons could be many, including a lower fat diet, more exercise, less beef, less obesity, more vegetables and seaweed. But researchers settled in on soybean products, including tofu and tempeh, as the primary protector against cancer. It has now been well established that regular consumption of soy products may lower the incidence of many forms of cancer.[58] While there are a rich collection of isoflavones, protease inhibitors and lectins in soybeans; researchers have focused on genistein as perhaps the principle cancer-protective bioflavonoid in soy.

Genistein may be able to:
◊ selectively kill cancer cells
◊ reduce the tumor growth capacity of sex hormones in both men and women
◊ induce programmed cell death (apoptosis) in cancer
◊ inhibit metastasis

◊ inhibit angiogenesis[59] (making of blood vessels from tumors)
◊ induce differentiation to help regulate proper cell growth.[60]

Genistein is one of the few agents on the planet earth that may be able to revert a cancer cell back to a normal healthy cell, called prodifferentiation.[61] Scientists have worked diligently to better understand the anti-cancer effects of protease inhibitors in soy.[62] Dr. Ann Kennedy spent 20 years at Harvard and now working at the University of Pennsylvania researching the extraordinary ability of the Bowman Birk Inhibitor (a protease inhibitor found in soy) to prevent and reverse cancer while also reducing the toxic effects of chemo and radiation on animals.[63]

Soy and breast cancer. Based on the fact that soy contains weak phytoestrogens that can induce infertility in zoo animals kept on a high soy diet, some experts have cautioned against the use of soy in estrogen/progesterone positive breast cancer. Tamoxifen is an estrogen binder drug that is given to women with estrogen positive breast cancer. Tamoxifen has a similar chemical structure to genistein, yet genistein does not have any of the toxic side effects of tamoxifen. Once again, Nature comes up with another brilliantly helpful molecule in genistein, which inhibits both breast and prostate cancer.[64] Genistein actually slows the growth of breast cancer cells in culture.[65] The macrobiotic diet uses large amounts of soy to help slow the growth of many cancers, including breast cancer. A fermented and concentrated soy product, Haelen 851, has been used successfully to reverse breast cancer. For more on this subject, refer to the explanation of ginseng, which also contains phytoestrogens, in Chapter 3.

There are over 10,000 different varieties of soybean that grow around the world (Glycine max L.). Genistein content can vary tremendously based upon variety of species, where harvested, and processing techniques. Therefore, ImmunoPower contains a guaranteed potency of soy genistein from soy protein at a 1:1000 ratio. 1000 milligrams of this soy protein is guaranteed to contain 1 mg of genistein. In order to obtain a therapeutic dose of genistein, ImmunoPower contains 6 grams of soy protein per scoop. This specially formulated protein also contains the proper ratio of essential amino acids and is highly digestible.

L-glycine 1 gm
Energizer, calmitive agent, detoxifier, controls fat levels in the blood, builds energy stores (glycogen) in the liver, helps in wound recovery and collagen synthesis.

Glycine's name reflects its sweet flavor. It is considered a non-essential amino acid, since it can be formed from the amino acids threonine and serine. Glycine has been included in ImmunoPower for several reasons:
◊ Acts as a preservative in foods
◊ Sweetening agent, since it tastes much like sugar, yet does not alter glycemic index

◊ May be converted into glutathione (see that section) for antioxidant and detoxification benefits

◊ May be converted in the body into Dimethylglycine (DMG, see that section)

◊ Works as a calming agent in the nervous system and also helps to improve spastic conditions[66] and muscular weakness.[67]

◊ Promotes collagen formation, thus possibly helping the body to encapsulate tumors

---

Glucaric acid (cal D glucarate) 500 mg
Improves detoxification in the gut and liver, escorts estrogen out of the system, may have anti-proliferative activity.

Calcium D-glucarate, or CDG, is such a non-toxic and potentially helpful substance for cancer patients that it is undergoing Phase I trials sponsored by the National Cancer Institute and held at Memorial Sloan Kettering Hospital in New York. D-glucaric acid is a substance found in certain fruits (oranges) and vegetables (broccoli, potatoes). CDG has been shown to encourage critical phase II detoxification pathways in the gut by inhibiting the counterproductive enzyme produced by intestinal bacteria, beta-glucuronidase.[68] Oral administration of CDG provided a 50% drop in beta-glucuronidase for 5 hours.[69] In animals fed CDG, serum estradiol levels were decreased (a good sign for breast cancer) by 23%.[70] Animals fed CDG experienced a 50-70% reduction in mammary cancers.[71] In cultured cancer cells, D-glucarate combined with retinoid (vitamin A analog) provided a synergistic inhibition of tumor growth.[72] When D-glucaric acid is bound to calcium, the resulting molecule, calcium D-glucarate, becomes a time-released version of glucaric acid in the gut, helping to detoxify poisons and hormones while dampening unregulated cell growth.

ENDNOTES

[1] . Haller, JS, Bull.NY Acad.Sci., vol.66, p.647, 1990

[2] . Danhof, IE, REMARKABLE ALOE, Omnimedicus Press, Grand Prairie, TX 1987

[3] . Lee, YC, Adv.Exp.Med.Biol., vol.228, p.103, 1984

[4] . Robson, MC, et al., J.Burn.Care Rehab., vol.3, p.157, 1982

[5] . Sheets, MA, et al., Mol.Biother., vol.3, p.41, 1991

[6] . Kahlon, JB, et al., Mol.Biother., vol.3, p.214, 1991

[7] . t'Hart, LA, et al., Planta.Med., vol.55, p.509, 1989

[8] . t'Hart, LA, et al., Int.J.Immunopharmacol., vol.12, p.427, 1990

[9] . Karaca, K., et al., Int.J.Immunopharmacol., vol.17, p.183, 1995

[10] . Kamasuka, T., et al., Gann, vol.59, p.443, 1968

[11] . Tizard, IR, et al., Mol.Biother., vol.1, p.290, 1989

[12] . Murray, RK, et al., HARPER'S BIOCHEMISTRY, p.648, Lange Medical, Stamford, CT 1996

[13] . Haas, EM, STAYING HEALTHY WITH NUTRITION, p.139, Celestial Arts, Berkeley, 1992

[14] . Reap, EA, et al., J.Lab.Clin.Med., vol.115, p.481, 1990

[15] . Graber, CD, et al., J.Infect.Dis., vol.143, p.101, 1982

[16] . Lane, IW, and L. Comac, SHARKS DON'T GET CANCER, Avery, Garden City, 1992

[17] . Langer, H. et al., Science, p.70, July 1976

[18] . Langer, R. et al., Proceedings National Academy of Sciences, vol.77, no.7, p.4331, July 1980

[19] . Lee, A., et al., Science, vol.221, p.1185, Sept.1983

[20] . Folkman, J, et al., Science, vol.235, p.442, Jan.1987

21. D'Amore, PA, Seminars in Thrombosis & Hemostasis, vol.14, p.73, 1988
22. Folkman, J., et al., Nature, vol.339, p.58, May 1989
23. Moses, MA, et al., Science, vol.248, p.1408, June 1990
24. Oikawa, T., et al., Cancer Letters, vol.51, p.181, 1990
25. Weidner, N., et al., New England Journal of Medicine, vol.324, p.1, Jan.1991
26. Folkman, J., Journal Clinical Oncology, vol.12, p.441, Mar.1994
27. Madden, JW, in SABISTON'S TEXTBOOK OF SURGERY, p.268, WB Saunders, Phila, 1972
28. Prudden, JF, et al., Seminars in Arthritis and Rheumatism, vol.3, p.287, Summer 1974
29. Prudden, JF, Journal of Biological Response Modifiers, vol.4, p.551, 1985
30. Durie, BGM, et al., Journal of Biological Response Modifiers, vol.4, p.590, 1985
31. Rosen, J, et al., Journal of Biological Response Modifiers, vol.7, p.498, 1988
32. Kinsella, J., et al., Crit.Care Med., vol.18, p.S94, 1990
33. Pizzini, RP, et al., Surgical Infection Society abstract, p.50, 1989
34. Cerra, FB, Am.J.Surg., vol.161, p.230, 1991; see also Cerra, FB, et al., Nutrition, vol.6, p.88, 1990; see also Lieberman, M., et al., Nutrition, vol.6, p.88, 1990
35. Aarons, S., et al., J.Surg.Onc., vol.23, p.21, 1983
36. Cameron, DE, et al., Am.J.Psychiatry, vol.120, p.320, 1963; see also Nodine, JH, et al., Am.J.Psychiatry, vol.123, p.1257, 1967
37. Newman, EA, et al., Amer.J.Physiol., vol.164, p.251, 1951
38. Pilch, YH, Am.J.Surg., vol.132, p.631, 1976
39. Michelson, AM, et al., Proc.Soc.Exper.Biol. Med., vol.179, p.1, 1985
40. Wiltrout, RH, et al., J.Biol.Resp.Mod., vol.4, p.512, 1985
41. Tomomatsu, H., Food Technology, p.61, Oct.1994
42. Fugiwara, S., et al., J.Japan Soc.Nutr.Food Science, vol.43, p.327, 1990
43. Qureshi, AA, et al., Am.J.Clin.Nutr., vol.53, p.1042S, 1991
44. Farrell, PM, et al., in MODERN NUTRITION IN HEALTH AND DISEASE, Shils, ME (eds), Lea & Febiger, Philadelphia, 1994
45. Komiyama, K., et al., Chem.Pharm.Bull., vol.37, p.1369, 1989
46. Tan, B., Nutrition Research, vol.12, p.S163, 1992
47. Azuine, MA, et al., Nutr. Cancer, vol.17, p.287, 1992
48. Bach, AC, et al., Am.J.Clin.Nutr., vol.36, p.950, 1982
49. Mascioli, EA, et al., J.Parenteral Enteral Nutr., vol.15, p.27, 1991
50. Jensen, GL, et al., J.Parenteral Enteral Nutr., vol.14, p.467, 1990
51. Maiz, A., et al., Metabolism, vol.33, p.901, Oct.1984
52. Brook, JG, et al., Biochem.Med.Metab.Biol., vol. 35, p.31, 1986
53. Gross, P, et al., NY State J.Med., vol.50, p.2683, 1950
54. Little, A., et al., J.Neurology, Neurosurgery & Psychiatry, vol.48, p.736, 1985
55. Jackson, IV, et al., Am.J.Psychiatry, vol.136, p.11, Nov.1979
56. Yokoyama, S, et al., Cancer Res., vol.45, p.2834, 1985
57. Zeisel, SH, et al., Fed Amer Soc Exper Biol., vol.5, p.2093, 1991
58. Messina, M., et al., J.Nat.Cancer Inst., vol.83, p.541, 1991
59. Fostis, T., et al., Proc. Natl. Acad.Sci., vol.90, p.2690, 1993
60. Boik, J., CANCER & NATURAL MEDICINE, p.184, Oregon Medical Press, Princeton, MN 1995
61. Watanabe, T., et al., Exp.Cell Res., vol.183, p.335, 1989; see also Constantinou, A., et al., Cancer Res., vol.50, p.2618, 1990
62. Hocman, G., Int.J.Biochem., vol.24, p.1365, 1992
63. Kennedy, AR, in ADJUVANT NUTRITION IN CANCER TREATMENT, p.129, Quillin, P. (eds), Cancer Treatment Research Foundation, Arlington Heights, IL 1994
64. Adlercreutz, H., et al., Lancet, vol.342, p.1209, Nov.1993
65. Peterson, G., et al., Biochem.Biophy.Res.Commun., vol.179, p.661, 1991; see also Zava, DT, et al., Nutrition & Cancer, vol.27, p.31, 1997
66. Davidoff, RA, Annals Neurology, vol.17, p.107, 1985
67. Braverman, ER, et al., HEALING NUTRIENTS WITHIN, p.238, Keats, New Canaan, CT 1987
68. Dwivedi, C, et al, Biochem.Med. & Metabolic Biol., vol.43, p.83, 1990
69. Dwivedi, C., et al., Biochem.Med.Metabol.Biol., vol.43, p.83, 1990
70. Walaszek, Z, et al., Carcinogenesis, vol.7, p.1463, 1986
71. Walaszek, Z, Cancer Letters, vol.54, p.1, 1990
72. Curley, RW, et al., Life Sciences, vol.54, p.1299, 1994

CHAPTER 8

THE POWER OF NUTRITIONAL SYNERGISM

★

synergism: the action of two or more substances to achieve an effect of which each is individually incapable

There are two primary lessons to be learned in nutritional synergism:

1) **ENHANCED EFFECTS.**
⇒ **Nutrient-nutrient combinations** augment each other to achieve greater healing capacity. Either vitamin C or essential fatty acids were able to inhibit the growth of melanoma in culture, yet when combined their anti-cancer activity was much stronger.[1]
⇒ **Nutrient-medicine combinations** help to protect the patient while selectively destroying the cancer cells. Maitake D-fraction inhibited tumor growth by 80% while the drug Mitomycin C inhibited tumor growth by 45%. Yet when both were given together, but at half the dosage for each, tumor inhibition was 98%. For more information on this concept, see chapter 9, in "nutrients reduce the toxicity from medical therapy".

2) **LOWER DOSES ARE REQUIRED** when nutrients are used synergistically. In animals with implanted tumors, vitamin C and B-12 together provided for significant tumor regression and 50% survival of the treated group, while all of the animals not receiving C and B-12 died by the 19th day.[2] C and B-12 seemed to form a cobalt-ascorbate compound that selectively shut down tumor growth. When vitamin C and K were added to cancer cells in culture, the dosage required to kill cancer cells dropped by 98% compared to the dosage required by either of these vitamins alone.[3] Combining vitamins C and K-3 against cultured human breast cancer cells allowed for inhibition of the cancer growth at doses 90-98% less than what was required if only one of these vitamins was used against the cancer.[4]

"No [nutrient] is an island, entire of itself; every [nutrient] is a piece of the continent, a part of the main." paraphrasing John Donne

---

Listening to the rapture of a symphonic orchestra, I was impressed with the complex synergistic nature of most aspects of our lives. No one and nothing operates in isolation. Both 20th century research and our multi-billion dollar pharmaceutical-based medical system are rooted in the concept of using a single agent to treat a single symptom. Unfortunately, life is much more complicated than that.

NEGATIVE SYNERGISM OF TOXINS

We know that barbiturates have a certain toxicity on the liver, which is synergistically enhanced when alcohol is consumed at the same time. We know that tobacco brings a major risk for lung cancer, as does asbestos exposure, yet when a person is exposed to both there is a 500% greater risk for lung cancer than what would have been expected by adding the two risks (1+1=2). Scientists recently found that pesticides amplify one another's toxicity by 500-1000 fold.[5] Thus, 1+1=500. This discovery of synergistic toxicity presents the chilling possibility that the 1.2 billion pounds of pesticides sprayed on our domestic food supply may not be as safe as we once thought.

In 1976, a study examined animals that were fed 2% of their diet as either red dye, sodium cyclamate or an emulsifier--all approved at the time by the Food and Drug Administration. Animals fed one food additive showed no harmful effects. Animals fed two of the food additives exhibited balding scruffy fur, diarrhea, and retarded weight gain. Animals fed all three additives all died within 2 weeks.[6] The take-home lesson is that poisons probably amplify each other's toxicity in logarithmic fashion. Given the cavalier spirit with which Americans have nonchalantly discarded and intentionally added toxins to our air, food and water supply; synergistic toxicity gives me an uneasy feeling about the future health of our nation.

POSITIVE SYNERGISM OF NUTRIENTS

While the prospects of synergistic toxicity are daunting, the prospects of synergistic nutritional healing may be the key to solving many of our health problems. Perusing any biochemistry textbook we find an abundance of synergistic nutritional relationships: calcium with magnesium with potassium with sodium; vitamin E with selenium; polyunsaturated fats with vitamin E; protein with B-6; and so on.

Antioxidants have surfaced as the "fire extinguishers" that minimize the cellular damage from reactive oxygen species, or free radicals. Yet, these antioxidants work in a hierarchy, not unlike a game of "hot potato", trying to pass along the unpaired electron until the energy dissipates. In this hierarchy, vitamin C recharges vitamin E. Biologists find this complex hierarchy of antioxidants consists of 20,000 bioflavonoids; 800 carotenoids; known essential vitamins, like C and E; conditionally essential vitamins, like lipoic acid and coenzyme Q; and endogenously synthesized antioxidants like superoxide dismutase (SOD) and glutathione peroxidase (GSH-Px). The possible combinations and permutations of antioxidants in the human body makes the combinations in the Rubik's cube look like mere child's play. When these antioxidants are all in their proper place in optimal amounts, we have a relatively impenetrable barrier against oxidative damage. Researching any one of these nutrients in isolation is overly simplistic and doomed to misleading results.

BETA-CAROTENE CAUSES LUNG CANCER?

YES

1994 Finnish study
29,000 smokers
beta 5-8 yrs
1996 CARET study
18,000 smoker/asbestos
30 mg beta 25,000 A
NO BENEFIT
1995 Phys Health Study
22,000 MDs
50 mg beta 12 yr

NO

Over 200 epidemiology studies show
fruits & veg lower risk
11 studies show beta protective
against lung ca
8+ studies show beta reverses
premalignant lesions
3 studies show beta improves
human cancer outcome
4 animal studies show beta cures ca
As sole nutrient, AOX can be PROX

RECOMMENDATIONS: Eat a diet rich in green & orange fruits & veg.
Take beta, mixed carot, other AOX. Don't smoke.

The National Cancer Institute reported in 1994 that beta-carotene supplements provided a slightly elevated risk for lung cancer in heavy smokers.[7] Yet other prominent researchers in nutrition and cancer have published papers showing that antioxidants, like beta-carotene, can become pro-oxidants in the wrong biochemical environment, such as the combat zone of free radicals generated by heavy tobacco use.[8] At the International Conference on Nutrition and Cancer, sponsored by the University of California at Irvine, held in July of 1997, there were several watershed presentations showing that one nutrient alone may be ineffective or counterproductive while a host of compatible nutrients in the proper ratio can be extremely effective at slowing or reversing cancer.

NUTRITIONAL SYNERGISM AGAINST CANCER

While vitamin C or K alone had mild anti-neoplastic activity against cancer cells in culture, when combined together these nutrients showed improved tumor cell destruction at 10 to 50 times lower dosages.[9] Other scientists found that vitamins C and B-12 have a synergistic action at slowing cancer growth in animal studies.[10] Apparently, the cobalt from the B-12 attaches to the ascorbic acid to form cobalt ascorbate, a selective toxin against cancer cells.

In another animal study, researchers found that DMBA-exposed animals all died. When provided a single chemopreventive nutrient (either selenium, magnesium, vitamin C, or

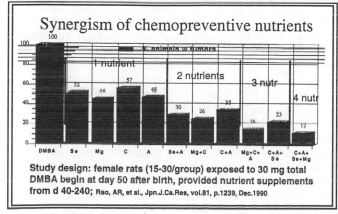

Synergism of chemopreventive nutrients

Study design: female rats (15-30/group) exposed to 30 mg total DMBA begin at day 50 after birth, provided nutrient supplements from d 40-240; Rao, AR, et al., Jpn.J.Ca.Res, vol.81, p.1239, Dec.1990

vitamin A), cancer incidence after DMBA exposure was cut in half. When two nutrients were combined, the cancer incidence was cut by 70%; with 3 chemopreventive nutrients the cancer incidence was 80%, and with 4 nutrients the cancer incidence was cut by 88%.[11]

Lamm and colleagues found that a multi-nutrient packet of vitamins A, E, C, B-6 and the mineral zinc cut cancer recurrence more than in half in bladder cancer patients treated with BCG.[12] A group of Finnish oncologists treated 18 non-randomized lung cancer patients with chemotherapy, radiation and a collection of nutrition factors. The anticipated outcome in this group of poor prognostic patients is 1% survival at 30 months after diagnosis. In these nutritionally supported lung cancer patients, 44% were still alive 6 years (72 months) after diagnosis with half of these surviving patients in remission.[13] Something in multi-nutrient synergism had provided a major boost over the anticipated outcome in these patients.

One of the brightest nutritional physicians of the 20th century, Abram Hoffer, MD, PhD and his colleague, twice Nobel laureate, Linus Pauling, PhD, tracked129 human cancer patients for over 11 years. Of the 31 patients who received only medical intervention for their cancer, the average lifespan was about 6 months. Of the remaining 98 patients who received a combination of medical and nutritional therapies, the average lifespan was about 6 years, a 1200% increase in lifespan, with poor responders (20%) somewhat offsetting exceptional responders (33%).[14]

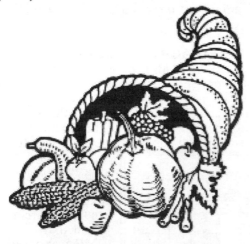

Based upon all of this very crucial ground work, I designed a synergistic collection of 65 (now 77) nutritional ingredients which all had some proven ability to bolster host defense mechanisms against cancer. This product, originally called Advanced Nutrition Composite and now called ImmunoPower, has been clinically tested in hundreds of cancer patients for nearly 3 years. The results have been astounding. Patients "sailing through" 2 bone marrow transplant procedures, which usually induces severe digestive and immune disturbances. Several patients who were considered "unsalvageable" who have had "no progress of the disease" while on this product for over 18 months. Many "poor prognostic" patients who have beat the odds and are in remission. Patients who maintain their energy levels and keep their hair throughout the most rigorous chemotherapy protocols. Most patients using this product report a substantial improvement in energy levels and quality of life while going through conventional chemo and radiation therapy. While this product is not sole therapy for advanced cancer, it is a remarkable step forward in the practical applications of supportive clinical nutrition for cancer patients.

EASY SCIENCE OR REALISTIC SCIENCE?

Our bodies are composed of around 60 trillion cells, working in synergistic unison. While our textbooks speak of around 50 essential nutrients for the human body, the number is probably much higher if the endpoint were "thriving" versus the Recommended Dietary Allowance goal of "surviving". Those nutrients work in synergism, not isolation. While mono-nutrient studies are easier to get funded, easier to statistically interpret, and more likely to lead to some drug patent application; these projects fail miserably at appreciating the grandiose complexities of the human body. Nutritional synergism is a biological law that we can either ignore, or capitalize on to improve outcome in a variety of disease states.

ENDNOTES

[1]. Gardiner, N, et al., Pros.Leuk., vol.34, p.119, 1988
[2]. Poydock, ME, Am.J.Clin.Nutr., vol.54, p.1261S, 1991
[3]. Noto, V., et al., Cancer, vol.63, p.901, 1989
[4]. Noto, V., et al., Cancer, vol.63, p.901, 1989
[5]. Arnold. SF, et al., Science, vol.272, p.1489, 1996
[6]. Ershoff, BH, Journal of Food Science, vol.41, p.949, 1976
[7]. Alpha tocopherol beta-carotene cancer prevention study group, New England Journal of Medicine, vol.330, p.1029, 1994
[8]. Schwartz, JL, Journal of Nutrition, vol.126, 4 suppl, p.1221S, 1996
[9]. Noto, V., et al., Cancer, vol.63, p.901, 1989
[10]. Poydock, ME, American Journal of Clinical Nutrition, vol.54, p.1266IS, 1991
[11]. Rao, AR, et al., Japanese Journal Cancer Research, vol.81, p.1239, Dec.1990
[12]. Lamm, DL, et al., Journal of Urology, vol.151, p.21, Jan.1994
[13]. Jaakkola, K., et al., Anticancer Research, vol.12, p.599, 1992
[14]. Hoffer, A., et al., Journal Orthomolecular Medicine, vol.5, no.3, p.143, 1990

CHAPTER 9

NUTRITION CAN IMPROVE OUTCOME IN CANCER TREATMENT

★

"A well-nourished cancer patient can better manage and beat the disease."

Nutrition is a low cost, non-toxic, and scientifically-proven helpful component in the comprehensive treatment of cancer. Adjuvant (helpful) nutrition and traditional oncology are synergistic, not antagonistic. The advantages in using an aggressive nutrition program in comprehensive cancer treatment are, in this critical order of importance:
⇒ 1) avoiding malnutrition
⇒ 2) reducing the toxicity of medical therapy while making chemotherapy and radiation more selectively toxic to the tumor cells
⇒ 3) stimulating immune function
⇒ 4) selectively starving the tumor
⇒ 5) nutrients acting as biological response modifiers to assist host defense mechanisms and improve outcome in cancer therapy.

THE NEED TO EXPLORE OPTIONS
President Richard Nixon declared "war on cancer" on December 23, 1971. Nixon confidently proclaimed that we would have a cure for cancer within 5 years, by the 1976 Bicentennial. However, by 1991 a group of 60 noted physicians and scientists gathered a press conference to tell the public "The cancer establishment confuses the public with repeated claims that we are winning the war on cancer... Our ability to treat and cure most cancers has not materially improved."[1] The unsettling bad news is irrefutable:
    -newly diagnosed cancer incidence continues to escalate, from 1.1 million Americans in 1991 to an anticipated 1.3 million in 1993
    -deaths from cancer in 1992 are projected at 520,000, up from 514,000 in 1991

-since 1950, the overall cancer incidence has increased by 44%, with breast cancer and male colon cancer up by 60% and prostate cancer by 100%

-for decades, the 5 year survival has remained constant for non-localized breast cancer at 18% and lung cancer at 13%

-only 5% of the $1.8-$2.4 billion annual budget for the National Cancer Institute is spent on prevention

-grouped together, the average cancer patient has a 50/50 chance of living another five years; which are the same odds he or she had in 1971

-claims for cancer drugs are generally based on tumor response rather than prolongation of life. Many tumors will initially shrink when chemo and radiation are applied, yet tumors often develop drug-resistance and are then unaffected by therapy.

-39% of women and 45% of men alive today are expected to develop cancer in their lifetime. By the turn of the century, cancer is expected to eclipse heart disease as the number one cause of death in America. It is already the number one fear.

John Bailar, MD, PhD, former editor of the Journal of the National Cancer Institute, confronts the NCI's unfounded enthusiasm with his article in the New England Journal of Medicine, "We are losing the war against cancer" and has shown that the death rate, age-adjusted death rate and both crude and age-adjusted incidence rate of cancer continues to climb in spite of efforts by the NCI. Non-whites are excluded from the NCI statistics for vague reasons. Blacks, urban poor, and the 11 million workers exposed to toxic substances have all experienced a dramatic increase in cancer incidence and mortality. Less than 10% of patients with cancer of the pancreas, liver, stomach and esophagus will be alive in five years.[2]

As a percentage of total annual deaths in America, cancer has escalated from 3% in 1900 to 22% of today's deaths. Given the limited successes in traditional cancer treatment, it is not surprising that 50% of all American cancer patients seek "alternative therapies", however vaguely that term is still defined. Unfortunately, there are no unqualified cures for all cancers in either conventional or alternative modalities. While the conventional therapies of chemotherapy, radiation, surgery, and biological therapies oftentimes do reduce tumor burden, these therapies do not change the underlying causes of the disease. In a recent pivotal paper from researchers published in the official journal of the American Society of Clinical Oncology, "the limits of the cancer killing model seem to have been reached...conventional antineoplastic approaches will play a role as debulkers...the strategy will change to one of reregulation."[3] Given the blatant failures of conventional cancer therapies, it is imperative that we examine optional and complementary therapies to assist the swelling ranks of American cancer patients. ImmunoPower is a crucial addition to the comprehensive cancer treatment of most cancer patients.

NUTRIENTS AS BIOLOGICAL RESPONSE MODIFIERS

In the early phase of nutrition research, nutrient functions were linked to classical nutrient deficiency syndromes: e.g. vitamin C and scurvy, vitamin D and rickets, niacin and pellagra. Today nutrition researchers find various levels of functions for nutrients. For example, let's look at the "dose dependent response" from niacin:

⇒20 milligrams daily will prevent pellagra
⇒100 mg becomes a useful vasodilator
⇒2000 mg is a hypocholesterolemic agent endorsed by the National Institutes of Health.

While 10 iu of vitamin E is considered the RDA, 800 iu was shown to improve immune functions in healthy older adults.[4] While 10 mg of vitamin C will prevent scurvy in most adults, the RDA is 60 mg, and 300 mg was shown to extend lifespan in males by an average of 6 years.[5]

The dietary requirement of a nutrient may well depend on the health state of the individual and what you are trying to achieve. In animal studies, 7.5 mg of vitamin E per kilogram of body weight was found to satisfactorily support normal growth and spleen to body weight ratio. Yet, consumption at twice that level of vitamin E was essential to prevent deficiency symptoms of myopathy and testis degeneration. Intake at 7 times base level of vitamin E was required to prevent red blood cell hemolysis. Intake of 27 times base level provided optimal T- and B-lymphocyte responses to mitogens.[6]

You can accelerate the rate of a reaction by increasing temperature, surface area, or concentration of substrates or enzymes. Clearly, above-RDA levels of nutrients can offer safe and cost-effective enhancement of metabolic processes, including immune functions. Therapeutic dosages of nutrients may be able to reduce tumor recurrence, selectively slow cancer cells, stimulate the immune system to more actively destroy tumor cells, alter the genetic expression of cancer, and more.

CAN NUTRITION HELP THE MALNOURISHED CANCER PATIENT?

A position paper from the American College of Physicians published in 1989 basically stated that TPN had no benefit on the outcome of cancer patients.[7] Unfortunately, this article excluded malnourished patients, which is bizarre, since TPN only treats malnutrition, not cancer.[8] Most of the scientific literature shows that weight loss drastically increases the mortality rate for most types of cancer, while also lowering the response to chemotherapy.[9] Chemo and radiation therapy are sufficient biological stressors alone to induce malnutrition.[10]

In the early years of oncology, it was thought that one could starve the tumor out of the host. Pure malnutrition (cachexia) is responsible for somewhere between 22% and 67% of all cancer deaths. Up to 80% of all cancer patients have reduced levels of serum albumin, which is a leading indicator of protein and calorie malnutrition.[11] Dietary protein restriction in the cancer patient does not affect the composition or growth rate of the tumor, but does restrict the patient's well being.[12]

Parenteral feeding improves tolerance to chemotherapeutic agents and immune responses.[13] Malnourished cancer patients who were provided TPN had a mortality rate of 11% while a comparable group without TPN feeding had a 100% mortality rate.[14] Pre-operative TPN in patients undergoing surgery for GI cancer provided general reduction in the incidence of wound infection, pneumonia, major complications and mortality.[15] Patients who were the most malnourished experienced a 33% mortality and 46% morbidity rate, while those patients who were properly nourished had a 3% mortality rate with an 8% morbidity rate.

In 20 adult hospitalized patients on TPN, the mean daily vitamin C needs were 975 mg, which is over 16 times the RDA, with the range being 350-2250 mg.[16] Of the 139 lung cancer patients studied, most tested deficient or scorbutic (clinical vitamin C deficiency).[17] Another study of cancer patients found that 46% tested scorbutic while 76% were below acceptable levels for serum ascorbate.[18] Experts now recommend the value of nutritional supplements, especially in patients who require prolonged TPN support.[19]

RATIONALE FOR USING ADJUVANT NUTRITION IN CANCER TREATMENT

1) Avoiding malnutrition. 40% or more of cancer patients actually die from malnutrition, not from the cancer.[20] Nutrition therapy is essential to arrest malnutrition.

2) Reducing the toxic effects of conventional medical treatment. Properly nourished patients experience less nausea, malaise, immune suppression, hair loss and organ toxicity than patients on routine oncology programs. Antioxidants, like beta carotene, vitamin C, vitamin E, and selenium appear to enhance the effectiveness of chemo, radiation, and hyperthermia while minimizing damage to the patient's normal cells; thus making therapy more of a "selective toxin." An optimally nourished cancer patient can better tolerate the rigors of cytotoxic therapy.

VITAMIN K. While in simplistic theory, vitamin K might inhibit the effectiveness of anticoagulant therapy (coumadin), actually vitamin K seems to augment the anti-neoplastic activity of coumadin. Patients with mouth cancer who were pre-treated with injections of K-3 prior to radiation therapy doubled their odds (20% vs. 39%) for 5 year survival and disease free status.[21] Animals with implanted tumors had greatly improved anti-cancer effects from all chemotherapy drugs tested when vitamins K and C were given in combination.[22] In cultured leukemia cells, vitamins K and E added to the chemotherapy drugs of 5FU (fluorouracil) and leucovorin provided a 300% improvement in growth inhibition when compared to 5FU by itself.[23] Animals given methotrexate and K-3 had improvements in cancer reversal with no increase in toxicity to the host tissue.[24]

VITAMIN C. Tumor-bearing mice fed high doses of vitamin C (antioxidant) along with adriamycin (pro-oxidant) had a prolonged life and no reduction in the tumor killing capacity of adriamycin.[25] Lung cancer patients who were provided antioxidant nutrients prior to, during, and after radiation and chemotherapy had enhanced tumor destruction and significantly longer life span.[26] Tumor-bearing mice fed high doses of vitamin C experienced an increased tolerance to radiation therapy without reduction in the tumor killing capacity of the radiation.[27]

FISH OIL. EPA improves tumor kill in hyperthermia and chemotherapy by altering cancer cell membranes for increased vulnerability.[28] EPA increases the ability of adriamycin to kill cultured leukemia cells.[29] Tumors in EPA-fed animals are more responsive to Mitomycin C and doxorubicin (chemotherapy drugs).[30] EPA and GLA were selectively toxic to human tumor cell lines while also enhancing the cytotoxic effects of chemotherapy.[31]

VITAMIN A & BETACAROTENE. There is a synergistic benefit of using vitamin A with carotenoids in patients who are being treated with chemo, radiation and surgery for common malignancies.[32] Beta-carotene and vitamin A together provided a significant improvement in outcome in animals treated with radiation for induced cancers.[33]

VITAMIN E. Vitamin E protects the body against the potentially damaging effects of iron and fish oil. Vitamin E deficiency, which is common in cancer patients, will accentuate the cardiotoxic effects of adriamycin.[34] The worse the vitamin E deficiency in animals, the greater the heart damage from adriamycin.[35] Patients undergoing chemo, radiation and bone marrow transplant for cancer treatment had markedly depressed levels of serum antioxidants, including vitamin E.[36] Vitamin E protects animals against a potent carcinogen, DMBA.[37] Vitamin E supplements prevented the glucose-raising effects of a chemo drug, doxorubicin[38] while improving the tumor kill rate of doxorubicin.[39] Vitamin E modifies the carcinogenic effect of daunomycin (chemo drug) in animals.[40]

NIACIN. Niacin supplements in animals were able to reduce the cardiotoxicity of adriamycin while not interfering with its tumor killing capacity.[41] Niacin combined with aspirin in 106 bladder cancer patients receiving surgery and radiation therapy provided for a substantial improvement in 5 year survival (72% vs. 27%) over the control group.[42] Niacin seems to make radiation therapy more effective at killing hypoxic cancer cells.[43] Loading radiation patients with 500 mg to 6000 mg of niacin has been shown to be safe and one of the most effective agents known to eliminate acute hypoxia in solid malignancies.[44]

SELENIUM. Selenium-deficient animals have more heart damage from the chemo drug, adriamycin.[45] Supplements of selenium and vitamin E in humans did not reduce the efficacy of the chemo drugs against ovarian and cervical cancer.[46] Animals with implanted tumors who were then treated with selenium and cis-platin (chemo drug) had reduced toxicity to the drug with no change in anti-cancer activity.[47] Selenium supplements helped repair DNA damage from a carcinogen in animals.[48] Selenium was selectively toxic to human leukemia cells in culture.[49]

CARNITINE. Carnitine may help the cancer patient by protecting the heart against the damaging effects of adriamycin.[50]

QUERCETIN. Quercetin reduces the toxicity and carcinogenic capacity of substances in the body[51] YET at the same time may enhance the tumor killing capacity of cisplatin.[52] Quercetin significantly increased the tumor kill rate of hyperthermia (heat therapy) in cultured cancer cells.[53]

GINSENG. Panax ginseng was able to enhance the uptake of mitomycin (an antibiotic and anti-cancer drug) into the cancer cells for increased tumor kill.[54]

⇒In both human and animal studies, nutrients improve the host tolerance to cytotoxic medical therapies while allowing for unobstructed death of tumor cells. Nutrition therapy makes medical therapy more of a selective toxin on the tumor tissue.

3) Bolster immune functions. When the doctor says: "We think we got it all." what he or she is really saying is: "We have destroyed all DETECTABLE cancer cells, and now it is up to your immune system to find and destroy the cancer cells that inevitably remain in your body." A billion cancer cells is about the size of the page number at the top of this page. We must rely on the capabilities of the 20 trillion cells that compose an intact immune system to destroy the undetectable cancer cells that remain after medical therapy. There is an abundance of data linking nutrient intake to the quality and quantity of immune factors that fight cancer.[55]

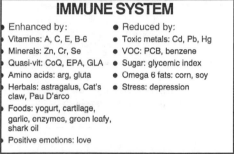

IMMUNE SYSTEM

▸ Enhanced by:
▸ Vitamins: A, C, E, B-6
▸ Minerals: Zn, Cr, Se
▸ Quasi-vit: CoQ, EPA, GLA
▸ Amino acids: arg, gluta
▸ Herbals: astragalus, Cat's claw, Pau D'arco
▸ Foods: yogurt, cartilage, garlic, enzymes, green leafy, shark oil
▸ Positive emotions: love

● Reduced by:
● Toxic metals: Cd, Pb, Hg
● VOC: PCB, benzene
● Sugar: glycemic index
● Omega 6 fats: corn, soy
● Stress: depression

4) Selectively starve the tumor. Tumors are primarily obligate glucose metabolizers, meaning "sugar feeders".[56] Americans not only consume about 20% of their calories from refined sucrose, but often manifest poor glucose tolerance curves, due to stress, obesity, low chromium and fiber intake, and sedentary

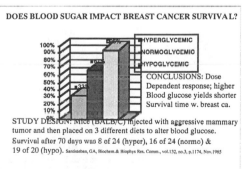

DOES BLOOD SUGAR IMPACT BREAST CANCER SURVIVAL?

HYPERGLYCEMIC
NORMOGLYCEMIC
HYPOGLYCEMIC

CONCLUSIONS: Dose Dependent response; higher Blood glucose yields shorter Survival time w. breast ca.

STUDY DESIGN: Mice (BALB/C) injected with aggressive mammary tumor and then placed on 3 different diets to alter blood glucose. Survival after 70 days was 8 of 24 (hyper), 16 of 24 (normo) & 19 of 20 (hypo). Santisteban, GA, Biochem.& Biophys Res. Comm., vol.132, no.3, p.1174, Nov.1985

lifestyles. In an animal study, there was a dose-dependent response: the more sugar from the diet, the quicker the breast cancer's killed the animals.

5) Anti-proliferative factors. Certain nutrients, like selenium, vitamin K, vitamin E succinate, and the fatty acid EPA, appear to have the ability to slow down the unregulated growth of cancer. Various nutrition factors, including vitamin A, D, folacin, bioflavonoids, and soybeans, have been shown to alter the genetic expression of tumors.

NUTRITION THERAPY IMPROVES OUTCOME IN CANCER TREATMENT

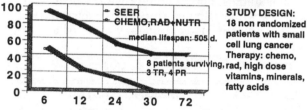

LUNG CANCER THERAPY with chemo, rad., & nutrition

STUDY DESIGN: 18 non randomized patients with small cell lung cancer Therapy: chemo, rad, high dose vitamins, minerals, fatty acids

"No side effects observed [from nutrients]." "Surviving patients started AOX treatment earlier than those who succumbed." "AOX treatment should start as early as possible in combination w. chemo and/or rad."
Jaakkola, K., et al., Anticancer Research, vol.12, p.599, 1992

Finnish oncologists used high doses of nutrients along with chemo and radiation for lung cancer patients. Normally, lung cancer is a "poor prognostic" malignancy with a 1% expected survival at 30 months under normal treatment.. In this study, however, 8 of 18 patients (44%) were still alive 6 years after therapy.[57] Oncologists at West Virginia Medical School randomized 65 patients with

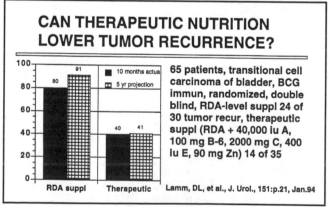

CAN THERAPEUTIC NUTRITION LOWER TUMOR RECURRENCE?

■ 10 months actual
▨ 5 yr projection

65 patients, transitional cell carcinoma of bladder, BCG immun, randomized, double blind, RDA-level suppl 24 of 30 tumor recur, therapeutic suppl (RDA + 40,000 iu A, 100 mg B-6, 2000 mg C, 400 iu E, 90 mg Zn) 14 of 35

Lamm, DL, et al., J. Urol., 151:p.21, Jan.94

transitional cell carcinoma of the bladder into either the "one-per-day" vitamin supplement providing the RDA, or into a group which received the RDA supplement plus 40,000 iu of vitamin A, 100 mg of B-6, 2000 mg of vitamin C, 400 iu of vitamin E, and 90 mg of zinc. At 10 months, tumor recurrence was 80% in the control group (RDA supplement) and 40% in the experimental "megavitamin" group. Five year projected tumor recurrence was 91% for controls and 41% for "megavitamin" patients. Essentially, high dose nutrients cut tumor recurrence in half.[58]

In a non-randomized clinical trial, Drs. Hoffer and Pauling instructed patients to follow a reasonable cancer diet (unprocessed food low in fat, dairy, and sugar), coupled with therapeutic doses of vitamins and minerals.[59] All 129 patients in this study received concomitant oncology care. The control group of 31 patients who did not receive nutrition support lived an average of less than 6 months. The group of

98 cancer patients who did receive the diet and supplement program were categorized into 3 groups:

Poor responders (n=19) or 20% of treated group. Average lifespan of 10 months, or a 75% improvement over the control group.

Good responders (n=47), who had various cancers, including leukemia, lung, liver, and pancreas; had an average lifespan of 72 months (6 years).

Good female responders (n=32), with involvement of reproductive areas (breast, cervix, ovary, uterus); had an average lifespan of over 10 years. Many were still alive at the end of the study.

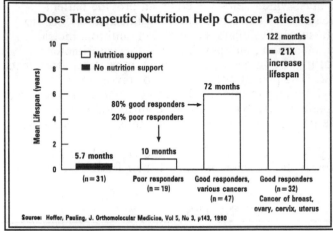

In examining the diet and lifespan of 675 lung cancer patients over the course of 6 years, researchers found that the more vegetables consumed, the longer the lung cancer patient lived.[60] Of the 200 cancer patients studied who experienced "spontaneous regression", 87% made a major change in diet, mostly vegetarian in nature, 55% used some form of detoxification and 65% used nutritional supplements.[61]

Researchers at Tulane University compared survival in patients who used the macrobiotic diet versus patients who continued with their standard Western lifestyle. Of 1467 pancreatic patients who made no changes in diet, 146 (10%) were alive after one year, while 12 of the 23 matched pancreatic patients (52%) consuming macrobiotic foods were still alive after one year.[62]

THE COMPONENTS OF A NUTRITIONAL ONCOLOGY PROGRAM

1) **Food.** If the gut works and if the patient can consume enough food through the mouth, then this is the primary route for nourishing the patient. The diet for the cancer patient should be high in plant food (grains, legumes, colorful vegetables, some fruit), unprocessed (shop the perimeter of the grocery store), low in salt, fat, and sugar, with adequate protein (1-2 grams/kilogram body weight).

2) **Supplements.** Additional vitamins, minerals, amino acids, food extracts (i.e. bovine cartilage), conditionally essential nutrients (i.e. fish, flax, and borage oil; Coenzyme Q-10), and botanicals (i.e. echinecea, golden seal, astragalus) can enhance the patient's recuperative powers. ImmunoPower is the most clinically-tested, cost-effective and convenient way to take nutritional supplements.

3) **Total parenteral nutrition** (TPN) There are many cancer patients who are so malnourished (weight loss of 10% below usual body weight within 1 month period and/or serum albumin below 2.5 mg/dl) that we must interrupt this deterioration with TPN. When the patient cannot or will not eat adequately, TPN can be an invaluable life raft during crucial phases of cancer treatment.

4) **Assessment**. It is important to determine the patient's general health and nutrient status, which helps the clinician provide patient-specific therapy. Means of assessment include: health history form to detect lifestyle risk factors, physician's examination, anthropometric measurements of height, weight, and percent body fat, calorimeter measurement of basal metabolic needs, and various other laboratory tests.

5) **Education**. The patient needs a sense of involvement and control in the therapy, which can improve his or her chances for recovery. Just as much as the patient's lifestyle may have contributed to the problem, a pro-active patient can help reverse the underlying causative factors.

6) **Research**. Those who advance the knowledge base have a responsibility to properly gather data and report their findings to the world.

ENDNOTES

[1]. Ingram, B., Medical Tribune, vol.33, no.4, p.1, Feb.1992
[2]. Squires, S, Washington Post, p.Z19, Dec.3, 1991
[3]. Schipper, H., et al., J.Clin.Oncology, vol.13, no.4, p.801, Apr.1995
[4]. Meydani, SN, et al, Vitamin supplementation enhances cell-mediated immunity in healthy elderly subjects, Am J Clin Nutr, 52,557-63, 1990
[5]. Enstrom, JE, et al., Vitamin C intake and mortality among a sample of the United States population, Epidem, 3, 3:194-6, 1992
[6]. Bendich, A, et al., Dietary vitamin E requirement for optimum immune response in the rat, J Nutr;116:675-681, 1986
[7]. Meta-analysis of survival in cancer patients using total parenteral nutrition, Ann Intern Med, 110, 9, 735-7, May 1989
[8]. Kaminsky, M. (ed.), Hyperalimentation: a Guide for Clinicians, Marcel Dekker, NY, Oct.1985, p.265
[9]. Dewys, WD, et al., Cachexia and cancer treatment, Amer J Med, 69, 491-5, Oct.1980
[10]. Wilmore, DW, Catabolic illness, strategies for enhancing recovery, N Engl J Med, 1991, 325:10:695-702
[11]. Dreizen, S., et al., Malnutrition in cancer, Postgrad Med, 87, 1, 163-7, Jan.1990
[12]. Lowry, SF, et al., Nutrient restriction in cancer patients, Surg Forum, 28, 143-9, 1977
[13]. Eys, JV, Total parenteral nutrition and response to cytotoxic therapies, Cancer, 43, 2030-7, 1979
[14]. Harvey, KB, et al., Morbidity and mortality in parenterally-nourished cancer patients, Cancer, 43, 2065-9, 1979
[15]. Muller, JM, et al., Nutritional status as a factor in GI cancer morbidity, Lancet, 68-73, Jan.9, 1982
[16]. Abrahamian, V., et al., Ascorbic acid requirements in hospital patients, JPEN, 7, 5, 465-8, 1983
[17]. Anthony, HM, et al., Vitamin C status of lung cancer patients, Brit J Ca, 46, 354-9, 1982
[18]. Cheraskin, E., Scurvy in cancer patients?, J Altern Med, 18-23, Feb.1986
[19]. Hoffman, FA, Micronutrient status of cancer patients, Cancer, 55, 1 sup.1, 295-9, Jan.1, 1985
[20]. Grant, JP, Nutrition, 6, 4, 6S, July 1990 suppl
[21]. Krishanamurthi, S., et al., Radiology, vol.99, p.409, 1971
[22]. Taper, HS, et al., Int.J.Cancer, vol.40, p.575, 1987
[23]. Waxman, S., et al., Eur.J.Cancer Clin.Oncol., vol.18, p.685, 1982
[24]. Gold, J., Cancer Treatment Reports, vol.70, p.1433, Dec.1986
[25]. Shimpo,K, Am.J.Clin.Nutr.54,1298S,1991
[26]. Jaakkola, K. Anticancer Res., 12, 599, 1992
[27]. Okunieff, P, Am.J.Clin.Nutr.54, 1281S, 1991
[28]. Burns, CP, et al., Nutrition Reviews, vol.48, p.233, June 1990

[29] . Guffy, MM, et al., Cancer Research, vol.44, p.1863, 1984
[30] . Cannizzo, F., et al., Cancer Research, vol.49, p.3961, 1981
[31] . Begin, ME, et al., J.Nat.Cancer Inst., vol.77, p.1053, 1986
[32] . Santamaria, L., et al., Nutrients and Cancer Prevention, p.299, Prasad, KN (eds), Humana Press, 1990
[33] . Seifter, E., et al., J.Nat.Cancer Inst., vol.71, p.409, 1983
[34] . Singal, PK, et al., Mol.Cell.Biochem., vol.84, p.163, 1988
[35] . Singal, PK, et al., Molecular Cellular Biochem., vol.84, p.163, 1988
[36] . Clemens, MR, et al., Am.J.Clin.Nutr., vol.51, p.216, 1990
[37] . Shklar, G., et al., J.Oral Pathol.Med., vol.19, p.60, 1990
[38] . Geetha, A., et al., J.Biosci., vol.14, p.243, 1989
[39] . Geetha, A., et al., Current Science, vol.64, p.318, Mar.1993
[40] . Wang, YM, et al., Molecular Inter Nutr.Cancer, p.369, , Arnott, MS, (eds), Raven Press, NY, 1982
[41] . Schmitt-Graff, A., et al, Pathol.Res.Pract., vol.181, p.168, 1986
[42] . Popov, Al, Med.Radiol. Mosk., vol.32, p.42, 1987
[43] . Kjellen, E., et al., Radiother.Oncol., vol.22, p.81, 1991
[44] . Horsman, MR, Radiotherapy Oncology, vol.22, p.79, 1991
[45] . Coudray, C., et al., Basic Res.Cardiol., vol.87, p.173, 1992
[46] . Sundstrom, H., et al., Carcinogenesis, vol.10, p.273, 1989
[47] . Ohkawa, K., et al., Br.J.Cancer, vol.58, p.38, 1988
[48] . Lawson, T., et al.,Chem.Biol.Interactions, vol.45, p.95, 1983
[49] . Milner, JA, et al., Cancer Research, vol.41, p.1652, 1981
[50] . Furitano, G, et al., Drugs Exp.Clin.Res., vol.10, p.107, 1984
[51] . Wood, AW, et al., in PLANT FLAVONOIDS IN BIOLOGY AND MEDICINE, p.197, Cody, V. (eds), Liss, NY, 1986
[52] . Scambia, G., et al., Anticancer Drugs, vol.1, p.45, 1990
[53] . Kim, JH, et al., Cancer Research, vol.44, p.102, Jan.1984
[54] . Kubo, M., et al., Planta Med, vol.58, p.424, 1992
[55]. Bendich, A, Chandra, RK (eds), Micronutrients and Immune Function, New York Academy of Sciences, 1990, p.587
[56]. Rothkopf, M, Fuel utilization in neoplastic disease: implications for the use of nutritional support in cancer patients, Nutrition, supp, 6:4:14-16S, 1990
[57]. Jaakkola, K., et al., Treatment with antioxidant and other nutrients in combination with chemotherapy and irradiation in patients with small-cell lung cancer, Anticancer Res 12,599-606, 1992
[58]. Lamm, DL, et al., Megadose vitamin in bladder cancer: a double-blind clinical trial, J Urol, 151:21-26, 1994
[59]. Hoffer, A, Pauling, L, Hardin Jones biostatistical analysis of mortality data of cancer patients, J Orthomolecular Med, 5:3:143-154, 1990
[60]. Goodman, MT, Vegetable consumption in lung cancer longevity, Eur J Ca, 28: 2: 495-499, 1992
[61]. Foster, HD, Lifestyle influences on spontaneous cancer regression, Int J Biosoc Res, 10:1:17-20, 1988
[62]. Carter, JP, Macrobiotic diet and cancer survival, J Amer Coll Nutr, 12:3:209-215, 1993

CHAPTER 10

HOW DOES NUTRITION AFFECT CANCER OUTCOME?
✯
NUTRIENTS AS BIOLOGICAL RESPONSE MODIFIERS

The following is a very brief overview of how nutrients affect the body's ability to recover from cancer. Remember that it takes 2-3 months for nutrition therapy to have time to change the underlying mechanisms of disease. For more detailed information and references, please see the following section "OTHER GOOD SOURCES OF INFORMATION ON NUTRITION AND CANCER".

IMMUNE STIMULANTS

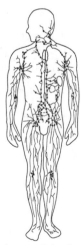

A healthy adult body includes around 60 trillion cells, of which nearly a third, or 20 trillion cells are immune factors. Among the primary aspects of the immune system are:

⇒ **Birth place**. The bone marrow generates most immune cells, primarily in the long bones, especially the ribs.

⇒ **Maturation**. Bone immune cells (B-cells) move into the thymus gland for maturation and activation, and are then called "T" cells.

⇒ **Gastro-intestinal tract**. 40% of the immune system surrounds the GI tract as lymph nodes, not only to absorb fat soluble nutrients (like essential fatty acids), and to protect against bacterial translocation (crossing of the intestinal barrier into the bloodstream by disease-causing bacteria) but also to stimulate the production of various immunoglobulins (IgA etc.) A healthy gut is a critical aspect of a healthy immune system.

⇒ **Filtering**. The immune cells move through the lymphatic ducts, not unlike the blood moving through the arteries and veins. Dead immune cells and invaders are filtered out of this "freeway" system in the spleen and lymph nodes.

⇒ **Quantity**. There are many factors that can influence the sheer numbers of immune warriors. Factors that will improve quantities of immune cells include:

⇒ **Quality**. Not all immune cells have the same level of ferocity against an invading tumor cell. Some immune cells become confused about "who to shoot at" and end up creating an autoimmune response (often called an allergic response), which imbalances the immune system and detracts from the critical task of killing cancer cells. Some nutrients provide the immune warriors with a protective coating, like an asbestos suit, so that the immune cell is not destroyed in the process of killing a cancer cell with some "napalm". Some nutrients provide the immune cells with more "napalm" or "bullets" in the form of granulocytes and nitric oxide.

Many components in ImmunoPower affect the ability of the immune system to recognize and destroy cancer cells and invading bacteria.

ALTER GENETIC EXPRESSION OF CANCER

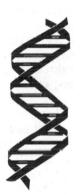

Cancer involves DNA that has "gone mad" or lost its ability to properly replicate and then die at the appropriate time. There are numerous checks and balances in the control of abnormal DNA. Nutrients, like folate and B-12, help to provide correct duplication of DNA. Nutrients, like vitamin D, help to squelch the growth of abnormal genetic fragments, or episomes. Nutrients, like vitamin A, actually have a receptor site on the DNA, without which cancer is likely to happen. Nutrition factors, like genistein from soy and oligomeric proanthocyanidins from bioflavonoids, can actually help a cancer cell to revert back to a normal healthy cell in the process of cell differentiation.

CELL MEMBRANE DYNAMICS

Most of the 60 trillion cells in an adult body are like "water balloons" floating in an ocean of extracellular fluid, in the sense that they are full of fluid and have a barrier that keeps them intact. This barrier, or cell membrane, has a 3 layered look with water soluble molecules on the outside and fatty tails toward the inside. This lipid bilayer gives rise to the ability of the cell to accept the proper nutrients along with oxygen, eliminate the hazardous toxins produced within the cell, and reject the circulating toxins and cancer cells that try to penetrate the cell membrane barrier. A healthy cell membrane is built from the essential fatty acids from fish oil (eicosapentaenoic acid), flax oil (alpha linolenic acid), evening primrose oil (gamma linolenic acid), lecithin (phosphatidylcholine), cholesterol and other nutrients. A defective cell membrane is built from hydrogenated fats (trans fatty acids), too much saturated fats, has been "tanned" by exposure to excess sugar floating through the bloodstream and various nutritional deficiencies. A healthy cell membrane allows the cell to "breathe" aerobically and expel waste products. Otherwise, cancer can be the result.

DETOXIFICATION

America's increasing incidence of cancer has closely paralleled our increasing exposure to cancer-causing substances in our environment. We consume toxins:

⇒ voluntarily through alcohol, drugs, and tobacco

⇒ involuntarily through industrial and agricultural pollutants that end up in the food, air and water supply

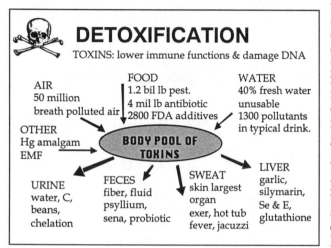

DETOXIFICATION

TOXINS: lower immune functions & damage DNA

AIR	FOOD	WATER
50 million breath polluted air	1.2 bil lb pest. 4 mil lb antibiotic 2800 FDA additives	40% fresh water unusable 1300 pollutants in typical drink.

OTHER
Hg amalgam
EMF

BODY POOL OF TOXINS

URINE water, C, beans, chelation	FECES fiber, fluid psyllium, sena, probiotic	SWEAT skin largest organ exer, hot tub fever, jacuzzi	LIVER garlic, silymarin, Se & E, glutathione

⇒ internally (endogenously) produced toxins from energy metabolism in the cell and bacterial fermentation in the gut.

We detoxify by eliminating waste products through urine, feces, sweat and liver detoxification. Nutrients assist each of these processes. The liver is a chemical detoxification "factory" in its ability to bind toxins (conjugate), split toxins (hydrolyze), and neutralize toxins through Phase I and Phase II enzyme pathways. These pathways are augmented with nutrients, like garlic, calcium D-glucarate, selenium, vitamin E, and glutathione.

In many people, cancer cannot be cured without the assistance of an aggressive detoxification program.

ACID & BASE BALANCE

Humans have a very specific need to maintain a proper pH balance. pH refers to "potential hydrogens" and is measured on a scale from 1 (very acidic) to 7 (neutral) to 14 (very alkaline, base). Foods that encourage a healthy pH are vegetables and other plant foods. Foods that encourage an unhealthy pH include beef, dairy and sugar. Proper breathing, exercise, and adequate water intake further improve pH to discourage cancer growth. Cancer cells give off lactic acid in anaerobic fermentation of foodstuffs. This Cori cycle generates a lower pH which then further compromises the cells ability to fight off the cancer. Acid foods (like tomatoes, citrus, and vinegar) help to create an "alkaline tide" which helps to discourage cancer and fungus growth.

CELLULAR COMMUNICATION
Cells communicate between each other, a.k.a. intercellular or "gap junction" communication, through ions that float in and out of pores in the cell membranes. Vitamin A and beta-carotene are among the crucial nutrients that encourage this "telegraph" system that keeps cells healthy and non-cancerous.

There is also evidence that communication exists within a cell (intracellular communication) through such nutrients as the glycoproteins in aloe vera.

PROSTAGLANDIN SYNTHESIS
Prostaglandins are hormone-like substances that are produced regionally within most cells and have an incredible influence on the functions that help us to beat cancer. Essentially, when our intake of simple carbohydrates (like sugar and easily digested starches) is high and our intake of fish oil and primrose oil is low, then emergency prostaglandins (PGE-2) are generated to augment cancer growth.

When our blood sugar levels are kept low (around 60 to 90 milligrams per deciliter) through a proper diet low in sweets, and when we eat enough fish oil and evening primrose oil, then the favorable prostaglandin of PGE-1 will:
⇒ stimulate immune activity
⇒ improve circulation through vasodilation
⇒ reduce the stickiness of cells which inhibits metastasis through platelet aggregation
⇒ help to produce estrogen receptors to dull the potential damage from circulating estrogen
⇒ and much more.

Only a concerted effort of dietary regulation and proper supplements can produce healthy prostaglandins to suppress cancer.

STEROID HORMONE ACTIVITY
Certain cancers that are very dependent on testosterone (prostate cancer) or estrogen (for breast, ovarian and cervical cancer). These hormones are not only produced by the gonads (testosterone) and ovaries (estrogen), but also produced by fat cells. Meaning that, the more body fat a person has, the higher the likelihood of generating more tumor-enhancing hormones. A calculated program to gradually reduce excess body fat is crucial in the treatment of hormone dependent tumors.

Also, a number of nutrition factors help to reduce the tumor-enhancing capacity of hormones, including fish oil, evening primrose oil, cruciferous sulforphane, calcium D-glucarate, and others.

BIOENERGETICS
AEROBIC VS ANAEROBIC
Cancer cells are anaerobic sugar feeders, while healthy cells are aerobic (oxygen-requiring) cells that can burn sugar, protein or fats. Professor Otto Warburg was awarded the Nobel prize in medicine in 1931

for his work in cell respiration and received a second Nobel prize in 1944 for his work in electron transfer. This brilliant researcher spent considerable time investigating the differences between healthy cells and cancer cells: "...the prime cause of cancer is the replacement of the respiration of oxygen in normal body cells by a fermentation of sugar."[1]

The more dense and anaerobic the mass of cancer, the more resistant it is to treatment, medical or otherwise. In order to beat cancer, one must make the body a well oxygenated aerobic organism. Proper breathing and exercise are crucial to generate an aerobic environment.

Also, there are nutrients, including Coenzyme Q-10, chromium GTF (glucose tolerance factor), thiamin, niacin, riboflavin, lipoic acid and others that enhance aerobic metabolism.

BACTERIA IN THE GUT

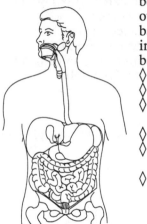

According to Nobel prize winner, Eli Metchnikoff, PhD, "death begins in the colon". There are more bacteria in our lower intestines than cells in our body. The bacteria in our gut either enhance or detract from immune functions and general health. Healthy bacteria (probiotics) help to:

◊ produce essential vitamins (like K and biotin)
◊ generate a critical immune factor IgA
◊ protect the gut mucosa against translocation of bacteria into the bloodstream
◊ improve the pH in the colon
◊ aid in digestion and absorption of essential nutrients
◊ reduce the carcinogenic by-products that are produced in the colon from putrefaction of fecal matter.

Healthy bacteria are encouraged by a diet low in sugar and meat and high in vegetables, whole grains, and active-cultured foods (like yogurt or soy tempeh). High fiber and fluid intake help this crucial balance of friendly bacteria. Fructo-oligosaccharides are special starches found in whole grains and onions (and ImmunoPower) that help to nourish the friendly bacteria (also in ImmunoPower).

PRO-OXIDANTS VS ANTIOXIDANTS

Our greatest enemy is oxygen, since it generates free radicals (a.k.a. pro-oxidants, reactive oxygen species) which can damage the delicate DNA, immune factors, and cell membranes. Yet our greatest ally is a well-oxygenated system. How, then, to balance this seeming paradox? A well-oxygenated (aerobic) system along with optimal protection from free radicals via antioxidants is the ideal combination for good health. Free radicals are an inherent aspect of generating energy (ATP) from foodstuff in the mitochondria. Free radicals are the weapons used by immune cells to kill cancer cells. So free radicals cannot be eliminated in the human body, but must be controlled or they turn into "forest fires" that devastate the cells.

A strategic blend of antioxidants can provide broad spectrum protection against damage from chemotherapy, radiation therapy, protecting the immune cells from their own poisons, and improving vigor in the cancer patient undergoing treatment. Vitamins C, E, beta-carotene, selenium, lipoic acid, lycopene, glutathione, tocotrienols, quercetin, Coenzyme Q, oligomeric proanthocyanidins from grape seed, curcumin, Ginkgo biloba, and green tea are in the ImmunoPower to provide complete protection from an entire hierarchy of antioxidants.

ANTI-PROLIFERATIVE AGENTS

While most nutritionists agree on the importance of growth (proliferative) nutrients, few nutritionists respect the importance for anti-proliferative nutrients. For every force in the body, there must be an opposing force to regulate that mechanism. There are agents that cause fluid loss from the kidneys (diuresis) and other agents that stem this fluid loss when it is excessive (anti-diuretic hormone). Just as there is a need for nutrients to augment growth, there is a need for nutrients to control excessive growth and shut down the process.

Selenium, fish oil, garlic, Cat's claw, Maitake D-fraction, vitamin E succinate, vitamin K, quercetin, genistein, and bovine cartilage all may assist the cancer patient in this manner.

ALTER TUMOR PROTECTIVE MECHANISMS

The tumor is a well-adapted parasite, which hides from the body's immune system by generating a "stealth" coating of human chorionic gonadotropin (HCG) which provides regional immune suppression. The cancer pretends to be a fetus, which then stops the attack by the immune system. High doses of niacin (B-3) as inositol hexanicotinate work to dissolve this "stealth" coating of the tumor. Additionally, digestive enzymes of protease can be beneficial in augmenting this dissolving of the tumor's protective coating. It is very difficult to include digestive enzymes in a mixture of protein powder (soy) without the enzymes adversely affecting the smell, taste, and shelf life of ImmunoPower. Adding protease enzymes to the ImmunoPower regimen would be a good idea, taking 2-3 tablets first thing in the morning and last thing at night on an empty stomach.

ENDNOTES

[1] . Levine, SA, et al., ANTIOXIDANT ADAPTATION, p.209, Biocurrents, San Leandro, CA 1986

CHAPTER 11

RATIONAL CANCER TREATMENT
✷
IF I HAD CANCER, WHAT WOULD I DO?

I would use an appropriate combination of:
1) restrained cytotoxic therapies to reduce tumor burden
2) an aggressive collection of naturopathic (cell restorative) therapies to bolster host defense mechanisms.

The combination of changing the underlying conditions that brought on the cancer (naturopathic) and attacking the cancer with therapies that kill cancer but do not harm the host (cytotoxic) can be incredibly effective.

Chemotherapy, radiation and surgery may be appropriate in certain cancers and for certain people. But make sure that the physician understands the concept of "restrained" medical therapies against cancer. I have worked with cancer patients who were exposed to 45 minutes of regional radiation to an esophageal cancer, which devastated the entire chest region and left the patient near dead. Other patients have gone through radical mastectomy when a lumpectomy would have been sufficient.

R̶x ATIONAL CANCER TREATMENT
synergism between naturopathy & restrained allopathy

NATUROPATHY/cell restorative	ALLOPATHIC/cytotoxic
nutrients (essential & non-essential)	Tributyrate/antineoplastons
oxygenation (exercise/breathing)	hydrazine sulfate (cachexia)
detoxification	Coley's toxins or IAT
psycho-neuroimmunology	oleander
hormonal/glandular balancing	cesium chloride
probiotic establishment	laetrile/amygdalin
digestive improvements	Cell Specific Cancer Ther.
magnets/energy medicine/chakras	IV proteolytic enzymes
spinal & cranial subluxation	surgery/chemo/rad TX
homeopathy	Ukrain or Metbal (Cellbal)
massage therapy	apheresis: TNF-i
botanicals (Essiac, Iscador)	urea/urine
	Govallo's vaccine

Other patients who received intensive systemic chemotherapy, when a more effective and non-toxic approach may be fractionated chemotherapy or intra-arterial infusion of chemo to the site of the tumor.

If you threw a hand grenade into your garage to get rid of the mice, then you may have accomplished to goal of killing the mice, but you don't have a garage anymore. Similarly, too many cancer patients are exposed to "maximum sub-lethal" therapies which may provide an initial "response" or tumor shrinkage, but in the end may reduce the quality and quantity of life for the cancer patient by suppressing immune functions, damaging the heart and kidneys and creating a tumor that is "drug resistant", or virtually bullet-proof.

NATUROPATHIC APPROACHES
Helping to reverse cancer by changing the underlying causes of the disease. Listed in approximate order of importance. Find a health care professional listed in Chapter 14 who will help you detect and solve these problems.

1) PSYCHO-SPIRITUAL.
Grief, loss of loved one, lack of purpose, depression, low self esteem, hypochondriasis as means of attention, need love for self and others, touching, be here now, sense of accomplishment, happiness, music, beauty, sexual satisfaction, forgiveness, etc..

2) TOXIC BURDEN.
INTAKE from:
> **Voluntary pollutants of drugs, alcohol, tobacco**
> **Involuntary toxins of:**

⇒ Food (1.2 billion lbs/yr pesticides on fresh produce, 2800 FDA-approved food additives, 5 million lbs/yr of antibiotics to grow animals faster, herbicides, fungicides, wax on produce, parasites, veterinarian drug residue, hormones.

⇒ Water. EPA estimates that 40% of fresh water in US is unusable. 1300 different chemicals in the average "EPA-approved" city drinking water. Chlorine and lead are most common, with many industrial volatile organic chemicals ending up in the drinking water. 60,000 chemicals in regular use, according to American Chemical Society, half of these in contact with humans. Farm runoff of herbicides, pesticides, fertilizer (nitrates combine with amino acids in stomach to form carcinogenic nitrosamines).

⇒ Air. 50 million Americans breath air that is dangerous for health. Smoking and second hand smoke are obvious. Millions of tons of known carcinogens produced annually and legally from paper mills, petrochemical refineries, burning of medical waste (generate dioxin from PVC). Crop dusting, diesel fumes, leaded exhaust, etc.

⇒ Industrial exposure. Workers in factories, vinyl industry, paper mills, refineries, asbestos, etc.

⇒ Other. Mercury amalgams, electro-magnetic fields from cellular phone antenna, high voltage power lines.

DETOXIFICATION (EXCRETION) VIA:

* Urine. Increase intake of clean water, vitamin C, beans (sulfur amino acids are chelators), garlic, chelation EDTA therapy.

* Feces. 50 billion bacteria/lb fecal matter. 40% of lymphoid tissue is surrounding the GI tract. Common constipation leads to toxic buildup, dysbiosis. Increase fluid, fiber, psyllium seed husk, sena, cascara sagrada, buckthorn, fructo-oligosaccharides, probiotics (lactobacillus, yogurt). Appropriate use of enemas, coffee enemas (every other day during intensive detox).

* Sweat. Skin is the largest organ of body, 2000 pores/square inch skin. Increase sweating through exercise, hot tubs, jacuzzi, sauna.

Hyperthermia can be useful. Bring core body temperature up to 102 F for 10 minutes/day. Do not use anti-perspirants.

* Liver. Most significant detoxifying organ of body, using conjugase (put together), oxidase, reductase, and hydrolase enzymes to neutralize poisons. Increase intake of glutathione (dark green leafy veg), silymarin, garlic, vitamin E, selenium.

* Other. Some chose chelation therapy, mercury amalgam removal, magnets to neutralize EMF pollution.

3) MALNUTRITION
MACRONUTRIENTS OF:
⇒ Carbohydrates (simple vs complex, glycemic index of foods, regulating prostaglandins through insulin & glucagon levels)

⇒ Fiber (soluble vs insoluble, adequate for regular bowel movements)

⇒ Fat: Useful include olive, canola, medium chain triglycerides, lecithin, fish oil, flax, borage, evening primrose, black current, hemp. Unhealthy fats include: too much fat (40% kcal vs 20%), hydrogenated, saturated, oxidized.

⇒ Protein: Proper quantity and quality necessary. Lean and clean protein found in chicken, fish, turkey, and beans. Vegetarians must match grains with legumes for complementary amino acids to create a high quality (biological value) protein.

⇒ Water. 2/3 of our body is water. Must consume high quality clean water throughout the day to improve hydration.

MICRONUTRIENTS OF:
⇒ Vitamins

⇒ Minerals

⇒ Ultra trace minerals

⇒ Minor dietary constituents (i.e. lycopenes from tomato, allicin from garlic, sulforaphane from cabbage)

⇒ Conditionally essential nutrients (i.e. Coenzyme Q-10, taurine, arginine, EPA).

Too much, too little, or an imbalance of any nutrient leads to malnutrition. Most malnutrition in US is via the cumulative effects of long term sub-clinical deficiencies.

---

4) EXERCISE.
Absolutely essential ingredient for health. A primary tool for detoxification, stabilizing blood glucose levels, improving digestion and regularity, proper oxygenation of tissue, stress tolerance, improving hormone output (i.e. growth hormone & DHEA), burning fatty tissue, eliminating harmful by-products (i.e. estrogen, uric acid).

5) BLOOD GLUCOSE
Average American consumes 20% of calories from refined white sugar, which is more of a drug than a food. Eat less sweet foods. Never eat anything sweet by itself. Chose fructose, honey, molasses, sucanat &

colorful fresh fruit. Exercise, stress, alcohol and drug intake all relate to maintenance of healthy blood glucose.

6) REDOX
There is an ongoing balance between pro-oxidants (free radicals) and anti-oxidants (like vitamin C and tocotrienols). Energy metabolism and immune system generate pro-oxidants, so does most degenerative diseases and the aging process. Anti-oxidants slow aging and oxidative destruction. Seeking balance.

7) IMMUNE DYSFUNCTIONS
Via toxic burden, stress, no exercise, poor diet, unbridled use of antibiotics and vaccinations, innoculations from world travellers, and less breast feeding. Many Americans have a weak immune system.

8) GLAND/ORGAN INSUFFICIENCY
As we age, many glands and organs produce less vital hormones and secretions.
* Stomach (hydrochloric acid)
* Pancreas (digestive enzymes)
* Thyroid (thyroxin)
* Adrenals (DHEA, cortisol)
* Thymus (thymic extract)
* Spleen (spleen concentrate)
* Joints (glucosamine sulfate)
* Pineal (melatonin)
* Pituitary (growth hormone).
     Replacing missing secretions often dramatically improves health.

9) MALDIGESTION
After lifetime of high fat, high sugar, overeating, too much alcohol, stress, drugs, indigestible foods (i.e. pizza); many Americans have poor peristalsis, insufficient stomach and intestinal secretions, damaged microvilli, imbalances of friendly (probiotic) vs unfriendly (anaerobic, pathogenic) bacteria. One must remove, repair, replace, re-inoculate. Food separation (combinations) may be of value for a brief time until the GI tract recuperates. Digestive enzymes and/or hydrochloric acid taken with meals may help.

10) CHRONIC INFECTIONS.
Candida albicans is very common in women, especially people who eat much sugar. Intestinal parasites and even liver flukes are common in the US. Use garlic, iodine, wormwood, walnut shell extract, cloves, and other purgatives with caution as vermifuge.

11) pH (potential hydrogens)
Acid alkaline balance (7.41 ideal in human veins) brought about by:
♦ proper breathing
♦ exercise (carbonic buffer from carbon dioxide in blood)

- diet (plant foods elevate pH, animal foods and sugar reduce pH)
- water (adequate hydration improves pH).
- other agents, such as cesium chloride, citric acid, sodium bicarbonate

12) HYPOXIA

Humans are aerobic organisms. All cells thrive when there is proper oxygenation to the tissue. Red blood cell production is dependent on iron, copper, B-6, folate, B-12, protein, & zinc. Adequate exercise and proper breathing help. Cofactors, like CoQ, B-vitamins improve aerobic energy metabolism in cell mitochondria. Fatty acids in diet dictate "membrane fluidity" of all cells and ability to absorb oxygen.

13) EFFECTS OF AGING.

By age 65, average American has eaten 100,000 lb (50 tons) of food. Poor diet accumulates in chronic sub-clinical malnutrition; such as calcium & osteoporosis, chromium & diabetes, vitamin E & heart disease, vitamin C and cancer. Toxins accumulate in fatty tissue and liver. Chronic exposure to unchecked pro-oxidants eventually creates arthritis, Alzheimer's, heart disease, stroke, cancer, etc. Organ reserve is used up in stress and poor diet. The Hayflick principle tells us that we have 55 cell divisions maximum in a lifetime. Once your "bank account" is empty, it is difficult to recover from serious disease. Errors in DNA replication become more common as we age. Telomeres become shortened. The risk for cancer doubles with every 5 years of age. 12% of US is over 65 yrs, but 67% of US cancer patients over 65. Gland/organ insufficiencies can be partially compensated. Ill health consequences of aging may be slowed down.

14) PHYSICAL ALIGNMENT

Spinal vertebrae must be in proper alignment. Chiropractic & osteopathic manipulations on spine, joints, skull plates can be helpful. Accidents, poor muscle tone, and aging create alignment problems. Exercise, inversion and physical manipulations may solve these problems.

15) ENERGY ALIGNMENT

Meridians, shakras, and energy pathways were discovered by acupuncturists. Use acupuncture, electro-acupuncture, and acupressure to correct these problems.

16) MECHANICAL INJURY

Chronic injury requires hyperplasia, or the growth of new cells. If not properly nourished, new cell growth can become erratic and error-prone, leading to arthritis, cancer, & Alzheimers.

SKILLS FOUND IN AN EFFECTIVE HEALTH CARE PROFESSIONAL

Compassion, Intuition, Knowledge, Experience, Judgment

CHAPTER 12

CLINICAL HIGHLIGHTS

★

PATIENTS WHO HAVE BENEFITTED FROM THE USE OF IMMUNOPOWER

REMEMBER, results will vary with the individual. None of the below results are guaranteed.

ImmunoPower currently is being used with excellent results by well-respected physicians who are treating many cancer patients:

Jesse Stoff, MD, 2122 N. Craycroft #112, Tucson, AZ 85712; phone 520-290-4516 fax-6403

Sandra Denton, MD, Alaska Medical Center, 3201 C St. #602, Anchorage, AK 99503, ph 907-563-6200

Michael Schachter, MD, Two Executive Blvd. #202, Suffern, NY 10901; phone 914-368-4700

Leonard Smith, MD, 720 SW 2nd Ave. #202, Gainesville, FL 32601; phone 352-378-6262

William LaValley, MD, Austin, TX 512-467-9396, or in Nova Scotia, Canada 902-275-2573

Contact these physicians if you are interested in more information regarding their treatment of cancer.

THANKS FROM A USER OF IMMUNOPOWER

"Thank you for your help in putting me in remission. I had stage 4 non-Hodgkin's lymphoma and your product help put me in remission. I used it on land and at sea and within six months I was in remission. D.S.

BEAT COLON CANCER

S.B. is a 52 year old male who was diagnosed in August of 1996 with stage 2 colon cancer. Chemotherapy was administered in October of 1996 and produced severe reactions. Patient ceased therapy. He was then told by his surgeon to spend 2 months getting his white cell count (immune system) elevated prior to having surgery to remove the golf ball size tumor mass in his colon. Began ImmunoPower August of 1997 for 2 months as sole therapy. Upon surgical removal of 17 cm (6.5 inches) mass in colon and 10 lymph nodes, there were no living cancer cells found in the pathology report. All of the cancer cells had become a calcified necrotic mass. When the body begins to destroy a cancer, this is the process. Hence, CAT scan X-rays may show the tumor mass to be the same size. Yet, either cancer is growing or dying. It rarely sits in a state of dormancy, unless being blasted by chemotherapy. Physicians were so surprised at this patient's outcome, that he was highlighted in a hospital tumor board presentation. As of December 1997, still in remission.

BEAT UNTREATABLE LUNG CANCER

P.S. is a 50 year old female diagnosed in April of 1992 with adenocarcinoma of the lungs. Surgery (lobectomy) & radiation eliminated the measurable tumor mass. Recurrence of the lung cancer in August of 1995 was considered inoperable, metastatic and untreatable. The patient was told "there is nothing more that we can do for you". She was given the anticipated life expectancy of 2 months. She began ImmunoPower as sole therapy in January of 1996. As of January, 1998, she has had no growth of tumors and no progression of disease. She works 40 hours/week, walks 3 miles per night & feels great. Remember, if cancer is not growing, then it is most likely being destroyed and calcified by the body.

STOPPED RECURRENCE OF SARCOMA

G.B. is a 48 year old male with multiple recurrent sarcoma in his abdomen. Each year for 5 years in a row, he was forced to have a surgical excision of a "football size" tumor from his abdomen region. He began ImmunoPower as sole therapy in October of 1996 following surgery. He has had no recurrence of tumor as of June 1997.

STABILIZED METASTATIC DISEASE

W.R. is 71 year old male with primary colon cancer diagnosed in November 1993. He had a colostomy to remove the tumor. He then had lung metastasis discovered in July of 1995 with a thoracotomy, or surgical removal of the tumor. He experienced new lung metastases in November of 1996, which were defined as inoperable. He began using ImmunoPower in December of 1996. His CAT scans as of January 1997, April 1997, and June of 1997 showed no growth of tumor (size 5x6x10 cm). Co-morbidity (other diseases) includes emphesema (quit smoking 1991), atrial fibrillation, tachycardia, and gall stones. He feels very good and has high praises for the value of ImmunoPower.

REVERSING PROSTATE CANCER

T.B. is a 69 year old male diagnosed with prostate cancer with metastasis to the bone in June of 1987. Initially, he employed primarily a vegetarian diet as sole therapy. His bone scans in June of 1988 showed no malignancy. "Several years later" he experienced a recurrence of prostate cancer after his dietary relapse. He began ImmunoPower in November of 1996 with PSA levels dropping from 630 to 2.6, then 5.3. His liver metastasis has been reduced. He says that he feels good.

BEAT REFRACTORY COLON CANCER

D.S. is a 45 year old male diagnosed with stage 3 colon cancer in January of 1996 with 3 of 5 lymph nodes positive. He was administered the chemo drug 5FU for 6 months but developed severe toxic reactions. 2 new nodes appeared on his CAT scan in September of 1996, thus he had failed chemotherapy. He began ImmunoPower as sole therapy in January of 1997. His CAT scans showed no malignancy as of April 1997 and again in December 1997. Feels great and praises the product.

STABILIZING MULTIPLE CANCERS

F.J. is a 65 year old male diagnosed in June of 1996 with stage 3 colon cancer. He was given levamisol chemotherapy which produced severe flu-like symptoms. He began ImmunoPower in October of 1996. Doctors and nurses were surprised at how he "sailed through therapy". CAT scans show no colon cancer as of July of 1997. In July of 1997 was given the diagnosis of indolent prostate cancer. He feels greats and works full time. He is very pleased with ImmunoPower.

SLOWS PROSTATE CANCER

H.E. is a 74 year old male diagnosed in February of 1996 with advanced prostate cancer, with Gleason's scale of 8 (10 is worst). Upon exploratory surgery, 1 lymph node was removed. Other lymph involvement was significant and non-resectable. His physician expected a rapid spread of malignancy with no therapy available to slow tumor growth. His PSA was 25 at that time. He began ImmunoPower July of 1996 along with hormone ablation injections. His PSA dropped to 0.9. He quit hormone shots October 1996 due to drastic side effects. His PSA rose to 6.0. After orchiectomy on April 1997, his PSA dropped to 0.4. He works full time, up to 14 hours per day and hikes 15 miles per weekend because he runs a retreat in the Rocky Mountains. His PSA has been below 1.0 for 6 months. He has no pain and good energy. He is very pleased with ImmunoPower.

SLOWING PROSTATE CANCER

R.J. is a 69 year old male diagnosed August 1990 with prostate cancer, followed by prostatectomy. In January 1997, his PSA levels rose to 1.4 and his home town physician wanted to begin radiation therapy. In January 1997, a surgical biopsy of his lymph nodes in upper chest region showed enlargement and atypia (possible spreading of prostate cancer). He began ImmunoPower at full dosage in January 1997 and lupron injections once each 90 days in March 1997. As of June 1997, his PSA levels were down to 0.6 and lymph nodes have returned to normal size. He is feeling good & working full time. He is very pleased with ImmunoPower.

CONQUERED BREAST CANCER

D.S. is a 61 year old female diagnosed in November of 1995 with Stage III breast cancer. Underwent radical mastectomy (1 breast) with 4 of 22 nodes found to have cancer. Two subsequent rounds of chemotherapy produced severe side effects--patient passed out within 5 minutes of beginning chemo. Told by oncologist that without chemo, D.S. had a 5% chance of survival. Discontinued therapy. February of 1997 went to different physician who possible disease in the remaining breast. Surgeon performed lumpectomy and there was no cancer in this tissue, as per the pathologist report. March 1997, she began ImmunoPower and a good diet as sole therapy. In June of 1997, she was found to have enlarged lymph nodes with possible disease. August 1997 checkup found these nodes to have disappeared. As of January 1998, no recurrence of disease. She is very pleased with the healing power of nutrition.

REVERSING INCURABLE CYTOMA

S.M. is a 44 year old male diagnosed in April of 1997 with a rare form of cancer (hemangiopericytoma) that had caused pain, weakness and numbness in his back and legs. Began 13 rounds of radiation therapy to spinal region which produced considerable relief from pain and weakness. May of 1997, CAT scans and liver biopsy found metastatic disease throughout pancreas, liver, kidneys, lungs and pressing on spinal cord. Physicians agreed in medical staff meeting that this condition is "refractory to all medical therapy and invariably fatal." Patient began aggressive nutrition program of diet and ImmunoPower, along with detoxification (coffee enemas), 3 months chemotherapy (FUDR) and extensive prayer. As of November 1997, CAT scans showed 50% shrinkage in tumors on pancreas, lungs & kidneys with elimination of tumors on liver. Throughout this rigorous chemotherapy treatment protocol, S.M.'s bloodwork was constantly normal, whereas one would expect declines in white cell count (leukopenia) and red blood cell count (anemia). As of January 1998, patient has had excellent quality of life with no limitations, other than mild fatigue following chemotherapy injection.

CONQUERED BREAST CANCER

G.R. is a 48 year old female diagnosed in October of 1995 with advanced breast cancer. After her bilateral radical mastectomy, doctors discovered 14 positive lymph nodes. Prognosis: less than 2 years to live, even with medical therapy. Patient began 6 rounds of chemo in her home town. Became violently ill. "Camped out in the bathroom" with nausea and vomitting. In June of 1996, went to another hospital where she refused chemo, but received 6 weeks of radiation therapy twice daily to the chest and underarm lymph nodes that were positive. At same time began an aggressive nutrition program including lean and clean meat (elk, deer, fish), lots of vegetables and water, abundant prayer, and a wide assortment of nutrition supplements. As of July 1996, she was considered "disease free". Began taking 1 dose per day of ImmunoPower in September of 1996 because it was so much more complete, convenient and economical than taking many individual nutrients. As of January 1998, she continues to be healthy with no disease detectable and excellent quality of life. She offers these words of encouragement to anyone facing advanced cancer: "You need to have a determination and a will to live. Fight the cancer."

CONQUERED ADVANCED BREAST CANCER

B.C. is a 39 year old female diagnosed in April of 1995 with advanced breast cancer. Began 3 different regimens of chemotherapy. All failed. Underwent bone marrow transplant January 1996, which also failed as the malignancy then spread to the spine and lungs. Began ImmunoPower and taxol May 1997 while also shifting from a complete vegan diet to including some lean and clean animal foods. In November 1997 and May 1998 all scans and x-rays showed no disease present. Has continued with ImmunoPower and shifted medical therapy from taxol to tamoxifen. Is very pleased to be in such good shape after so many poor report cards on her breast cancer condition.

CONQUERED PROSTATE & COLON CANCER

F.J. is a 66 year old male diagnosed in June of 1996 with colon cancer. Underwent surgical resection of half of colon, then began 6 months of chemotherapy of 5FU and levamisole. Became very ill with first few treatments of levamisole. Began ImmunoPower August 1996 and never had another negative reaction to the levamisole. Diagnosed in May of 1997 with localized prostate cancer. Underwent brachytherapy only. As of May 1998 is cancer free. Since beginning ImmunoPower, all laboratory values have been in normal range.

CHAPTER 13
★
INSURANCE REIMBURSEMENT

Health insurance companies have two primary goals:

1) Keep the customer satisfied. Provide reasonable financial reimbursement for medically necessary and scientifically supported therapies.

2) Keep the stockholders satisfied. Produce a reasonable profit margin from gross revenue.

ImmunoPower can assist the insurance company in meeting both of these goals. ImmunoPower has been shown in extensive clinical experience to provide measurable improvements in quality and quantity of life and chances for a complete remission in many cancer patients. Most importantly, ImmunoPower may reduce complications of

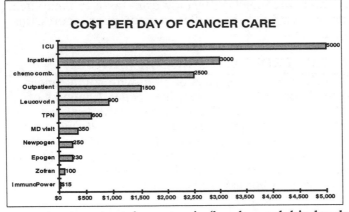

cancer treatment, such as anemia (low hemoglobin levels, treated with Epogen), leukopenia (reduced immune cell count, treated with Newpogen), nausea (treated with Zofran) and other common side effects of medical treatment which require expensive drugs to counter the side effects of chemo. Please see the chapter on "Clinical Highlights" of successful users of ImmunoPower, as well as the following letters from physicians using ImmunoPower and an insurance company who reimbursed their client for ImmunoPower (then called the Advanced Nutrition Composite).

ImmunoPower will likely provide cancer patients with fewer complications, fewer infections, greater energy levels, less medication required and less chance for "medical emergencies" to arise. ImmunoPower is good for the customer (cancer patient) and cost effective for the health insurance company. If ImmunoPower keeps the cancer patient out of the hospital for 1-2 days, then it has paid for itself for a full year. The following 2 letters are from physicians who have used ImmunoPower with good success.

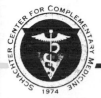

SCHACHTER CENTER FOR COMPLEMENTARY MEDICINE

A Holistic & Comprehensive Approach To Health Care Since 1974

December 7, 1997

Patrick Quillin, Ph.D., RD, CNS
Box 700512
Tulsa OK 74170

Dear Patrick:

Just a short note to let you know that I'm excited about your development of the Immunopower supplement for cancer patients. As you know, I've used this formula (previously known as Advanced Nutritional Composite or ANC) in some cancer patients and have found it to be very helpful either as an adjunct to conventional treatment or in some cases as a substitute for conventional treatment. For example one woman with breast cancer and a few lymph nodes involved was recommended to have radiation and chemotherapy. Since she and her husband were not particularly impressed with the therapeutic results of radiation and chemotherapy in this type of situation, she decided to use an immune enhancing alternative treatment program instead. ANC was the focal point of this treatment approach. It has now been a few years since she has been on this program. Not only has she had not a breast cancer recurrence, but she reports feeling very well and is extremely pleased at her decision to forego the side effects and risks of radiation and chemotherapy.

I believe that a strong nutritional program, including support from the nutrients present in Immunopower will result in much better therapeutic results in all cancer patients, whether or not they accompany this treatment with conventional therapy. In the long run, this treatment should be cost effective. Hopefully, insurance companies will soon realize the importance of this approach in helping their subscribers and also their bottom line.

You may use this letter with insurance companies to help them understand the benefits and cost effectiveness of supporting Immunopower for cancer patients.

Sincerely,

Michael B. Schachter MD

Michael B. Schachter, MD

Executive Boulevard • Suite 202 • Suffern, New York 10901-4184 • (914) 368-4700 • FAX (914) 368-4727
http://www.mbschachter.com/ • E-mail: office@mbschachter.com

LEONARD SMITH, M.D., P.A.

General & Vascular Surgery
Nutritional Medicine

720 S. W. 2nd Avenue, Suite 202   (352) 378-6262
Gainesville, Florida 32601   (352) 378-0779 FAX

December 3, 1997

Patrick Quillin, PhD, RD, CNS, Director
Rational Healing Institute
Box 700512
Tulsa, Oklahoma 74170

Dear Patrick:

I want to congratulate you on the production of your product
Immunopower. I feel that you have created an excellent combination
of immunostimulants, antioxidants and other micronutrients that
synergistically work to create balance in the immune system that is
necessary for patients dealing with cancer. I have had many of my
patients on this product for several months and I am pleased to say
I am happy with the results. Most people seem to tolerate it and
are pleased that they only have to take the 1 scoop of powder and
1 package of capsules three times a day and know that they have
covered all of their micronutritional requirements.

Since I know you are using high quality products and many of these
products are quite expensive on their own, I certainly understand
why this product is relatively expensive compared to many other
supplements that patients find in health food stores. Despite the
cost, I believe that Immunopower will be cost effective for
insurance reimbursement since I find that my cancer patients using
Immunopower have fewer infections, fewer side effects from
chemotherapy and are less likely to be hospitalized. These
improvements in symptomatology and morbidity make the product
effective for the cancer patients and thereby cost effective for
the insurance companies. I am encouraged by the results I have
obtained with my patients using this product and I am pleased to
endorse the use and insurance reimbursement of the Immunopower for
cancer patients.

Thanks again for this wonderful contribution, and I look forward to
seeing you at the nutritional meetings in the upcoming year.

Sincerely,

Leonard O. Smith, M.D.

LOS/ss

APPENDIX
✯
NUTRITIONALLY-ORIENTED DOCTORS

PHYSICIANS WHO USE NUTRITION AS PART OF CANCER TREATMENT

ZIP CODE, NAME, CREDENTIALS, ADDRESS, CITY, STATE, PHONE, FAX

08648 Charles Simone MD, 123 Franklin Corner Rd, Lawrenceville, NJ 609-896-2646
10019 Emanuel Revici MD, 200 W. 57th St., #402, New York, NY 212-246-5122
10022 Robert Atkins MD, 152 E. 55th St. New York, NY 212-758-2110
10901 Michael Schachter MD, Two Executive Blvd, #202, Suffern NY 914-368-4700
23507 Vincent Speckhart MD, 902 Graydon Ave, #2, Norfolk, VA 804-622-0014
30342 Stephen Edelson MD, 3833 Roswell Rd #110, Atlanta, GA 404-841-0088
33133 Victor Marcial-Vega MD, 4037 Poinciana Av, Coconut Grove,FL 305-442-1233
60008 Jack Taylor DC, 3601 Algonquin Rd, #801, Rolling Meadows, IL 847-222-1192
60201 Keith Block MD, 1800 Sherman Ave, #515, Evanston, IL 847-492-3040
80303 Robert Rountree MD, 4150 Darley Ave, #1, Boulder, CO 303-499-9224
85712 Jesse Stoff MD, 2122 N Craycroft Rd, #112, Tucson, AZ 520-290-4516
89502 Douglas Brodie MD, 309 Kirman Ave, #2, Reno, NV 702-324-7071
89502 James Forsythe MD, 75 Pringle Way, #909, Reno, NV 702-826-9500
89502 John Diamond MD, 4600 Kietzke Ln, M-242, Reno, NV 702-829-2277
91910 Lawrence Taylor MD, 1000 Cordova Court, Chula Vista, CA 888-422-7434
92143 Ernesto Contreras MD, P.O. Box 43-9045, San Ysidro, CA 800-700-1850
92154 Ger. Rubio MD, 555 Saturn Blvd #B, M/S 432, San Diego,CA 619-267-1107
97209 Tori Hudson ND, 2067 NW Lovejoy, Portland, OR 503-222-2322
97214 Martin Milner ND, 1330 SE 39th Ave, Portland, OR 503-232-1100
98105 Patrick Donovan ND, 5312 Roosevelt Way NE, SeattleWA 206-525-8015
98199 Dan Labriola ND, P.O. Box 99157, Seattle, WA 206-285-4993
V8T 4E5 Abram Hoffer MD, 2727 Quadra, #3, Victoria, BC CANADA 250-386-8756
W1N1AA Etienne Callebout MD, 10 Harley St., London CANADA 44-171-467-8312

HEALTH CARE PROFESSIONALS WHO USE NUTRITION AS PART OF THEIR GENERAL PRACTICE

*The following health care professionals include Medical Doctors (MD), Doctors of Chiropractic (DC), Naturopathic Doctors (ND), and Doctors of Osteopathy (DO) who have the training and experience to assist you with your health care needs. While every effort has been made to ensure the accuracy and completeness of this list, inclusion here does not constitute an endorsement from the author or publisher.

00731, Milva Vega Garcia, ND, Ave Fagot #81, Ponce, PR, ph. 787-840-3793
00824, Lynda Clark, ND, Box 25479, Christiansted, USVI, ph. 340-773-4594
00924, Efrain Rodriguez, ND, Calle Lodi 571, Urb. Luarca, Rio Piedres, PR, ph. 787-751-4682
01002, Amherst Family Health Ctr., 12 Dickinson St., Amherst, MA, ph. 413-253-2300, fax 256-0464
01060, Barry D. Elson, MD, 52 Maplewood, Old South St., Northhampton, MA, ph. 413-584-7787
01060, Northampton Wellness Assoc., 52 Maplewood, Northampton, MA, ph. 413-584-7787, fax -7778
01370, Teri Kerr, RD, 304 Shelburne Center Rd., Shelburne Falls, MA, ph. 413-625-2745, -9619
01506, Robert F. Barnes, DO, 3489 E. Main Rd., Fredonia, NY, ph. 716-679-3510, fax -3512

01523, Maharishi Med Ctr., 679 George Hill Rd., Lancaster, MA, ph. 800-290-6702, fax 508-368-0674
01583, Thomas LaCava, MD, 360 W. Boylston St. #107, W Boylston, MA, ph. 508-854-1380, fax -1377
01583, Vera Jackson, MD, 360 W. Boylston St. #107, West Boylston, MA, ph. 508-854-1380
01609, Jodie Tonelli-Chapin, ND, 232 Chandler, Worcester, MA, ph. 508-754-2707
01742, Janet Beaty, ND, 747 Main St., Concord, MA, ph. 508-287-5352
01824, Paul Rajcok, ND, 6 Courthouse Lane #16, Chelmsford, MA, ph. 978-452-3776
01852, Svetlana Kaufman, MD, 24 Merrimack St. #323, Lowell, MA, ph. 508-453-5181
01950, Barbara S. Silbert, DC, 172 State St. #1, Newburyport, MA, ph. 508-465-0929
01950, Barbara Silbert, DC, ND, 172 State St. #1, Newburyport, MA, ph. 978-465-0929
02062, Comp Psychiatric Res, Inc., 49 Walpole St. #2, Norwood, MA, ph. 617-551-8181, 332-9936
02126, Ruben Organesov, MD, 1601 Blue Hill Ave. #7, Mattapan, MA, ph. 617-296-5710
02134, Commonwealth Chelation Ctr., 39 Brighton Ave., Allston, MA, ph. 617-254-2500, fax 783-1519
02134, Ruben Oganesov, MD, 39 Brighton Ave., Boston, MA, ph. 617-783-5783, fax, -1519
02140, Marino Ctr. for Health, 2500 Massachusetts Ave., Cambridge, MA, ph. 617-661-6225, fax-492-2002
02144, John Bordiuk, MD, 55 Davis Square, Somerville, MA, ph. 617-628-9900, fax -1064
02146, Judith K. Shabert, MD, 125 Rockwood St., Brookline, MA, ph. 617-738-0370
02146, Shiva Barton, ND, 1152 Beacon St., Brookline, MA, ph. 617-277-4150
02161, Carol Englender, MD, 1126 Beacon St., Newton, MA, ph. 617-965-7770, fax -7378
02161, Jeanne Hubbuch, MD, 1126 Beacon St., Newton, MA, ph. 617-965-7770, fax -7378
02167, Lynn Hsu, ND, 824 Boylston St. #101, Chestnut Hill, MA, ph. 617-739-1001
02169, Geffin Falken, ND, 1073 Hancock St. #103, Quincy, MA, ph. 617-448-0095
02174, Glenn Rothfeld, MD, 180 Mass. Ave. #303, Arlington, MA, ph. 781-641-1901, fax -3963
02178, Joan-Ellen Macredis, ND, 63 Moraine St. #18, Belmont, MA, ph. 617-489-9835
02193, Barry Taylor, ND, 270 Winter St., Weston, MA, ph. 781-237-8505
02339, Richard Cohen, MD, 51 Mill St #1, Hanover, MA, 617-829-9281, fax -0904
02360, Anne McClenon, ND, 116 Court St., Plymouth, MA, ph. 508-830-1644
02360, Elizabeth Wotton, ND, 116 Court St., Plymouth, MA, ph. 508-830-1644
02630, Michael Janson, MD, 275 Milway, Barnstable, MA, ph. 508-362-4343, fax -1525
02630, Peter Glidden, ND, PO Box 1300, Barnstable, MA, ph. 508-362-7089
02653, Maria Perillo, ND, 62-A Cranberry Hwy, Orleans, MA, ph. 508-255-8686
02720, Paul Giordano, DC, ND, 101 President Ave., Fall River, MA, ph. 508-324-9999
02879, Peter Himmel, MD, 321 Main St., Wakefield, RI, ph. 401-783-6777, fax -6752
02906, Jill Sanders Stanard, ND, 469 Angell St., Providence, RI, ph. 401-455-0546
03038, Keith D. Jorgensen, MD, 44 Birch St. #304, Derry, NH, ph. 603-432-8104
03104, Shirley Snow, ND, 755 Straw Hill, Manchester, NH, ph. 603-644-4525
03246, Liam McClintock, ND, 401 Gilford Ave. #250, Gilford, NH, ph. 603-524-9261
03257-1999, Savely Yurkovsky, MD, 12 Newport Rd., New London, NH, ph. 603-526-2001
03264, Inst Naturopathic Health, 572 Tenney Mt. Hwy., Plymouth, NH, ph. 603-536-4888, fax 927-4309
03301, Christine Kuhlman, ND, 35 West St., Concord, NH, ph. 603-224-0000
03301, Pamela Herring, ND, 46 S. Main St., Concord, NH, ph. 603-228-0407
03431, Michele C. Moore, MD, 103 Roxbury St. #302, Keene, NH, ph. 603-357-2180
03444, Nina Iselin, ND, Main St., Dublin, NH, ph. 603-563-7066
03755, Maureen Williams, ND, 45 Lynne Rd., Ste. 210A, Hanover, NH, ph. 603-643-4818
03801, James D'Adamo, DC, ND, 44-46 Bridge St., Portsmouth, NH, ph. 416-968-0496
03801, Kristy Fassler, ND, 500 Market St. #1F, Portsmouth, NH, ph. 603-427-6800
03801, Leon Hecht III, ND, 500 Market St. #1F, Portsmouth, NH, ph. 603-427-6800
03833, Carole Robinson, ND, PO Box 887, Exeter, NH, ph. 603-772-1800
03903, Dayton Haigney, MD, 46 Dow Hwy., Eliot, ME, ph. 207-384-2828
03908, Dayton Haigney, MD, 21 Liberty St., South Berwick, ME, ph. 207-384-2828
04011, Julie Taylor, ND, 171 Park Row, Brunswick ME, ph. 207-798-3993
04011, Richard Maurer, ND, 34 Cumberland St., Brunswick, ME, ph. 207-721-8400
04011, Sarah Ackerly, ND, 171 Park Row, Brunswick ME, ph. 207-798-3993
04096, Women to Women, One Pleasant St., Yarmouth, ME, ph. 207-846-6163
04101, Devra Krassner, ND, 4 Milk St., Portland, ME, ph. 207-773-2517
04101, Priscilla Skerry, ND, 4 Milk St., Portland, ME, ph. 207-772-5227
04281, Kenneth E. Hamilton, MD, PA, 52 High St., South Paris, ME, ph. 207-743-9295, fax -0540
04347, Janet Ballard, ND, 220 Water St. #3, Hallowell, ME, ph. 207-621-4100
04401, Laura Bridgman, ND, 142 Hammond St. #5, Bangor, ME, ph. 207-941-0981
04785, Joseph Cyr, MD, 47 Main St., Van Buren, ME, ph. 207-873-7721, fax -7724
04843, Laralee Jasper-Litov, ND, 35 Harden Ave., Camden, ME, ph. 207-236-0036
04901, Arthur B. Weisser, DO, 184 Silver St., Waterville, ME, ph. 207-873-7721, -7724
05055, Susan Kowalsky, ND, PO Box 851, Norwich, VT, ph. 802-649-1064
05201, Kathleen Audette, ND, 185 North St., Bennington, VT, ph. 802-442-7000
05301, Grace Urological, Inc., 194 Canal St., Brattleboro, VT, 802-257-4265
05401, Donna Powell, ND, 41 Main St., Burlington, VT, ph. 802-863-7099
05401, Molly Fleming, ND, 41 Main St., Burlington, VT, ph. 802-863-7099
05452, Charles Anderson, MD, 175 Pearl St., Essex Junction, VT, ph. 802-879-6544

05482, Lorilee Schoenbeck, ND, 2 Harbor Rd., Shelburne, Vt., ph. 802-985-8250
05482, William Warnock, ND, 2 Harbor Rd., Shelburne, VT, ph. 802-985-8250
05602, Bernie Noe, ND, 73 Main St. #41, Montpelier, VT, ph. 802-229-2038
05602, Donna Caplan, ND, 28 E. State St., Montpelier, VT, ph. 802-229-2635
05602, Lydia Faesy, ND, 73 Main St. #41, Montpelier, VT, ph. 802-229-2038
06001, Nancy Mazur, ND, PO Box 1644, Avon, CT, ph. 860-675-1011
06040, Optimum Health, 483 West Middle Turnpike #309, Manchester, CT, ph. 860-643-5101
06082, Amy Rothenberg, ND, 115 Elm St., Enfield, CT, ph. 203-763-1225
06082, Lucia Coletta, ND, 139 Hazard Ave. #3, Enfield, CT, ph. 860-749-1941
06082, Paul Herscu, ND, 115 Elm St. #210, Enfield, CT, ph. 203-763-1225
06333, Whitney Miller, ND, 126 Boston Post Rd., East Lynne, CT, ph. 860-691-1166
06355, Deirdre O'Connor, ND, 12 Roosevelt Ave., Mystic, CT, ph. 860-572-9566
06410, Central Connecticut Chiropractic, 391 Highland Ave. Rt. 10, Cheshire, CT, ph. 203-272-3239
06418, Christine Girard-Couture, ND, 130 Division St., Derby, CT, ph. 203-732-1138
06437, Tammy Alex, ND, 35 Boston St. #4, Guilford, CT, ph. 203-453-0122
06440, Kathleen Riley, ND, 31 Hawleyville Rd., Hawleyville, CT, ph. 203-426-2306
06450, Meriden Chiropractic Group, 74 South Broad St., Meriden, CT, ph. 203-235-0171, fax 630-3611
06457, Enrico Liva, ND, 87 Bernie O'Rourke Dr., Middletown, CT, ph. 860-347-8600
06457, Jacqueline Germain, ND, 87 Bernie O'Rourke Dr., Middletown, CT, ph. 860-347-8600
06457, Keli Samuelson, ND, 87 Bernie O'Rourke Dr., Middletown, CT, ph. 860-347-8600
06457, Michael Kane, ND, 87 Bernie O'Rourke Dr., Middletown, CT, ph. 860-347-8600
06460, Alan R. Cohen, MD, 67 Cherry St., Milford, CT, ph. 203-877-1936, fax –2228
06470, Deep Brook Center, 46 West St., Newtown, CT, ph. 203-426-4553
06475, Cathryn Flanagan, ND, 12 Spencer Plains Rd., Old Saybrook, CT, ph. 860-399-1212
06477, Mark A. Breiner, DDS, 325 Post Road #3A, Orange, CT, ph. 203-799-6353, fax 795-2749
06477, Robban A. Sica, MD, 325 Post Rd. #2A, Orange, CT, ph. 203-799-7733, fax –3560
06488, Andrew Rubman, ND, 900 Main St. S., Southbury, CT, ph. 203-262-6755
06497, Michael Petreycik, ND, PO Box 747, Stratford, CT, ph. 203-333-8916
06518, James Sensenig, ND, 2558 Whitney Ave., Hamden, CT, ph. 203-230-2200
06518, Robin Ritterman, ND, 2558 Whitney Ave., Hamden, CT, ph. 203-230-2200
06610, Tadeusz A. Skowron, MD, 50 Ridgefield Ave. #317, Bridgeport, CT, ph. 203-368-1450
06614, Jennifer Brett, ND, 998 Nichols Ave., Stratford, CT, ph. 203-377-1525
06757, Kent Chiropractic Health Ctr., PC, 25 N Main St. #6, Kent, CT, ph. 860-927-4455, fax -4463
06790, Jerrold N . Finnie, MD, 333 Kennedy Dr., Torrington, CT, ph. 860-489-8977
06790, Michelle Pouliot, ND, 118 Mijun Ave., Torrington, CT, ph. 860-482-4730
06790, Robert Murphy, ND, 118 Migeon Ave., Torrington, CT, ph. 860-482-4730
06798, Debra Gibson, ND, 51 Sherman Hill Rd., Woodbury, CT, ph. 203-266-4007
06804, Sherry Stemper, ND, 18 Old Route 7, Brookfield, CT, ph. 203-740-7745
06810, Harold Ofgang, ND, 57 North St. #323, Danbury, CT, ph. 203-798-0533
06820, Sandoval Melim, ND, 1500 Boston Post Rd., Darien, CT, ph. 206-656-6635
06820, Susanna Reid, ND, 1500 Boston Post Rd., Darien, CT, ph. 203-656-6635
06820, Victoria Zupa, ND, 762 Post Rd., Darien, CT, ph. 718-275-6599
06851, Ahmed N. Currim, 148 East Ave. #1L, Norwalk, CT, ph. 203-853-1339, fax -866-4616
06851, Daniel Heller, ND, 112 Main St., Norwalk, CT, ph. 203-845-0734
06851, Marvin Schweitzer, ND, 1 Westport Ave., Norwalk, CT, ph. 203-847-2788
06854, Christopher Fabricius, ND, 21 Ann, Ste. AC-1, Norwalk, CT, ph. 203-299-0143
06877, George P. Zabrecky, MD, 31 Bailey Ave., Ridgefield, CT, ph. 203-894-8370, fax 431-6167
06877, Warren M. Levin, MD, 31 Bailey Ave., Ridgefield, CT., ph. 203-894-8370, fax 431-6167
06880, Gabriele Kallenborn, ND, 61 Edgewater Commons Lane, Westport, CT, ph. 203-454-5989
06880, Howard Fine, ND, 4 Cross Hwy., Westport, CT, ph. 203-221-0216
06880, Lawrence Caprio, ND, 830 Post Road E, Westport, CT, ph. 203-226-4167
06880, Marie A. DiPasquale, MD, 29 Old Hill Farms Rd., Westport, CT, ph. 203-226-1719
06880, Sidney M. Baker, MD, 40 Hillside Rd., Weston, CT, ph. 203-227-8444, fax -8443
06880, Thomas T. Brunoski, MD, 4 Ivy Knoll, Westport, CT, ph. 203-454-5963, fax 221-1522
06883, Pearlyn Goodman-Herrick, ND, 21 Trails End Rd., Weston, CT, ph. 203-227-5534
06905, Peter D'Adamo, ND, 2009 Summer St., Stamford, CT, ph. 203-348-4800
07003, Majid Ali, MD, 320 Belleville Ave., Bloomfield, NJ, ph. 201-586-4111
07003, R. Russomanno, MD, 350 Bloomfield Ave. #1, Bloomfield, NJ, ph. 201-748-9330, fax -6985
07024, Gary Klingsberg, DO, 1355 15th St. #200, Fort Lee, NJ, ph. 201-585-9368
07024, Gary Klingsberg, DO, 1355 15th St. #200, Fort Lee, NJ, ph. 201-585-9368
07040, Donald Brown, ND, 180 Wyoming Ave., Maplewood, NJ, ph. 973-762-0840
07041, James Neubrander, MD, 96 Millburn Ave. #200, Millburn, NJ, ph. 201-275-0234, fax -1646
07042, Plastic Surgery Ctr., Montclair, NJ, ph. 201-746-3535, fax -4385
07052, Faina Munits, MD, 51 Pleasant Valley Way, West Orange, NJ, ph. 201-736-3743
07055, Jose R. Sanchez-Pena, MD, 124 Gregory Ave. #201, Passaic, NJ, ph. 201-471-9800, fax -9240
07065, Dr.'s Choice, 1082 St. George Ave., Rahway, NJ, ph. 908-388-4787, fax -4380
07080, Mark Friedman, MD, PA, 2509 Park Ave. #2D, S. Plainfield, NJ, ph. 908-753-8622, fax -0141

07423, Irene Catania, ND, 119 First St., Ho-Ho-Kus, NJ, ph. 201-444-4900
07450, Constance Alfano, MD, 104 Chestnut, Ridgewood, NJ, ph. 201-444-4622
07470-3493, Homeopathy Ctr. of New Jersey, 746 Valley Rd., Wayne, NJ, ph. 201-694-7711
07512, Boro Chiropractic, 79 Union Boulevard, Totowa, NJ, ph. 201-904-0997, fax -9055
07601, Robin Leder, MD, 235 Prospect Ave., Hackensack, NJ, ph. 201-525-1155
07628, Jack Larmer, ND, 34 Bussell Ct., Dumont, NJ, ph. 201-385-7106
07675, Joseph Spektor, MD, 54 Indian Dr., Woodcliff Lake, NJ, ph. 201-307-0633
07701, Family Chiro Ctr, 746 Sycamore Ave., Shrewsbury/Tinton Fa, NJ, ph. 908-530-0405, fax -4195
07702, David Dornfield, DO, 167 Ave. at the Common #1, Shrewbury, NJ, ph. 908-389-6455, fax -6365
07702, Neil Rosen, DO, 167 Avenue at the Common #1, Shrewsbury, NJ, ph. 908-389-6455, fax -6365
07748, David Dornfeld, DO, 18 Leonardville Rd., Middletown, NJ ph. 908-671-3730, fax 706-1078
07748, Neil Rosen, DO, 18 Leonardville Rd., Middletown, NJ, ph. 908-671-3730, fax 706-1078
07834, Majid Ali, MD, 95 E. Main St., Denville, NJ, ph. 973-586-4111, fax –8466
07840, Robert A. Siegel, MD, 2-B Doctors Park, Hackettstown, NJ, ph. 908-850-1810
07940, Howard C. Weiss, MD, 28 Walnut St., Madison, NJ, ph. 201-301-1770, fax -9445
07962, New Health Initiatives, 95 Mt. Kemble Ave., Morristown, NJ, ph. 973-971-4610, fax 290-7582
08003, Allan Magaziner, DO, 1907 Greentree Rd, Cherry Hill, NJ, ph. 609-424-8222, fax –2599
08034, Brian Karlin, DO, 1916 Old Cuthbert Rd. #A-1, Cherry Hill, NJ, ph. 609-429-3335
08043, Lifeline Medical Ctr., 1600 S. Burntmill Rd., Voorhees, NJ, ph. 609-627-5600
08092, Robert D. Miller, DO, 196 Main St., West Creek, NJ, ph. 609-296-4643, fax -3393
08203, Michael J. Dunn, Jr., MD, Brigantine Town Ctr., Brigantine, NJ, ph. 609-266-2473
08225, Barry D. Glasser, MD, Rt. 9 & Mill Rd., Northfield, NJ, ph. 609-646-9600
08234, E.Andujar, MD, 3003 English Cr Ctr. #210, Egg Harbor Township, ph. 609-646-2900, fax -3436
08332, Charles H. Mintz, MD, 10 E. Broad St., Millville, NJ, ph. 609-825-7372, fax 327-6588
08502, Amwell Health Ctr., 450 Amwell Rd., Belle Mead, ph. 908-359-1775
08540, Leonid Magidenko, MD, 212 Commons Way #2, Princeton, NJ, ph. 609-921-1842, fax -6092
08559, Stuart H. Freedenfeld, MD, 56 S. Main St., Stockton, NJ, ph. 609-397-8585, fax –9335
08648, C. Simone, MD, 123 Franklin Corner Rd., Lawrenceville, NJ, ph. 609-896-2646, fax 883-7173
08701, Ivan Krohn, MD, 117 E. County Line Rd., Lakewood, NJ, ph. 908-367-2345, fax -2727
08816, P. Gilbert, DDS, 123 Dunhams Corner Rd, East Brunswick, NJ, ph. 732-754-7946, fax 254-0287
08837, C. Y. Lee, ME, 952 Amboy Ave., Edison, NJ, ph. 908-738-9220, fax -1187
08837, C.Y. Lee, MD, 952 Amboy Ave., Edison, NJ, ph. 732-738-9220, fax –0363
08837, Dr. Richard B. Menashe, 15 S. Main St., Edison, NJ, ph. 732-906-8866, fax -0124
08837, Ralph Lev, MD, 15 S. Main St., Edison, NJ, ph. 908-738-9220, fax -1187
08837, Richard B. Menashe, DO, 15 S. Main St., Edison, NJ, ph. 732-906-8866, fax –0124
08854, Laurence Rubenstein, DO, 10 Plainfield Ave., Piscataway, NJ, ph. 908-469-1155, fax 457-9420
08873, Marc Condren, MD, 15 Cedar Grove Lane #20, Somerset, NJ, ph. 908-469-2133
08873, Marc Condren, MD, 7 Cedar Grove Lane #20, Somerset, NJ, ph. 732-469-2133, fax 464-9777
08879, Center for Head & Facial Pain, 2045 Rt. 35 S., South Amboy, NJ, ph. 908-727-5000, fax -5497
10001, Sheila George, MD, 226 W. 26th St. 5th Floor, New York, NY, ph. 212-924-5900, fax -7600
10011, Scott Gerson, MD, 13 W. Ninth St., New York, NY, ph. 212-505-8971, fax 677-5397
10016, Achieving Total Health, 274 Madison Ave. #402, NY, NY, ph. 212-213-6155, fax -6188
10016, Michael Teplitsky, MD, 31 E. 28th St., New York, NY, ph. 212-679-3700, fax -9730
10016, Nancy Weiss, MD, 109 E. 36th St., New York, NY, ph. 212-683-8105
10016, Nicholas J. Gonzalez, MD, 36 E. 36 St., New York, NY, ph. 212-213-3337, fax –3414
10016, Robert Faylor, MD, 377 Park Ave. S. #33, New York, NY, ph. 212-679-6717, fax -6714
10016, Ronald Hoffman, MD, 40 E. 30th St. 10th Floor, New York, NY, ph. 212-779-1744, fax -0891
10016, Ronald L. Hoffman, MD, 40 E. 30 St., 10th Floor, New York, NY, ph. 212-779-1744, fax –0891
10019, Carol Goldstein, DC, 850 7th Ave. #602, New York, NY, ph. 212-489-9396, fax -8164
10019, Physicians For Complementary Med, 24 W. 57th St. #701, NY, NY, ph. 212-397-5900, fax -6054
10019, Robin Leder, MD, 159 W. 53rd St. #18-D, New York, NY, ph. 212-333-2626
10019, Serafina Corsella, MD, 200 W. 57 St., New York, NY, ph. 212-399-0222
10021, Jay Lombard, DO, 133 E. 73rd St., New York, NY, ph. 212-861-9000
10021, Leo Galland, MD, 133 E. 73rd St., New York, NY, ph. 212-861-9000
10021, Martin Feldman, MD, 132 E. 76th St., New York, NY, ph. 212-744-4413, fax 249-6155
10021, Richard Ash, MD, 860 Fifth Ave., New York, NY, ph. 212-628-3113, fax 249-3805
10021, Richard N. Ash, MD, 860 Fifth Ave., New York, NY, ph. 212-628-3113, fax 249-3805
10021, Strang Cancer Prevention Ctr., 428 E. 72nd St., New York, NY, ph. 212-410-3820, fax 794-4958
10021, Tom Bolte, MD, 133 E. 73rd St., New York, NY, ph. 212-861-9000, fax 516-897-8386
10021, Woodson C. Merrell, MD, 44 E. 67 St., New York, NY, ph. 212-535-1012, fax –1172
10022, Frederick Mindel, DC, 133 E. 58th St. #505, New York, NY, ph. 212-223-8683, fax -8687
10022, Robert C. Atkins, MD, 152 E. 55 St., New York, NY, ph. 888-ATKINS-8, fax 212-355-8874
10022, Warren M. Levin, MD, 18 E. 53 St., New York, NY, ph. 212-838-9100, fax –8803
10023, Teresa Rossi, ND, 310 W. 72 St. #1-G, New York, NY, ph. 212-580-3333, fax –3759
10023, Tristate Healing Ctr., 175 W. 72nd St., New York, NY, ph. 212-362-9544, fax 769-3566
10024, Edward S. Cheslow, MD, 107 W. 82nd St. #103, New York, NY, ph. 212-362-0449
10024, Katherine H. Leddick, 25 Central Park West, New York City, NY, ph. 212-875-1770

10025, Holistic Health Center, 229 W. 97th St., New York, ph. 212-932-2381, fax -1363
10025, Ostrow Inst. for Pain Mgmt., 250 W 100th St. #317, NY, NY, ph. 212-838-8265, fax 752-5140
10038, Carol O. Ellis, MD, 11 John St. #603, New York, NY, ph. 212-227-2462, fax 809-6549
10128, Firshein Ctr. Comprehensive Med, 1230 Park Ave. #1B, NY, NY, ph. 212-860-0282, fax -0276
1018, Sally Ann Rex, DO, 1343 Easton Ave., Bethlehem, PA, ph. 215-866-0900
10312, Napoli Chiropractic, 611 Lamoka Avenue, Staten Island, NY, ph. 718-967-0300, fax -0300
10458, Shashikant Patel, MD, 405 E. 187th St., Bronx, NY, ph. 718-365-7777, fax -1179
10459, Richard Izquiredo, MD, 1070 Southern Blvd. Lower Level, Bronx, NY, ph. 212-589-4541
10460, Uttam L. Munver, MD, 1963-A Daly Ave., Bronx, NY, ph. 718-991-8300
10509, J. C. Kopelson, MD, 221 Clock Tower Commons, Brewster, NY, ph. 914-278-6800, fax -6897
10509, Jeffrey Kopelson, MD, 221 Clock Twr Commons, Brewster, NY, ph. 914-278-6800, fax -6897
10530, Gary Young, DC, 234 N. Central Park #204, Hartsdale, NY, ph. 914-683-1777, fax –8951
10538, Monica Furlong, MD, 29 Rockwood Dr., Larchmont, NY, ph. 914-834-2742
10543, Healing Partners, 921 W. Boston Post Rd., Mamaroneck, NY, ph. 914-381-7687, fax -0942
10543, Monica Furlong, MD, 921 W. Boston Post Rd., Mamaronerck, NY, ph. 914-381-7687, fax -0942
10549, Henry C. Sobo, MD, 213 Main St., Mt. Kisco, NY, ph. 914-241-7030, fax –7038
10566, Joel Edman, 2 Rence Fate, Courtlandt Manor, NY, ph. 914-528-7878, fax -7991
10901, Bruce Oran, DO, DC, Two Executive Blvd. #202, Suffern, NY, ph. 914-368-4700, fax -4727
10901, Michael B. Schacter, MD, 2 Executive Blvd. #202, Suffern, NY, ph. 914-368-4700, fax –4727
10941, Optimal Health Medical Assoc., P.L.L.C., 825 Rt. 211 East, Middletown, NY, ph. 914-344-3278
10950, David Drier, DC, PO Box 198, Monroe, NY, ph. 914-774-7378, fax –1357
10962, Neil L. Block, MD, 60 Dutch Hill Rd., Orangeburg, NY, ph. 914-359-3300
11001, Robert A. Kornfeld, DPM, 153 Tulip Ave., Floral Park, NY, ph. 516-326-1170, fax –2055
11024, Mary F. DiRico, MD, 1 Kingsport Rd., Great Neck, NY, ph. 516-466-5245
11040, Sun F. Pei, DO, 1 Fairfield Lane, New Hyde Park, NY, ph. 516-775-5285
11042, Lakeville OB-Gyn, 2001 Marcus Ave., Lake Success, NY, ph. 516-488-2757, fax -3940
11106, Albert W. Winyard III, MD, 23-35 Broadway, Astoria, NY, ph. 212-249-0903
11204, Pavel Yutsis, MD, 1309 W. 7th St., Brooklyn, NY, ph. 718-259-2122, fax -3933
11204, Yelena Shvarts, MD, 1309 W. 7th St., Brooklyn, NY, ph. 718-259-2122, fax -3933
11210, Brooklyn Ctr. of Holistic Med, 2515 Avenue M, Brooklyn, NY, ph. 718-258-7882, fax 692-4175
11210, Jean Grandoit, ND, 2176 Nostrand Ave., Brooklyn, NY, ph. 718-859-3222, fax –0653
11218, A. F. Chu-Fong, MD, 185 Prospect park SW #102, Brooklyn, NY, ph. 718-438-6565, fax -1361
11219, Tova Rosen, MD, 5001 - 14th Ave. #A-7, Brooklyn, NY, ph. 718-435-9695
11228, Morris Westfried, 7508 15th Ave., Brooklyn, NY, ph. 718-837-9004
11229, Asya Benin, MD, 2116 Avenue P, Brooklyn, NY, ph. 718-338-1616
11230, Tsilia Sorina, MD, 2026 Ocean Ave., Brooklyn, NY, ph. 718-375-2600
11235, Michael Telpistky, MD, 415 Oceanview Ave., Brooklyn, NY, ph. 718-769-0997, fax 646-2352
11358, Ronald B. Keys, 13 06 159th St., Flushing, NY, ph. 718 160 3966, fax 3966
11377, Fire Nihamin, MD, 39 - 65 52nd St., Woodside, NY, ph. 718-429-0039, fax -6965
11548, D'Brant Chiropractic, 55 Northern Blvd., Greenvale, NY, ph. 516-484-4897, fax -1964
11554, C. L. Calapai, DO, 1900 Hempstead Turnpike, East Meadow, NY, ph. 516-794-0404, fax -0332
11557, Kelly Cohen, ND, 1431 Vlan Ave., Hewlett, NY, ph. 212-995-5379
11559, Mitchell Kurk, MD, 310 Broadway, Lawrence, NY, ph. 516-239-5540, fax 371-2919
11577, Rachlin Centre, 10 Power House Rd., Roslyn Heights, NY, ph. 516-625-6884, fax -6294
11590, Savely Yurkovsky, MD, 309 Madison St., Westbury, NY, ph. 516-333-2929
11717, Juan J. Nolasco, MD, 78 Wicks Rd #1, Brentwood, NY, ph. 516-434-4840
11743, Serafina Corsella, MD, 175 E. Main St., Huntington, KY, ph. 516-271-0222, fax –5992
11746, Michael Fass, MD, A-Plaza 680 East, Huntington Station, NY, ph. 516-549-4607
11777, Roseann Nenninger, ND, 109 Randall Ave., Port Jefferson, NY, ph. 516-331-0161
11777, Steve Nenninger, ND, 109 Randall Ave., Port Jefferson, NY, ph. 516-331-0161
11784, Pernice Chiropractic, 301 Mooney Pond Rd., Seldem, NY, ph. 516-736-1000, fax -1023
11787, Michael Jardula, MD, 60 Terry Road, Smithtown, NY, ph. 516-361-3363
11788, Vincent C. Parry, DO, 236 Northfield Rd., Hauppauge, NY, ph. 516-724-2233
11792, Ashley Lewin, ND, 27 Locust St., Wading River, NY, ph. 516-929-3950
11797, Nutrition Works, 814 Woodbury Rd., Woodbury, NY, ph. 516-364-4441, fax -2602
11803, Thomas K. Szulc, MD, 720 Old Country Rd., Plainview, NY, ph. 516 931 1133, fax 1167
11959, Lewis S. Anreder, MD, 33 Montauk Hwy. Quogue, NY, ph. 516-653-6000, fax 288-8208
12203, K. A. Bock, MD, FACAM, 10 McKown Road #210, Albany, NY, ph. 518-435-0082, fax -0086
12572, Janet Draves, ND, 8 Knollwood Rd., Rhinebeck, NY, ph. 914-876-3993, fax -5365
12572, Kenneth Bock, MD, 108 Montgomery St., Rhinebeck, NY, ph. 914-876-7082, fax –4615
12901, Adirondack Preventive Center, 50B Court St., Platsburgh, NY, ph. 518-561-2023, fax 561-2042
13039, ADIO Health Systems, 8129 Rt. 11, Cicero, NY, ph. 315-699-5000
13205, Jennifer S. Daniels, MD, 3100 S. Salina St., Syracuse, NY, ph. 315-475-3393
13662, Robert W. Snider, MD, 284 Andrews St., Massena, NY, ph. 315-764-7328, fax –5699
13820, Richard J. Ucci, MD, 521 Main St., Oneonta, NY, ph. 607-432-8752, fax 431-9641
13850, Acup & Chinese Herbal Med, 1020 Vestal Pkwy East, Vestal, NY, ph. 607-754-6043, fax -6150
14063, Robert F. Barnes, DO, 3489 E. Main Rd., Fredonia, NY, ph. 716 679 3510, fax 3512

14092, Donald M. Fraser, MD, 5147 Lewiston Rd., Lewiston, NY, ph. 716-284-5777
14217, Doris J. Rapp, MD, 2757 Elmwood Ave., Buffalo, NY, ph. 716-875-5578, fax -5399
14224, James H. Matthews, MD, 721 Center Rd., West Seneca, NY, ph. 716-675-4012, fax –4646
14225, Allergy & Environmental Health Ctr., 65 Wahrie Dr., Buffalo, NY, ph. 716-833-2213, fax -2244
14301, Paul Cutler, MD, 652 Elmwood Ave., Niagara Falls, NY, ph. 888-233-3762, fax 716-284-5159
14733, Reino Hill, MD, 230 W. Main St., Falconer, NY, ph. 716-665-3505
15012, Laurie D. Pavtis, DC, 1035 Broad Ave., Belle Vernon, PA, ph. 724-929-4250, fax –4214
15203, Pain Release Clinic, 1320 E. Carson St., Pittsburgh, PA, ph. 412-431-7246, fax 488-3039
15215, Christiane Siewers, MD, 35 Freeport Rd., Pittsburgh, PA, ph. 412-782-2992, fax –3108
15237, David Goldstein, MD, 9401 McKnight Rd #301B, Pittsburgh, PA, ph. 412-366-6780, fax –8644
15237, Paul Del Bianco, MD, 9401 McKnight Rd. #301-B, Pittsburg, PA, ph. 412-366-6780
15317, Dennis J. Courtney, MD, 4198 Washington Road #1, McMurray, PA, ph. 412-941-1193
15522, Bill Illingwirth, DO, 120 W. John St., Bedford, PA, ph. 814-623-8414
15601, Alfonso S. Arevalo, MD, 100 W. Point Dr., Greensburg, PA, ph. 412-836-6041
15601, Ralph A. Miranda, MD, RD 12, Box 108, Greensburg, PA, ph. 724-838-7632, fax 836-3655
15644, R. Christopher Monsour, MD, 70 Lincoln Way East, Jeannette, PA, ph. 412-527-1511
15666, Mamduh El-Attrache, MD, 20 E. Main St., Mt. Pleasant, PA, ph. 412-547-3576
16066, Donald Mantell, MD, 6505 Mars Rd., Cranberry Twp, PA, ph. 412-776-5610, fax –5612
16125, Roy E. Kerry MD, 17 Sixth Ave., Greenville, PA, ph. 412-588-2600
16146, Andrew Baer, MD, 92 West Connelly Blvd., Sharon, PA, ph. 412-346-6500
16335, Total Health Med, 505 Poplar St. Room PG02, Meadville, PA, ph. 814-337-7429, fax -5476
17011, Brian Freeman, ND, 3913 Market St., Camp Hill, PA, ph. 717-730-9066
17022, Dennis Gilbert, DO, 50 N. Market St., Elizabethtown, PA, ph. 717-367-1345, fax -6616
17055, John M. Sullivan, MD, 1001 S. Market St. #B, Mechanicsburg, PA, ph. 717-697-5050, fax -3156
17403, Kenneth E. Yinger, DO, 1561 E. Market St., York, PA, ph. 717-848-2544
17522, Michael Reese, ND, 4233 Oregon Pike, Ephrata, PA, ph. 717-859-4222
17701, Francis M. Powers, Jr., MD, 1100 Grampian Blvd., Williamsport, PA, ph. 717-326-8203
17701, Gregory Pais, ND, 837 Washington Blvd., Williamsport, PA, ph. 717-320-0747
17837, George C. Miller II, MD, 3 Hospital Dr., Lewisburg, PA, ph. 717-524-4405, fax 523-8844
18013, Francis J. Cinelli, DO, 153 N. 11th St., Bangor, PA, ph. 610-588-4502, fax -6928
18103, Frederick Burton, MD, 321 E. Emmaus Ave., Allentown, PA, ph. 610-791-2452, fax -9974
18104, Erik VonKiel, DO, 501 N. 17 St. #201, Allentown, PA, ph. 215-776-7639, fax 434-7040
18201, Arthur L. Koch, DO, 57 West Juniper St., Hazleton, PA, ph. 717-455-4747
18229, Edward D. Manzanella, MD, HC2 Box 2043, Jim Thorpe, PA, ph. 717-325-8393, fax –8029
18235, P. Jayalakshmi, MD, 330 Breezewood Rd., Lehighton, PA, ph. 215-473-7453
18253, K.R. Sampathachar, MD, 330 Breezewood Rd., Lehighton, PA, ph. 215-473-7453
18301, Brett Coryell, DC, 1 Village Center, East Stroudsburg, PA, ph. 717-223-7211, fax –7545
18335, Healthplex Medical Center, Rt. 209, Marshalls Creek, PA, ph. 800-228-4673, fax 717-223-7355
18411, Steven Nemeroff, ND, 3 Abington – Executive Park, Clarks Summit, PA, ph. 717-585-4040
18644, Family Chiropractic Center, 131 W. 8th St., Wyoming, PA, ph. 717-693-9393, fax -2703
18702, William N. Clearfield, DO, 318 S. Franklin St., Wilkes Barre, PA, ph. 717-824-0953
18821, Kristin Stiles, ND, 310 Main St., Great Bend, PA, ph. 717-879-2828
18910, Julia M. Duane, MD, PO Box 10, Bedminster, PA, ph. 215-795-2935
18923, Harold H. Byer, MD, PhD, 5045 Swamp Rd. #A-101, Fountainville, PA, ph. 215-348-0443
18940, Michael DiPalma, ND, 2700 S. Eagle Rd., Newton, PA, ph. 215-579-1300
18944, Robert Jenkins, DC, 800 Chestnut St., Perkasie, PA, ph. 215-453-9998
18951, Harold Buttram, MD, 5724 Clymer Rd., Quakertown, PA, ph. 215-536-1890
18951, William G. Kracht, DO, 5724 Clymer Rd., Quakertown, PA, ph. 215-536-1890
18966, Suvarna Hannah, ND, 3463 Norwood Place, Holland, PA, ph. 215-579-0409, fax 504-1094
19020, Robert J. Peterson, DO, 2169 Galloway Road, Bensalem, PA, ph. 215-579-0330
19023, Health Achievement Ctr., 112 S. 4th St., Darby, PA, ph. 610-461-6225, fax 583-3356
19040, Bartley L. Stein, 38 Maurice Lane, Hatboro, PA, ph. 800-213-6331, fax 215-674-3857
19041, C. G. Maulfair Jr., DO, FACAM, 600 Haverford Rd. #200, Haverford, PA, ph. 800-733-4065
19047, George Danielewski, MD, 142 Bellevue Ave., Penndel, PA, ph. 215-757-4455
19056, Joseph A. Maxian, DO, 56 Highland Park Way, Livittown, PA, ph. 215-945-0707, fax -9120
19063, Arthur K. Balin, MD, 110 Chesley Dr., Media, PA, ph. 610-565-3300, fax –9909
19064, Joseph Bellesorte, DO, 930 W. Sproul Rd., Springfield, PA, ph. 610-328-3000
19064, Walter Schwartz, DO, 471 Baltimore Pike, Springfield, PA, ph. 610-604-4800, fax –4815
19067, Center for Natural Medicine, 303 Floral Vale Blvd., Yardley, PA, ph. 215-860-1500
19072, Andrew Lipton, DO, 822 Montgomery Ave #315, Narbeth, PA, ph. 610-667-4601
19087, Joan Michelland, Lac, 700 Knox Road, Wayne, PA, ph. 610-687-8595
19095, Preventive medicine Group, 1442 Ashbourne Rd., Wyncote, PA, ph. 215-886-7842, 887-1921
19102, Robert A. Smith, MD, 1420 Locust St. #200, Philadelphia, PA, ph. 215-545-2828
19111, Quinlan Alternative Medicine Ctr., 7301 Hasbrook Ave., Philadelphia, PA, ph. 215-722-7200
19115, Larry S. Hahn, DO, 9892 Bustleton Ave. #301, Philadelphia, PA, ph. 215-464-4111
19116, Maura Galperin, MD, 824 Hendrix St., Philadelphia, PA, ph. 215-677-2337
19118, Brij Srivastava, MD, 3309 N. Friend St., Philadelphia, PA, ph. 215-634-1920

19144, Frederick Burton, MD, 69 W. Schoolhouse Ln., Philadelphia, PA, ph. 215-844-4660
19147, Sarah M. Fisher, MD, 706 S. Second St., Philadelphia, PA, ph. 215-627-8401, fax -7227
19148, Brian Karlin, Do, 2500 S. Sheridan St., Philadelphia, PA, ph. 215-465-5583
19148, Joseph Steingard, MD, 2601 S. 12th St., Philadelphia, PA, ph. 215-389-6461
19148, Mark Tests, DO, 2601 S. 12th St., Philadelphia, PA, ph. 215-389-6461
19151, K.R. Sampathachar, MD, 6366 Sherwood Rd., Philadelphia, PA, ph. 215-473-4226
19348, Nicholas D'Orazio, MD, 100 E. State St. 2nd Floor, Kennett Square, PA, ph. 610-444-7224
19562, Conrad G. Maulfair, DO, 403 N. Main St., Topton, PA, ph. 800-733-4065, fax 610-682 9781
19808, Chrysalis Natural Medicine, 1008 Milltow Rd., Wilmington, DE, ph. 302-994-0565, fax 995-0653
19810, Vincent Vinciguerr, DC, 1800 Naamans Road, Wilmington, DE, ph. 302-475-3200
19966, G. Yossif, MD, PhD, 559 E. Dupont Hwy., Millsboro, DE, ph. 800-858-3370, fax 302-934-7949
20002, Ali Safayan, MD, 1020 Mass. Ave. NE, Washington, DC, ph. 202-546-6163, fax 244-1340
20008, Andrea Sullivan, ND, 4601 Connecticut Ave. NW #6, Washington, DC, ph. 202-244-4545
20008, Andrew Baer, MD, 4123 Connecticut Ave., N.W., Washington, DC, ph. 202-363-8770
20008, G. H. Mitchell, MD, 2639 Connecticut Ave., N.W. #C-100, Washington, DC, ph. 202-265-4111
20008, George Mitchell, MD, 2639 Connecticut Ave. NW, Washington, DC, ph. 202-265-4092
20008, John C. Williams, NMD, 5039 Conn. Ave. NW, Washington, DC, ph. 202-686-7130, fax -7165
20008, Michelle Cochran, ND, 4820 Reno Rd. NW, Washington, DC, ph. 202-237-0717
20015, A Rosemblat, MD, 5225 Wisconsin Ave., N.W. #401, Wash, DC, ph. 202-237-7000, fax -0017
20016, Monique Lai, ND, 4801 Wisconsin Ave. NW, Washington, DC, ph. 202-244-1310
20016, Susan McConnell, 3006 Arizona, Washington, DC, ph. 202-966-3061
20036, J. Philip Shambaugh Jr., DC, 1900 L St. NW #204, Washington, DC, ph. 202-452-0060
20105, Norman W. Levin, MD, PO Box 107, Aldie, VA, ph. 703-260-3484
20164, Oscar G. Rasussen, Ph. 118 Avondale Dr., Sterling, VA, ph. 703-450-1640, fax -1630
20165-5843, Joan Walters, ND, 277 Terrie Dr., Sterling, VA, ph. 703-430-2310, fax -3405
20708, Paul V. Beals, MD, 9101 Cherry Lane #205, Laurel, MD, ph. 301-490-9911, fax 202-986-3255
20808, Paul V. Beals, MD, 9101 Cherry Lane #205, Laurel, MD, ph. 301-490-9911
20850, David G. Wember, MD, 26 Guy Ct., Rockville, MD, ph. 301-424-4048, fax 294-0854
20850, Zidi Berger, MD, 9707 Medical Center Dr., Rockville, MD, ph. 301-279-0488, fax 309-0435
20852, Bruce Rind, MD, 11140 Rockville Pike #520, Rockville, MD, ph. 301-816-3000, fax -0011
20852, Norton Fishman, MD, 11140 Rockville Pike #520, Rockville, MD, ph. 301-816-3000
20852, Norton L. Fishman, MD, 11140 Rockville Pike #600, Rockville, MD, ph. 301-816-0500
20895, Dana Godbout Laake, 11223 Orleans Way, Kensington, MD, ph. 301-933-5919
20895, Healing Matters, 3700 Washington St., Kensington, MS, ph. 301-942-9024, fax 946-9035
21117, Willow Moore, DC, ND, 10806 Reisters Town Rd. #1E, Owingsmills, MD, ph. 410-356-4600
21133, Arnold Brenner, MD, 8622 Liberty Plaza Mall, Randalistown, MD, ph. 410-922-1133, fax -9740
21146, Linda Ciotola, 692 Ritchie Hwy. #100, Severna Park, MD, ph. 410-544-6168
21207, Univ. of Maryland Compl Med, 2200 Kernan Dr., Baltimore, MD, ph. 410 448 6871, fax 6875
21208-3905, Ronald Parks, MD, 3655B Old Court Rd #19, Baltimore, MD, ph. 410-486-5656
21209, Binyamin Rothstein, DO, 2835 Smith Ave. #203, Baltimore, MD, ph. 410-484-2121, fax -0338
21209-2023, Acupuncture Clinic, 6719 Newstead Lane, Baltimore, MD, ph. 410-823-7793, fax -7793
21211, Lisa P. Battle, MD, 3100 Wyman Park Dr., Baltimore, MD, ph. 410-338-3059
21403, Cheryl Brown-Christopher, MD, 1419 Forest Dr. #202, Annapolis, MD, ph. 410-268-5005
21742, Giselle Lai, ND, 1305 Pennsylvania Ave., Hagerstown, MD, ph. 301-714-0500
21742, Steven Sinclair, ND, 1305 Pennsylvania Ave., Hagerstown, MD, ph. 301-714-0500
21903, A.P. Cadous, MD, 2324 W. Joppa Rd. #100, Baltimore, MD, ph. 410-296-3737, fax -0650
22001, E. Abdelhalim, MD, Rt. 40 W, 39070 John Mosby Hwy. Aldie, VA, ph. 703-327-2434, fax -2729
22001, N. W. Levin, MD, Rt. 50 W. 39070 John Mosby Hwy. Aldie, VA, ph. 703-327-2434, fax -2729
22003, Andrew Baer, MD, 7023 Little River Turnpike, Annandale, VA, ph. 703-941-3606
22041, Sohini Patel, MD, 5201 Leesburg Pike #301, Falls Church, VA, ph. 703-845-8686, fax -2661
22041, Sophini P. Patel, MD, 5201 Leesburg Pike #301, Falls Church, VA, ph. 703-845-8686, fax -2661
22044, A.M. Rosemblat, MD, 6316 Castle Pl. #200, Falls Church, VA, ph. 703-241-8989, fax 532-6247
22070, Patrick J. McNally, DC, 150 Elden St. #210, Herndon, VA, ph. 703-481-1616, fax -3474
22070, Philip Golinsky, DC, 1110-D Elden St. #206, Herndon, VA, ph. 703-904-9666, fax 471-4548
22304, Marie Steinmetz, MD, 5249 Duke St. #309, Alexandria, VA., ph. 703-823-5770, fax -9394
22831, Harold E. Huffman, MD, PO Box 197, Hinton, VA, ph. 540-867-5242, fax -9381
22831, Harold Huffman, MD, P.O. Box 197, Hinton, VA, ph. 703-867-5242
22974, Helga Fallis, ND, PO Box 1065, Troy, VA, ph. 804-589-1668
23093, David G. Schwartz, MD, 101 Woolfolk Ave., Louisa, VA, ph. 540-967-2050, fax -1623
23093, David G. Schwartz, MD, P.O. Box 532, Louisa, VA, ph. 540-967-2050
23112, Peter C. Gent, DO, 11900 Hull St., Midlothian, VA, ph. 804-379-1345
23185, The HEALTH. Center, 487 McLaws Circle #1A, Williamsburg, VA, ph. 757-656-6363, fax - 6363
23451, Stephanie Story, ND, PO Box 1087, Virginia Beach, VA., ph. 757-428-7979
23452, Nelson M. Karp, MD, 460 S. Independence Blvd., Virginia Beach, VA, ph. 704-497-3439
23454, Robert A. Nash, MD, 921 First Colonial Rd. #1705, Virginia Beach, VA, ph. 804-422-1295
23462, Robert Nash, MD, 5589 Greenwich Rd. #175, Virginia Bch, VA, ph. 757-490-9311, fax -9266

23507, Vincent J. Speckhart, MD, 902 Graydon Ave., Norfolk, VA, ph. 757-622-0014, fax –9808
23507, Vincent Speckhart, MD, 902 Graydon Ave., Norfolk, VA, ph. 804-622-0014
23518, Med Acupuncture Clinic, 3607 N. Military Hwy., Norfolk, VA, ph. 757-853-7434, fax 855-5215
23970, Frederick C. Sturmer, Jr., MD, 416 Durant St., South Hill, VA, ph. 804-447-3162
24179, Ralph Greenway, DDS, 1246 Chestnut Mountain Dr., Vinton, VA, ph. 540-890-3665
24378, E. M. Cranton, MD, Ripshin Rd. - Box 44, Trout Dale, VA, ph. 540-677-3631, fax -3843
24378, Eduardo Castro, MD, 799 Ripshin Rd., Trout Dale, VA, ph. 540-677-3631, fax –3843
24378, W. C. Douglass, Jr. MD, Ripshin Rd. - Box 44, Trout Dale, VA, ph. 540-677-3631, fax -3843
25301, Steve M. Zekan, MD, 1208 Kanawha Blvd. E, Charleston, WV, ph. 304-343-7559
25601, R.L. Toparis, DO, 20 Hospital Dr. Doctors Park, Logan, WV, ph. 304-792-1662
25601, Thomas A. Horsman, MD, 20 Hospital Dr. Doctors Park, Logan, WV, ph. 304-792-1624
25801, Michael Kostenko, DO, 114 E. Main St., Beckley, WV, ph. 304-253-0591
25801, Prudencio Corro, MD, 251 Stanaford Rd., Beckley, WI, ph. 304-252-0775
26651, John R. Ray, DO, 3029 Webster Road, Summersville, WV, ph. 304-872-6583
27103, Walter Ward, MD, 1411 B Plaza West Rd., Winston Salem, NC, ph. 910-760-0240
27510, Dennis W. Fera, MD, 103 Weaver St., Carrboro, NC, ph. 919-933-4303, fax –4354
27510, Susan Delaney, ND, 301 Weaver St., Carrboro, NC, ph. 919-932-6262
27511, Joan Nielsen, MD, 875 Walnut St. #370, Cary, NC, ph. 919-467-3686, fax 469-2971
27512, Priscilla Evans, ND, PO Box 69, Cary, NC, ph. 919-604-2235
27513, Loghman Zaiim, MD, 1817 N. Harrison Ave., Cary, NC, ph. 919-677-8383, fax -8380
27607, John Pittman, MD, 4505 Fair Meadow Lane #211, Raleigh, NC, ph. 919-571-4391, fax -8968
27607, Preeta Kuhlman, ND, Blue Ridge Plaza #203, Raleigh, NC, ph. 919-781-3978
27607, Tim Kuhlman, ND, Blue Ridge Plaza #203, Raleigh, NC, ph. 919-781-3978
27609, NC Prev & Wellness Med Ctr., 4016 Barrett Dr. #210, Raleigh, NC, ph. 919-787-0084, fax -0170
27705, Integrated Health Care, 112 Smoft Ave., Ourham, NC, ph. 919-286-7755, fax -7754
27820, Bhaskar D. Power, MD, 1201 E. Littleton Road, Roanoke Rapids, NC, ph. 919-535-1411
27870, Gen. Hlth Ctr., 1201 E. Littletown Rd., Roanoke Rapids, NC, ph. 919-535-1412, fax 567-5000
28203, Jay Wrigley, ND, 1201 East Blvd., Charlotte, NC, ph. 704-332-1201
28210, S. Charlotte Chiro. Center, Inc. 10701 - G Park Rd., Charlotte, NC, ph. 704-544-8844, fax -8631
28226, Leang Eap, ND, 6548 Carmel Rd. #124, Charlotte, NC, ph. 704-544-8681
28315, Keith E. Johnson, MD, 1111 Quewhiffle, Aberdeen, NC, ph. 919-281-5122
28387, Keith E. Johnson, MD, 1852 US Hwy One South, Southern Pines, NC, ph. 910-695-0335
28604, Charles Wiley, MD, P.O. Box 307, Banner Elk, NC, ph. 704-898-6949, fax -6950
28677, John W. Wilson, MD, Plaza 21 North, Statesville, NC, ph. 704-876-1617
28677, Ron Rosedale, MD, Plaza 21 North, Statesville, NC, ph. 704-876-1617
28711, James Biddle, MD, 465 Crooked Creed Rd., Black Mountain, NC, ph. 704-669-7762, fax -4255
28801, Caroline Ctr. for Metabolic Med., 49 Zillicoa St., Asheville, NC, ph. 704-252-5545, fax 281-3055
28801, Greenspan Chiropractic Clinic, 261 Asheland Ave., Asheville, NC, ph. 704-252-1882, fax -1417
28801, Stephen Barrie, MD, 63 Zilicoa St., Asheville, NC, ph. 828-253-0621
28805, Mary James, ND, 27 Spring Hollow Circle, Asheville, NC, ph. 828-253-0621
28806, Eileen W. Wright, MD, 1312 Patton Ave., Asheville, NC, ph. 704-252-9833, fax 255-8118
28806, John Wilson, MD, 1312 Patton Ave., Asheville, NC, ph. 800-445-4762, fax 704-876-0640
28806, Ron Rosedale, MD, 1312 Patton Ave., Asheville, NC, ph. 800-445-4762, fax 704-876-0640
28806, Stephen Blievernicht, MD, 1312 Patton Ave., Asheville, NC, ph. 704-252-9833, fax 255-8118
29169, James M. Shortt, MD, SC, 2228 Airport Road, Columbia, SC, ph. 800-992-8350
29169, Theodore C. Rozema, MD, 2228 Airport Rd., Columbia, SC, ph. 800-992-8350
29304, Ctr. for Compl.Health & Ed., 404 Hope Mills Rd., Fayetteville, NC, ph. 910-423-4086, fax -2930
29336, Lad Santiago, DC, PO Box 755, Fairforest, SC, ph. 864-595-1395
29340, William King, DDS, 715 Logan St., Gaffney, SC, ph. 864-489-8921
29352, Ted Rozema, MD, 1000 Rutherford Rd., Landrum, SC, ph. 864-457-4141, fax –4144
29356, Scott Brand, DC,103 S. Poplar Ave., Landrum, SC, ph. 864-457-5124
29406, Arthur M. LaBruce, 9275-G Medical Plaza Dr., Charleston, SC, ph. 803-572-1771
29407, Palmetto Orthod & TMJ, 712 St. Andrews Blvd., Charleston, SC, ph. 803-556-8930, fax -0742
29412, Peter Kfoury, DC, 354 Folly Rd.#1, Charleston, SC, ph.803-795-9333
29418, Judy Kameoka, MD, 3815 W. Montague Ave. #200, Charleston, SC, ph. 803-760-0770
29420, Ctr. Occup & Env Med. 7510 Nortforest Dr., N. Charleston, SC, ph. 803-572-1600, fax -1795
29566, David Croland, DO, 4326 Baldwin Ave., Little River, SC, ph. 803-249-6755, fax -3323
29575, Donald W. Tice, DO, 4301 Dick Pond Rd., Myrtle Beach, SC, ph. 803-215-5000, fax -5005
29687, Albert S. Anderson, MD, 3110 Wade Hampton Blvd., Taylors, SC, ph. 864-244-9020, fax -9044
30014, Gloria Freundlich, DO, 4122 Tate St., Covington, GA, ph. 770-787-0880
30060, Ralph C. Lee, MD, 110 Lewis Dr. #B, Marietta, GA, ph. 770-423-0064, fax -9827
30080, M. Truett Bridges, Jr., 1751 Point Pleasant, Smyrna, GA, ph. 770-436-0209, fax 444-9596
30120, Steven Garber, DC, 861 JFH parkway, Cartersville, GA, ph. 770-386-7707, fax 387-2414
30130, James L. Bean, MD, 4575 Piney Grove Dr., Cuming, GA, ph. 770-887-9418
30240, CliniCare Medical Center, 302 S. Greenwood St., LaGrange, GA, ph. 706-884-8360
30247, Pleasant Hill Chiropractic Ctr, 830 Pleasant Hill Rd., Lilburn, GA, ph. 770-925-9955, 923-0200
30303, Lavonne M. Painter, MD, 99 Butler St. S.E., Atlanta, GA, ph. 404-730-1491

30306, John Davis, ND, 1241 Virginia Ave. NE #C-4, Atlanta, GA, ph. 404-325-7734
30307, David Epstine, DO, 427 Moreland Ave. #100, Atlanta, GA, ph. 404-525-7333, fax, 521-0084
30309, Piedmont Hospital, 1968 Peachtree Road, NW, Atlanta, GA, ph. 404-605-3319, fax -1702
30309, William E. Richardson, MD, 1718 Peachtree St. NW #552, Atlanta, GA, ph. 404-607-0570
30337, D. Robert Howard, MD, 1650 Virginia Ave., College Park, GA, ph. 404-761-9500, fax -6995
30338, Bernard Miaver, MD, 4480 N. Shallowford Rd., Atlanta, GA, ph. 770-395-1600
30341, Mark Stallman, MD, 3201 Henderson Mill Rd. #10A, Atlanta, GA, ph. 770-934-2993
30342, Stephen B. Edelson, MD, 3833 Roswell Rd., Atlanta, GA, ph. 404-841-0088, fax -6416
30360, Milton Fried, MD, 4426 Tilly Mill Rd., Atlanta, GA, ph. 770-451-4857, fax 404-451-8492
30503, Kathryn Herndon, MD, 530 Spring St., Gainesville, GA, ph. 404-503-7222
30525, William J. Lee, MD, P.O. Box 229, Clayton, GA, ph. 706-782-4044
30701, Patricia Tygrett, DO, P.O. Box 1988, Calhoon, GA, ph. 706-625-5204
31088, Terril J. Schneider, MD, 205 Central Dr. #19, Warner Robins, GA, ph. 912-929-1027
31201, James T. Alley, MD, 380 Hospital Dr. #125, Macon, GA, ph. 912-745-1575, -1974
31322, Carlos Tan, MD, 4 Pooler Prof. Plaza, Pooler, GA, ph. 912-748-6631
31416, Joseph Marshall, DC, 411 Stephenson Ave., Savannah, GA, ph. 912-352-4832, fax -4833
31525, Ralph G. Ellis Jr., MD, 3945 Darien Hwy, Brunswick, GA, ph. 912-280-0304, fax -0601
31701-1875, Thomas C. Paschal, MD, 715 W. Third Ave., Albany, GA, ph. 912-438-9002
31730, Olive Gunter, MD, 24 N. Ellis St., Camilla, GA, ph. 912-336-7343, fax -7400
32084, St. Augustine Phys As. 419-A Anastasia Blvd., St. Augustine, FL, ph. 904-824-8353, fax -5705
32134, George Graves, DO, 11512 Country Road 316, Ft. McCoy, FL, ph. 352-236-2525, fax -8610
32159, Nelson Kraucak, MD, 8923 N.E. 134th Ave., Lady Lake, FL, ph. 904-750-4333
32174, Hana T. Chaim, DO, 595 W. Granada Blvd. #D, Ormond Beach, FL, ph. 904-672-9000
32216, John Mauriello, MD, 4063, Salisbury Road #206, Jacksonville, FL, ph. 904-296-0900, fax -8346
32216, Stephen Grable, MD, 4205 Belfort Rd. #3075, Jacksonville, FL, ph. 904-296-4977
32244, Psychotherapy Center, 6037 Longchamp Dr., Jacksonville, FL, ph. 904-771-8934
32250, Beaches Healthcare Center, 831-C N. Third St., Jacksonville Beach, FL, ph. 904-241-9680
32257, Mandarin Chiro. Ctr, 9891-2 San Jose Blvd. #2, Jacksonville, FL, ph. 904-262-8600, fax -3899
32317, Royce V. Jackson, MD, 1630-A N. Plaza Dr., Tallahassee, FL, ph. 904-656-8846, fax 671-2921
32405, James W. DeRuiter, MD, 2202 State Ave #311, Panama City, FL, ph. 904-747-4963, fax -1271
32405, Naima Abdel-Ghany, MD, PhD, 340 W. 23rd St. #E, Panama City, FL, ph. 904-763-7689
32524, Ward Dean, MD, P.O. Box 11097, Pensacola, FL, ph. 904-484-0595
32570, William Watson, MD, 5536 Stewart St. N.W., Milton, FL, ph. 904-623-3863, fax -2201
32605, G. G. Feussner, MD, 6717 N.W. 11th Pl. #D, Gainesville, FL, ph. 352-331-7303, fax 332-8732
32605, Leonard Smith, MD, 720 SW 2nd Ave. #202, Gainesville, FL, 352-378-6262, fax -0779
32646, Carlos F. Gonzales, MD, 7991 S. Suncoast Blvd., Homosasso, FL, ph. 352-382-8282
32708, Peter D. Hsu, DO, 116 W. SR 434, Winter Springs, FL, ph. 407-327-3322, fax -3324
32714, W. Clinic, 195 S. Westmonte Dr. #'s H I I, Altamonte Springs, FL, ph 407-862-8834, fax -5951
32716, Peter D. Hsu, DO, 1650 Ocean Shore Blvd., Ormond, Beach, FL, ph. 904-441-1477
32746, Campbell Douglass III, MD, 101 Timberlachen Circle #101, Lake Mary, FL, ph. 407-324-0888
32750, Bixon Chiropractic Center, 242 W. Hwy 434, Longwood, FL, ph. 407-834-2226
32750, Donald Colbert, MD, 1908 Boothe Cl., Longwood, FL, ph. 407-331-7007, fax -5777
32751, Eileen M. Wright, MD, 340 N. Maitland Ave. #100, Maitland, FL, ph. 407-740-6100
32751, Jack E. Young, MD, 341 N. Maitland Ave. #200, Maitland, FL, ph. 407-644-2729, fax -1205
32751, Joya L. Schoen, MD, 341 Maitland Ave. #200, Maitland, FL, ph. 407-644-2729, fax -1205
32763, Travis L. Herring, MD, 106 W. Fern Dr., Orange City, FL, ph. 904-775-0525, fax -3911
32765, Roy Kupsinel, 1325 Shangri-La Lane, Oviedo, FL, ph. 407-365-6681, fax 1834
32778, David Frerking, DC, 915 E. Alfred St., Tavares, FL, ph.352-343-9275
32778, James Coy, MD, 204 Texas Ave., Tavares, FL, ph. 904-742-7344
32789, James Parsons, MD, 8303 2699 Lee Rd., Winter Park, FL, ph. 407-528-3399
32792, Center Altern. Ther, 305 N. Lakemont Ave., Winter Park, FL, ph. 407-647-0077, fax -1923
32803, Inst. Pain Care & Fmly Hlth, 2224 E. Concord St., Orlando, FL, ph. 407-896-3005, fax -3066
32803, Humberto N. Arias, MD, 604 N. Bumby St., Orlando, FL, ph. 407-894-3050
32803, Way to Natural Health, 500 N. Mills Ave., Orlando, FL, ph. 407-841-4581, fax 843-2342
32804, Kenneth Hoover, MD, 2909 N. Orange Ave. #108, Orlando, FL, ph. 407-897-6002
32901, Rajiv Chandra, MD, 20 E. Melbourne Ave., Melbourne, FL, ph. 407-951-7404, fax -1610
32903, Glen Wagner, MD, 121 6th Ave., Indialantic, FL, ph. 407-723-5915, fax 724-0287
32907, Neil Ahner, MD, 1663 Georgia St., Palm Buy, FL, ph. 407-729-8581, fax -6079
32953, James Parsons, MD, 5 Minna Lane #201, Merritt Island, FL, ph. 407-452-0332
32958, C. Health Innovations, P.A., 600 Schumann Dr., Sebastian, FL, ph. 561-388-5554, fax -2410
32958, Peter Holyk, MD, 680 Jordan Ave., Sebastian, FL, ph. 407-388-1222
32960, John Song, MD, 1360 U.S. 1 #1, Vero Beach, FL, ph. 904-569-3566
33009, Phys Med S, 1140 E. Hallandale Beach Blvd. #A, Hallandale, FL, ph. 954-456-1311, fax -1473
33020, Herbert Padell, DO, 210 S. Federal Hwy. #302, Hollywood, FL, 954-922-0470, fax 921-5555
33020, S. Marshall Fram, MD, 1425 Arthur St. #211, Hollywood, FL, ph. 954-925-3140
33026, Eric Rosenkrantz, MD, 1551 N. Palm Ave., Pembroke Pines, FL, ph. 954-432-8511
33063, Keith Latham, Lac, 2650 Aloe Avenue, Coconut Creek, FL, ph. 954-973-7880

33064, Anthony J. Sancetta, DO, 3450 Park Central Blvd. N., Pompano Beach, FL, ph. 954-977-3700
33064, D Roehm, MD, 3400 Park Central Blvd. N. #3450, Pompano Bch, FL, ph. 305-977-3700, -0180
33064, Fariss D. Kimbell, Jr., MD, 3450 Park Central Blvd. N., Pompano Beach, FL, ph. 305-977-3700
33133, Victor A. Marcial-Vega, MD, 4037 Poinciana Ave., Miami, FL, ph. 305-442-1233, fax 445-4504
33134, Maria Vega, MD, 2916 Douglas Rd., Coral Gables, FL, ph. 304-442-1233
33139, Perfect Health Center, 901 Pennsylvania Ave. #203, Miami Beach, FL, ph. 305-538-1064
33155, Herbert Pardell, DO, 7980 Coral Way, Miami, FL, ph. 305-267-5790, fax -5855
33160, Martin Dayton, MD, 18600 Collins Ave., N. Miami beach, FL, ph. 305-931-8484, fax 936-1845
33162, S DiMauro, MD, 16666 N.E. 19th Ave. #101, N. Miami Bch, FL, ph. 305-940-4848
33176, Ear, Nose & Throat, 9805 WE 87th Ave., Stanley Cannon, MD, ph. 305-279-3020, fax -1751
33176, Joseph G. Godorov, DO, 9055 S.W. 87th Ave. #307, Miami, FL, ph. 305-595-0671
33179, Med Ctr, 1380 NE Miami Gardens Dr. #225, N. Miami Bch, FL, 305-949-4259, fax -947-2713
33179, Don S. Poster, MD, 1380 NE Miami Gardens Dr. #235, N. Miami Beach, FL, ph. 954-432-4518
33180, Herbert Pardell, DO, 19044 NE 29 Ave., Aventura, FL, ph. 305-705-0345, fax –0437
33180, Ntrl Hlth Institutes America, 19044 NE 29th Ave., Aventura, FL, ph. 305-705-0345, fax -0437
33304, Adam Frent, DO, 2583 E. Sunrise Blvd., Ft. Lauderdale, FL, ph. 313-425-0235, fax -9003
33314, Jonah Botknecht, DO, 6200 Stirling Rd, Davie, FL, ph. 954-964-6774
33316, Bruce Dooley, MD, 500 S.E. 17th St., Fort Lauderdale, FL, ph. 305-527-9355, fax -4167
33316, Malik Ahmad, MD, 1525 S. Andrews Ave #9, Ft. Lauderdale, FL, ph. 954-522-7111, fax –3422
33319, Arthritis Consulting Serv., 4620 N. State St. Rd 7 #206, Ft. Lauderdale, FL, ph. 800-327-3027
33319, Inst Med, 7200 W. Commercial Blvd. #210, Ft Lauderdale, FL, ph. 954-748-4991, fax -5022
33334, Bern. Chiro Ctr., 997 E. Oakland Park Blvd., Ft. Lauderdale, FL, ph. 954-565-4440, fax -5312
33401, Ember Carianna, ND, 1900 S. Olive Ave., W. Palm Beach, FL, ph. 561-835-6821
33406, J Medlock, DDS, 2326 S. Congress Ave. #1D, W. Palm Beach, FL, ph. 561-439-4620, fax -6704
33409, A. Court, MD, 2260 Palm Bch Lakes Blvd. #213, W Palm Bch, FL, ph. 561-684-8137,
33432, R. Willix, Jr. MD, 1515 S. Federal Hwy. #306, Boca Raton, FL, ph. 561-362-0724, fax -9924
33461, S. Pinsley, DO, 2290 - 10th Ave. N. #605, Lake Worth, FL, ph. 407-547-2264, fax 220-7332
33477, Neil Ahner, MD, 1080 E. Indiantown Rd., Jupiter, FL, ph. 407-744-0077, fax -0094
33486, Eric Hermansen, MD, 951 N.W. 13th St. #4B, Boca Raton, FL, ph. 407-392-4920, fax -4979
33487, A. Sancetta, DO, 7300 N. Federal Hwy. #104, Boca Raton, FL. ph. 800-995-9453
33487, L. Haimes, MD, 7300 N. Federal Hwy. #107, Boca Raton, FL, ph. 407-994-3868, fax 997-8998
33510, Carol Roberts, MD, 1209 Lakeside Dr., Brandon, FL, ph. 813-661-3662
33556, Bay Area Psy. Consultants, 13949 Friendship Ln, Odessa, FL, ph. 813-920-3014, fax 376-0078
33603, Edwin Muniz, NMD, 4809 N. Armedia Ave. #221, Tampa, FL, ph. 813-877-0427, fax 685-1992
33606, Eugene Lee, MD, 1804 W. Kennedy Blvd. #1, Tampa, FL, ph. 813-251-3089, fax -5668
33613, J. Ethridge, MD, 13615 Bruce Downs Blvd. #113, Tampa, FL, ph. 813-971-9850, fax -9817
33629, D. Carrow, MD, 3902 Henderson Blvd. #206, Tampa, FL, ph. 813-832-3220, fax 282-1132
33702, Ray Wunderlich, MD, 1152 94th Ave. N., St. Petersburg, FL, ph. 813-822-3612, fax -578-1370
33733, Intl Institute Reflexology, 5650-1st Ave. N., St. Petersburg, FL, ph. 813-343-4811, fax 381-2807
33743, Daniel S. Stein, MD, P.O. Box 49072, St. Petersburg, FL, ph. 813-864-6116
33760, Donald J. Carrow, MD, 4908-A Creekside Dr., Clearwater, FL, ph. 813-573-3775, fax –4489
33803, S. Todd Robinson, MD, 4406 S. Florida Ave. #30, Lakeland, FL, ph. 941-646-5088
33813, Robinson Family Clinic, 4406 S. Florida Ave., Lakeland, FL, ph. 941-646-5088, fax -7534
33907, Alters Chiro. & Natural Health Ctr., 33 Barkley Cl., Ft. Myers, FL, ph. 941-939-7645, fax -2644
33912, Gary L. Pynckel, DO, 3840 Colonial Blvd. #1, Ft. Myers, FL, ph. 941-278-3337, fax –3702
33937, Richard Saitta, MD, 1010 N. Barfield Dr., Marco Island, FL, ph. 813-642-8488
33940, David Perlmutter, MD, 800 Goodlette Road N. #270, Naples, FL, ph. 813-262-8971
33940, Myron B. Lezak, MD, 800 Goodlette Road N. #270, Naples, FL, ph. 941-649-7400, fax -6370
33948, James Dussault, ND, 1720 El Jobean Rd., Port Charlotte, FL, ph. 941-255-3988
33980, Health Altern. Inc., 22959 Bayshore Road, Port Charlotte, FL, ph. 941-766-1800, fax 255-0009
34102, Myron B. Lezak, MD, 800 Goodlette Rd. #270, Naples, FL, ph. 941-649-7400, fax –6370
34103, Joel Ferdinand Lopez, MD, 4035 10 St. N., Naples, FL, ph. 941-434-8853, fax –7311
34205, J. Ossorio, MD, 101 River Front Blvd. #150, Bradenton, FL, ph. 941-748-8704, fax 741-8066
34207, Center for Holsitic Medicine, 810 53d Ave. West, Bradenton, FL, ph. 941-727-7722, fax -7711
34208, Eteri Melnikov, MD, 116 Manatee Ave. East, Bradenton, FL, ph. 941-748-7943
34236, Thomas McNaughton, MD, 1521 Dolphin St., Sarasota, FL, ph. 941-965-6273, 365-4269
34239, Joseph Ossorio, MD, 2345 Bee Ridge Rd #5, Sarasota, FL, ph. 941-921-1412
34285, James A.L. Dussault, ND, 200 N. Tamaimi Trail, Venice, FL, ph. 941-496-8187, fax 627-4230
34429, Azeal Borromeo, MD, 700 S.E. 5th Terrace #7, Crystal River, FL, 904-795-4711, fax -7559
34471, John Podlaski, DC, 2721 SE 23rd Ave., Ocala, FL, ph.352-867-1015
34601, Holistic Health Clinic of Brooksville, 10443 N. Broad St., Brookville, FL, ph. 352-544-0047
34652, Michael H. Beilan, DO, 5211 U.S. Hwy. 19 N #200, New Port Richey, FL, ph. 813-842-3111
34683, Palm Harbor Ctr for Funct. Med, 2939 Alt. 19 N., Palm Harbor, FL, ph. 813-787-0706, fax -0734
34684, Glenn Chapman, MD, 34621 U.S. Hwy. #19-N, Palm Harbor, FL, ph. 813-786-1661
34695, Ctr. Holistic Medicine, 105 N. Bayshore Dr., Safety Harbor, FL, ph. 813-724-0135, fax -0129
34952, Ricardo V. Barbaza, MD, 1874 SE Port St. Lucie Blvd., Port St. Lucie, FL, ph. 561-335-4994
34972, Muzaffar Husain, MD, 1300 N. Parrott Ave., Okeechobee, FL, ph. 941-763-8000, fax –8212

34977, Sherri W. Pinsley, DO, 7000 SE Federal Hwy #302, Stuart, FL, ph. 407-220-1697
34994, Jason P. Schwartz, DC, 915 E. Ocean Blvd. #2, Stuart, FL, ph. 800-749-3651, fax 561-286-2649
34994, Neil Ahmer, MD, 705 N. Federal Hwy., Stuart, FL, ph. 407-692-9200, fax -9888
35226, Gus J. Prosch, Jr., MD, 759 Valley St., Birmingham, AL, ph. 205-823-6180, fax -6000
35661, Deborah Carter, ND, 503 State St. #3, Muscle Shoals, AL, ph. 256-386-9858
35801, George Gray, MD, 521 Madison St. #100, Huntsville, AL, ph. 205-534-1676, fax -0926
36117, Teresa Allen, DO, 7203 Copperfield Dr., Montgomery, AL, ph. 334-273-0904, fax -0905
36251, Robert B. Andrews, Jr., DO, 544 E. First Ave., Ashland, AL, ph. 205-354-2131
36547, New Beginnings Med. Grp., 1404 W. 1st St., Gulf Shores, AL, ph. 334-968-6515, fax -6756
36818, Pravinchandra Patel, MD, P.O. Drawer DD, Coldwater, MS, ph. 601-622-7011
37087, William Strauss, DC, 115 Castle Heights Ave. N., Lebanon, TN, 615-444-5335
37205, Stephen L. Reisman, MD, 28 White Bridge Rd., Nashville, TN, ph. 615-356-4244, fax -9741
37303, H. Joseph Holliday, MD, 1005 W. Madison Ave., Athens, TN, ph. 423-744-7540
37311, Cleveland Care First, 1995 Keith St, NW, Cleveland, TN, ph. 423-472-2273
37404, William B. Findley, MD, 1404 Dodds Ave., Chattanooga, TN, ph. 423-622-5113
37405, Robert Burkich, MD, 707 Signal Mtn. Rd., Chattanooga, TN, ph. 423-266-4474, fax -4464
37415, Charles C. Adams, MD, 3739 Hixson Pike, Chattanooga, TN, ph. 423-875-0999, fax 825-6875
37862, Ratcliff Chiropractic Office, 826 Middle Creek Rd., Sevierville, TN, ph. 615-453-1390
37923, James Carlson, DO, 509 N. Cedar Bluff Rd., Knoxville, TN, ph. 423-691-2961
38024, Lynn A. Warner, MD, 503 E. Tickel #3, Dyersburg, TN, ph. 901-285-4910
38119, Jerre Minor Freeman, MD, 6485 Poplar Ave., Memphis, TN, ph. 901-278-4432
38774, Robert Hollingsworth, MD, 901 Forrest St., Selby, MS, ph. 601-398-5106
39128, Internal Med Specialists, 201 N. Buffalo Dr., Las Vegas, NV, ph. 702-242-2737, fax 255-3170
39564, James H. Waddell, MD, 1520 Government St., Ocean Springs, MS, ph. 601-875-5505
40059, Kirk D. Morgan, MD, 9105 US Hwy 42, Prospect, KY, ph. 502-228-0156, fax -0512
40207, Eye Disease Prevention Task Force, 902 Dupont Rd. #200, Louisville, KY, ph. 800-852-7540
40222, Inner Light Consultants, Inc., 305 N. Lyndon Lane, Louisville, KY, ph. 502-429-8835, fax -8835
40391, Dewitt Garrett, DC, 221 Al Fan Ct., Winchester, KY, ph. 606-737-0529
40403, Edward K. Atkinson, MD, 448 Calico Rd., Berea, KY, ph. 606-925-2252
42025, 42025, Charles Leon Bolton, DC, 200 E. 12th St., Benton, KY, ph. 502-527-0994, fax -0994
42101, John C. Tapp, MD, 414 Old Morgantown Rd., Bowling Green, KY, ph. 502-781-1483
42501, Stephen S. Kiteck, MD, 600 Bogle St., Somerset, KY, ph. 606-677-0459
43017, Donn Griffith, NMD, 3859 W. Dublin-Granville Rd., Dublin, OH, ph. 614-889-2556
43065, William D. Mitchell, DO, 10401 Sawmill Parkway, Powell, OH, ph. 614-761-0555
43068, Active Life Family Chiro. Center, 7509 E. Main St. #104, Reynoldsburg, OH, ph. 614-866-5158
43220, M. Ayur-Veda, 3250 W. Henderson Rd. #202, Columbus, OH, ph. 614-451-0677, 293-5984
43224, David C. Korn, DO, 3278 Maize Rd., Columbus, OH, ph. 614-268-6170
43230, P. Chiro, Hunter's Ridge Mall, 336 S. Hamilton Rd, Gahanna, OH, ph. 614-471-5442, fax -5462
43348, Paul Bonetzky, DO, One Aries Ctr., Russels Point, OH, ph. 513-843-5000
43537, Elizabeth C. Christenson, MD, 219 W. Wayne St., Maymee, OH, ph. 419-893-8438, fax -1465
43623, James C. Roberts, Jr., MD, 4607 Sylvania Ave., Toledo, OH, ph. 419-882-9620, fax -9628
44052, Robert Stevens, DO, 2160 Reid Ave., Lorain, OH, ph. 216-246-3993
44060, Concord Chiropractic, 9841 Johnnycake Ridge Road, Mentor, OH, ph. 216-354-6767, fax -6919
44094, L. M. Porter, MD, 36001 Euclid Ave. #A-10, Willoughby, OH, ph. 216-942-5838, fax -1337
44113, Robert B. Casselberry, MD, 2132 W. 25th St., Cleveland, OH, ph. 216-771-5855, fax -4534
44124, Pain Relief & Med. Health Ctr., 5576 Mayfield Rd., Lyndhurst, OH, ph. 216-460-1880, fax -1832
44130, Radha Baishnab, MD, 7225 Old Oak Park Blvd. #2B, Cleveland, OH, ph. 216-234-8080
44131, John M. Baron, DO, 4807 Rockside Rd. #100, Cleveland, OH, ph. 216-642-0082, fax -1415
44145, Derrick Lonsdale, MD, 24700 Center Ridge Rd. #317, Westlake, OH, ph. 440-835-0104
44145, Douglas Weeks, MD, 24700 Ctr Ridge Rd, Cleveland, OH, ph. 216-835-0104, fax 871-1404
44145, James P. Frackelton, MD, 24700 Center Ridge Rd. #317, Westlake, OH, ph. 440-835-0104
44313, Josephine C. Aronica, MD, 1867 W. Market St., Akron, OH, ph. 330-867-7361, fax 869-7392
44320, Francis J. Waickman, MD, 544 "B" White Point Dr., Akron, OH, ph. 216-867-3767, fax -4857
44410, John L. Baumeier, DO, Inc., 1645 State Rte. 5, Cortland, OH, ph. 330-638-3026, fax -3704
44425, James P. Dambrogio, DO, 212 N. Main St., Hubbard, OH, ph. 216-534-9737, fax -9739
44460, William Z. Kolozsi, MD, 2380 Southeast Blvd., Salem, OH, ph. 216-337-1152
44511, J. Ventresco, Jr., DO, 3848 Tippecanee Road, Youngstown, OH, ph. 330-792-2349, fax -6415
44709, Robert C. Purdy, DPM, 206 21st St. NW, Canton, OH, ph. 330-455-6419, fax -6427
44718, Jack E. Slingluff, DO, 5850 Fulton Rd., NW, Canton, OH, ph. 330-494-8641
45231, Holistic Health Ctr., 800 Compton Rd #24, Cincinnati, OH, ph. 513-521-5333, fax -5334
45241, Ted Cole, DO, 9678 Cincinnati-Columbus Rd., Cincinnati, OH, ph. 513-779-0300
45244, David C. Black, DC, 502 Old St. Rt. 74, Cincinnati, OH, ph. 513-528-6112, fax -6112
45246, Leonid Macheret, MD, 375 Glensprings, Dr. #400, Cincinnati, OH, ph. 513-851-8790
45380, Charles W. Platt, MD, 552 South West St., Versailles, OH, ph. 513-526-3271
45410, Gary A. Dunlop, DO, 2640 St. Charles Ave., Dayton, OH, ph. 937-253-6741, fax -2431
45459, John Boyles, MD, 7076 Corporate Way, Centerville, OH, ph. 937-438-2909, fax 434-7413
45505, Narinder K. Saini, MD, 1911 E. High St., Springfield, OH, ph. 513-325-1155

45742, Essence of Life Ministries, Rt. 1, Box 172, Little Hocking, OH, ph. 614-989-2300
45817, Jay Nielsen, MD, 122 Thurman St. #248, Bluffton, OH, ph. 419-358-4627, fax -1855
45817, L. Terry Chappell, MD, 122 Thurman St., Bluffton, OH, ph. 419-358-4627, fax -1855
45879, Don K. Snyder, MD 11573 State Route 11, Paulding, OH, ph. 419-399-2045
46077, Robert C. Brooksby, DO, 1500 W. Oak St. #400, Zionsville, IN, ph. 317-873-3321
46131, Merrill Wesemann, MD, 251 E. Jefferson, Franklin, IN, ph. 317-736-6121
46158, Norman E. Whitney, DO, 492 S. Indiana St., Mooresville, IN, ph. 317-831-3352
46208, Gary L. Moore, MD, 3351 N. Meridian St. #202, Indianapolis, IN, ph. 317-923-8978, fax -8982
46220, Laurence Webster, MD, 6801 Lake Plaza Dr. Ste. B-208, Indianapolis, IN, ph. 317-841-9046
46227, David A. Darbo, MD, 2124 E. Hanna Ave., Indianapolis, IN, ph. 317-787-7221
46236-8923, Kevin Cantwell, MD, 11715 Fox Rd. #400-227, Indianapolis, IN, ph. 317-870-9360
46250, David A. Darbro, MD, 7168 Graham Rd. #180, Indianapolis, IN, ph. 317-913-3000, fax -1000
46322, Cal Streeter, DO, 9635 Saric Ct., Highland, IN, ph. 219-924-2410, fax -9079
46383, Brian McGuckin, DC, 3201 N. Calumet, Valparaiso, IN, ph.219-531-1234
46383, Myrna D. Trowbridge, DO, 850 - C Marsh St., Valparaiso, IN, ph. 219-462-3377
46385, Myrna D. Trowbridge, DO, 850-C Marsh St., Valparaiso, IN, ph. 219-462-3377, fax 464-4530
46404, Family Medicine & Wellness Ctr., 3300 W. 15th Ave., Gary, IN, ph. 219-944-3100, fax, 3110
46514, Douglas W. Elliott, MD, 1506 Osolo Rd. #A, Elkhart, IN, ph. 219-264-9635
46601, Anne L. Kempf, DC, 1202 Lincoln Way East, South Bend, IN, ph. 219-232-5892, fax 237-0910
46601, Keim T. Houser, MD, 515 N. Lafayette, Blvd., South Bend, IN, ph. 219-232-2037
46616, David E. Turner, DO, 336 W. Navarre St., South Bend, IN, ph. 219-233-3840
46703, Tri-State Chiropractic Clinic, 2014 N. Wayne St., Angola, IN, ph. 219-665-3106
46750, Huntington General Practice, 941 E. Etna Ave., Huntington, IN, ph. 219-356-9400, fax 356-4254
46805, Joseph P. Fiacable, MD, 2426 Lake Avenue, Fort Wayne, IN, ph. 219-423-3304
46962, Marvin D. Dziabis, MD, 300 W. Seventh St., North Manchester, IN, ph. 219-569-2274
47129, George M. Wolverton, MD, 647 Eastern Blvd., Clarksville, IN, ph. 812-282-4309, fax 283-8299
47130, George Wolverton, MD, 647 Eastern Blvd., Clarksville, IN, ph. 812-282-4309
47355, David Chopra, MD, P.O. Box 636, Lynn, IN, ph. 317-874-2411
47394, Oscar Ordonex, MD, 400 S. Oak, Winchester, IN, ph. 317-584-6600
47714, Harold T. Sparks, DO, 3001 Washington Ave., Evansville, IN, ph. 812-479-8228, fax -7327
48017, Gurudarshan S. Khalsa, MD, 450 S. Main St., Clawson, MI, ph. 248-288-9200
48018, Albert J. Scarchilli, DO, 30275 13 Mile Rd., Farmington Hills, MI, ph. 810-626-7544
48043, June DeStefano, DO, 263 5B Gratiot, Mt. Clemens, MI, ph. 810-465-7514
48080, Adam Frent, DO, 23550 Harper Ave., St. Clair Shores, MI, ph. 810-779-5700, fax -9296
48094, James Ziobron, DO, 58060 Van Dyke, Washington, MI, ph. 810-781-6523
48103, Lynn J. Chandler, PhD, 3599 Delhi Overlook, Ann Arbor, MI, ph. 313-663-7616
48104, Glenn Miller, DC, 1054 S. Main St., Ann Arbor, MI, ph. 313-995-2124
48104, Suzie Zick, ND, 111 N. First, Ste. 1, Ann Arbor, MI, ph. 734-994-6315
48176, John G. Ghuneim, MD, 420 Russell #204, Saline, MI, ph. 313-429-2581, fax -3955
48188, Jarmina Ramirez-Salcedo, MD, 2038 Otter Pond Ln., Canton, MI, ph. 313-397-5842
48203, E. M. Gidney, MD, 12850 Woodward Ave., Highland park, MI, ph. 313-869-5070, fax -5072
48304, Med. Ctr., 1520 N. Wdward Ave.#210, Bloomfield Hills, MI, 888-264-8211, fax 810-203-0321
48310, AlternaCare, PC, 37300 Dequindre #201, Sterling Heights, MI, ph. 810-268-0228
48322, Ellen Kahn, PhD, 7001 Orchard Lake Road #330A, West Bloomfield, MI, ph. 248-737-8780
48331, Farmington Med Ctr., 30275 W. 13 Mile Rd., Farmington Hills, MI, ph. 810-626-7544, fax -9698
48334, Mary E. Short, DO, 30275 13 Mile Rd., Farmington Hills, MI, ph. 810-626-7544
48345, Wahagn Agbabian, DO, PC, 28 N. Saginaw #1105, Pontiac, MI, ph. 248-334-2424, fax -2924
48346, Nedra Downing, DO, 5639 Sashabaw Rd., Clarkston, MI, ph. 810-625-6677, fax -5633
48451, Marvin D. Penwell, DO, 319 S. Bridge St., Linden, MI, ph. 313-735-7809
48451, Thomas A. Padden, DO, 16828 Bridge St., Linden, MI, ph. 313-432-1010, fax -9080
48532, Preventive and Family Care Ctr., 1044 Gilbert St., Flint, MI, ph. 810-733-3140, fax -5623
48532, The Fatigue Clinic of Michigan, G-3494 Beecher Rd, Flint, MI, ph. 810-230-7855
48532, William M. Bernard, DO, 1044 Gilbert St., Flint, MI, ph. 810-733-3140
48706, Parveen A. Malik, MD, 808 N. Euclid Ave., Bay City, MI, ph. 517-686-3760
48838, Longevity Ctr. of W. Michigan, 420 S. Lafayette, Greenville, MI, ph. 616-754-3679, fax -8968
48910, Dallas Chiropractic Clinic, 1505 W. Holmes Rd., Lansing, MI, ph. 517-882-0251
49004, Eric Born, DO, 100 Maple St., Parchment, MI, ph. 616-344-6183
49085, Jagir S. Judge, MD, 2550 Niles Rd., St. Joseph, MI, ph. 616-429-1085, fax -2202
49201, J. Daniel Clifford, MD, 300 W. Washington #270, Jackson, MI, ph. 517-787-9510
49240, Grass Lake Med Ctr., 12337 E. Michigan Ave., Grass Lake, MI, ph. 517-522-8403, fax -4275
49512, Tammy Geurkink-Born, DO, 3700 52nd St. SE, Grand Rapids, MI; ph 616-656-3700, fax -3701,
49709, Atlanta Medical Clinic, 12394 State St., Atlanta, MI, ph. 517-785-4254, fax -2273
49870, F. Michael Saigh, MD, 411 Murray Rd W. U.S. 2, Norway, MI, ph. 906-563-9600
50124, Ballard Chiropractic Office, 602 Main St. #370, Huxley, IA, ph. 515-597-3636
50314, Jacqueline Stoken, MD, DO, 411 Laurel #3300, Des Moines, IA, ph. 515-247-8400
50501, Calisesi Chiropractic Clinic, 24 S. 14th St., Ft. Dodge, IA, ph. 515-576-2183, fax -2336
51105, Horst G. Blume, MD, 700 Jennings St., Sioux City, IA, ph. 712-252-4386

52157, Gary Bowden, DC, Box C, McGregor, IA, ph.319-873-3404
52402, Robert J. Klein, DO, 1652 42nd St. NE, Cedar Rapids, IA, ph. 319-395-0223
52807, David Nebbeling, DO, 622 E. 38th St., Davenport, IA, ph. 319-391-0321, fax -5741
53018, Carol Ucbclacker, MD, 1760 Milwaukee St., Delafield, WI, ph. 414-646-4600, fax -4215
53027, Edward G. Holtman, DC, 315 S. Sumner St., Hartford, WI, ph. 414-673-5650
53186, Donald Bergman, DC, 161 W. Sunset Dr., Waukesha, WI, ph. 414-549-0606, fax -9121
53218, Milwaukee Pain Clinic, 6529 W. Fond du Lac Ave., Milwaukee, WI, ph. 414-464-7246
53226, J. Robertson, Jr. DO, 1011 N. Mayfair Rd. #301, Milwaukee, WI, ph. 414-302-1011, fax -1010
53226, Jerry N. Yee, DO, 2505 N. Mayfair Rd., Milwaukee, WI, ph. 414-258-6282
53226, Robert R. Stocker, DO, 2505 N. Mayfair Rd., Milwaukee, WI, ph. 414-258-5522
53965, Robert S. Waters, MD, 320 Race St., Wisconsin Delle, WI, ph. 608-254-7178, fax 253-7139
54022, Diane Diegel, Lac, 186 County Road U, River Falls, WI, ph. 715-425-0333, fax -2273
54311, Eleazar M. Kadile, MD, 1538 Bellevue St., Green Bay, WI, ph. 920-468-9442, fax -9714
54456, Bahri O. Grungor, MD, 216 Sunset Pl., Neillsville, WI, ph. 715-743-3101
54521, Kevin Branham, DC, 5680 Cloverland Dr., Eagle River, WI, ph.715-479-9066
54601, Lifespring Health Service, 216 S. 23rd St., La Crosse, WI, ph. 608-785-0038, fax -0038
54759, Bernie Finch, DC, 9410 Cedar Dr., Pepin, WI, ph.715-442-2016
54806, Craig Gilbaugh, DC, 1022 Lake Shore Dr.E., Ashland, WI, ph. 715-682-5333
55082, Sandra Spore, DC, 14727 N. 60th St., Stillwater, MN, ph.651-439-1013
55102, Helen Healy, ND, 905 Jefferson Ave. #202, St. Paul, MN, ph. 612-222-4111
55102, Phyllis Goldin, MD, 311 Ramsey, St. Paul, MN, ph. 612-227-3067
55104, Amrit Devgun, ND, 658 Selby Ave., Second Floor, St. Paul, MN, ph. 612-227-1803
55405, Wiliam Lyden, DC, 2526 Hennepin Ave. S., Minneapolis, MN, ph.612-374-5332
55407, John Hauser, ND, 3016 Portland Ave., Minneapolis, MN, ph. 612-824-7585
55410, Andrew Lucking, ND, 5032 Xerxes Ave. S., Minneapolis, MN, ph. 612-926-1549
55431, Johnathon Williams, DC, 2501 W. 84th St., Bloomington, MN, ph.612-888-4777
55441, Jean Eckerly, MD, 10700 Old County Rd. 15, Minneapolis, MN, ph. 612-593-9458, fax –0097
55441, M. Dole, MD, 10700 Old Country Rd 15 #350, Minneapolis, MN, ph. 612-593-9458, fax -0097
55805, Duluth Clinic, 400 E. 3rd St., Duluth, MN, ph. 218-722-8364, fax 725-3067
56303, Karla Lilleberg, ND, 1521 Nothway Dr. #110, St. Cloud, MN, ph. 320-203-8266
56308, Kristi Hawkes, ND, 1413 Broadway, Alexandria, MN, ph. 320-762-4295
56379, Sauk Rapids Chiropractic, 220 N. Benton Dr., Sauk Rapids, MN, ph. 320-255-1309, fax -0464
56716, Biermaier Chiro Clinic, 1226 University Ave., Crookston, MN, ph. 218-281-6311, fax -6312
57006, Bommersbach, DC, 1611 6th St., Brookings, SD, ph. 605-692-7888
57069, Harold J. Fletcher, MD, 28 E. Cherry, Vermillion, SD, ph. 605-624-2222
57104, Lauri Aesoph, ND, 717 S. Duluth Ave., Sioux Falls, SD, ph. 605-339-9080
57201, Mary Goepfert, MD, P.O. Box 513, Watertown, SD, ph. 605-882-4664
57301, Harvey & Associates, 409 E. 11th, Mitchell, SD, ph. 605-996-4533
57301, Roger Prill, DC, 1501 N. Main St., Mitchell, SD, ph.605-995-0293
57325, Theodore R. Matheny, MD, 1005 S. Sanborn St., Chamberlain, SD, ph. 605-734-6958
57730-9703, Dennis R. Wicks, MD, HCR 83, Box 21, Custer, SD, ph. 605-673-2689
58201, Richard H. Leigh, MD, 2134 Library Cl., Grand Forks, ND, ph. 701-775-5527, fax -2539
58701, Brian E. Briggs, MD, 718 SW 6, Minot, ND, ph. 701-838-6011, fax –5055
59068, Oliver B. Cooperman, MD, P.O. Box 707, Red Lodge, MT, ph. 406-446-3055
59101, Arthritis & Osteoporosis Ctr., 1239 N. 28th St., Billings, MT, ph. 800-648-6274
59101, Margaret Beeson, ND, 328 Grand Ave., Billings, MT, ph. 406-259-5096
59101, Roberta Bourgon, ND, 328 Grand Ave., Billings, MT, ph. 406-259-5096
59102, David C. Healow, MD, 1242 N. 28th #1001, Billings, MT, ph. 406-252-6674
59108, Richard A. Nelson, MD, 1001 S. 24th West #202, Billings, MT, ph. 406-656-7416
59405, Mona Morstein, ND, 518 Ninth St. S., Great Falls, MT, ph. 406-727-6680
59474, Robert Stanchfield, MD, 925 Oilfield Ave., Shelby, MT, ph. 406-434-5595, fax -2701
59601, Bruce T. Smith, MD, 111 N. Jackson #4J, Helena, MT, ph. 406-449-3636
59601, Michael Bergkamp, ND, 516 Fuller Ave., Helena, MT, ph. 406-442-2091
59601, Nancy Aagenes, ND, 330 Eleventh Ave., Helena, MT, ph. 406-442-8508
59645, Daniel J. Gebhardt, MD, 12 E. Main, White Sulphur Spring, MT, ph. 406-547-3384
59715, Elisabeth Kirchhof, ND, 203 Haggerty Lane, Bozeman, MT, ph. 406-586-8244, fax –2396
59729, Michael Lang, ND, Box 1473, Ennis, MT, ph. 406-682-5040
59801, M. Public Health Partners, 1637 S. Higgins, Missoula, MT, ph. 406-542-3400, fax 728-1830
59801, Nancy Dunne-Boggs, ND, 715 Kensington #24A, Missoula, MT, ph. 406-728-8544
59802, Jamison Starbuck, ND, 210 N. Higgins #222, Missoula, MT, ph. 406-549-0005
59802, Sarah Lane, ND, 210 N. Higgins #222, Missoula, MT, ph. 406-549-0005
59840, Hillery Daily, ND, 413 State St., Hamilton, MT, ph. 406-375-0167
59840, Timothy Binder, DC, ND, 173 Blodgett Camp Rd., Hamilton, MT, ph. 406-363-4044
59901, Ann Waltz, ND, 322 Second Ave. W., Ste. B, Kalispell, MT, ph. 406-756-0308
59937, Steve Gordon, ND, 333 Baker Ave., Whitefish, MT, ph. 406-863-9300
60004, Kingsley Medical Center, 3401 N. Kennicott Ave., Arlington Heights, IL, ph. 800-255-7030
60005, Terrill K. Haws, DO, 121 S. Wilke Rd #111, Arlington Heights, IL, ph. 847-577-9457, fax -8601

60008, Center BioEnergetic Med, 1811 Hicks Rd., Rolling Meadows, IL, ph. 847-934-1100, fax -0548
60013, Michael Shery, PhD, 121 Brookbridge, Gary, IN, ph. 800-516-1445, fax 847-639-0869
60014, Gary Oberg, MD, 31 N. Virginia St., Crystal Lake, IL, ph. 815-455-1990, fax -6780
60014, James McGinn, DC, 318 Memorial St., #200, Crystal, Lake, IL, ph.815-455-1910
60025, Edward R. Karp, 1969 John's Drive, Glenview, IL, ph. 847-998-6611, fax 564-4162
60031, Mark Fredrick, DC, 3930 Washington St.#B, Gurnee, IL, ph.847-662-1612
60045, Julie Martin, ND, 273 Market Square #14, Lake Forest, IL, ph. 847-735-9142
60046, Bergin, Jeffrey, DC,619 Greenbriar Ln, Lindenhurst, IL, ph.847-356-0619
60067, Susan K. Busse, MD, 909 E. Palatine Rd., Palatine, IL, ph. 847-776-2111, fax -1711
60076, John H. Olwin, MD, 9631 Gross Point Rd., Skokie, IL, ph. 817-676-4030
60091, Eileen Laurence, MD, 1132 Michigan Ave., Wilmette, IL, ph. 847-256-4123, fax -4473
60098, John R. Tambone, MD, 102 E. South St., Woodstock, IL, ph. 815-338-2345
60099, Timothy Birdsall, ND, 2520 Elisha Ave., Zion, IL, ph. 847-872-6067
60104, Stephen Boudro, DC, 4407 Butterfield Rd., Bellwood, IL, ph.708-544-2700
60108, Old Town Chiro Ctr, 125 S. Bloomingdale Rd #7, Bloomingdale, IL, ph. 630-893-7313, fax -7453
60108, William Epperly, MD, 245 S. Gary Ave. #105, Bloomingdale, IL, ph. 630-893-9661, fax -5665
60134, Richard Hrdlicka, MD, 302 Randall Rd. #206, Geneva, IL, ph. 630-232-1900, fax -7971
60137, Christina Nicholson, DC, 3 S. 250 Cypress Dr., Glen Ellyn, IL, ph.630-889-6695
60148, David Wickes, DC, 200 E. Roosevelt Rd., Lombard, IL, ph.630-889-6603
60148, William, Hogan, DC, 233 S. Craig Pl., Lombard, IL, ph.630-889-6522
60149, Grant Iannelli, DC, 200 E. Roosevelt, Rd., Lombard, IL, ph.630-889-6836
60187, Frank Strehl, DC, 111 E. Cole Ave., Wheaton, IL, ph.630-653-5780
60190, Pauline Harding, MD, 27 W. 281 Geneva Rd., Winfield, IL, ph. 630-653-9900, fax -8147
60194, Anthony Pantanella, DC, 1175 N. Barrington Rd., Hoffman Estates, IL, ph.847-885-1131
60194, Joseph Mercola, MD, 1443 W. Schaumburg Rd., Schaumburg, IL, ph. 847-985-1777, fax -0693
60201, Evanston Holistic Ctr., 1629 Orrington Ave., Evanston, IL, ph. 847-733-9900, fax -0105
60301, Biochem. Nutr, 715 Lake St #106, Oak Park, IL, ph. 708-383-3800, fax -3445
60301, Caring medical & Rehab. Svcs., 715 lake St. #600, Oak Park, IL, ph. 708-848-7789, fax -7763
60301, Paul J. Dunn, MD, 715 Lake St. #106, Oak Park, IL, ph. 708-383-3800, fax -3445
60301, Ross A. Hauser, MD, 715 Lake St. #600, Oak Park, IL, ph. 708-848-7789, fax -7763
60402, Cameo Chiropractic, Inc., 6929 Roosevelt Rd., Berwyn, IL, ph. 708-788-4950, fax -4953
60408, Braidwood Family Medical, 233 E. Reed St., Braidwood, IL, ph. 815-458-6700, fax -6705
60423, Briar House, 8504 Stuenkel Rd., Frankfort, IL, ph. 815-469-8385
60430, Frederick Weiss, MD, 3207 W. 184th St., Homewood, IL, ph. 708-334-7000
60457, Linda Ehlers, DC, 8700 W. 95th St. #3, Hickory, Hills, IL, ph.708-598-9028
60477, Holistic Health Chiropractic, 16543 Oak Park Ave., Tinley Park, IL, ph. 708-429-1670
60506, Thomas L. Hesselink, MD, 888 S. Edgelawn Dr., Aurora, IL, ph. 708-844-0011, fax -0500
60554, H.B. De Bartolo, Jr., MD, 11 DeBartolo Dr., Sugar Grove, IL, ph. 708-859-1818, fax -2021
60563, Naperville Holistic, 1280 Iroquois Ave. #200, Naperville, IL ph. 630-369-1220, fax -1639
60603, Alan F. Bain, MD, 104 S. Michigan Ave. #705, Chicago, IL, ph. 312-236-7010
60611, Cancer Prevention Coalition, Inc., 520 N. Michigan #410, Chicago, IL, 0ph. 312-467-0600
60612, Theodore Johnson, DC, 1615 W. Warren Blvd, Chicago, IL, ph.312-733-6490
60614, David Edelberg, MD, 990 W. Fullerton Ave. #300, Chicago, IL, ph. 773-296-6700, fax -1131
60641, Jan Radzik, MD, 5544 W. Belmont Ave., Chicago, IL, ph. 773-205-7744
60643, Hugh Jenkins, DC, 2148 W. 95 St., Chicago, IL, ph. 773-445-6800
60656, Laurence Grey, MD, ND, 5528 N. Chester Ave. #1N, Chicago, IL, ph. 905-725-7000
60659, Razvan Rentea, MD, 3525 W. Peterson #611, Chicago, IL, ph. 773-583-7793, fax -7796
60914, Douglas Stam, DC, 396 N.Belle Aire, Bourbonnais, IL, 815-933-7391
61008, M. Paul Dommers, MD, 554 S. Main St., Belvidere, IL, ph. 815-544-3112
61081, Thomas Jensen, DC, 2002, E. 5th St., Sterling, IL, ph.815-626-7100
61101, Maculan Chiropractic Clinic, 1005 S. Main St., Rockford, IL, ph. 815-965-3212, fax 969-8110
61252, Terry W. Love, DO, 2610 - 41st St., Moline, IL, ph. 309-764-2900
61265, Karla Sue Kruse, DC, 615 22nd Ave., Moline, IL, ph. 309-762-0979, fax -4950
61265, Pamela Taylor, ND, Fifth Ave. Bldg. #706, Moline, IL, ph. 309-797-3271
61548, Midwest Hlth Renewal Ctr., 205 S. Englewood Dr., Metamora, IL, ph. 309-367-2321, fax -2324
62656, David Hepler, DC, Box 507, Lincoln, IL, ph.217-735-4451
63017, Edward Bietto, MD, 15119 Chamisal Dr., Chesterfield, MO, ph. 314-532-4112
63033, Tipu Sultan, MD, 11585 W. Florissant, Florissant, MO, ph. 314-921-7100
63080, Ronald H. Scott, DO, 131 Meredith Lane, Sullivan, MO, ph. 314-468-4932
63084, Clinton C. Hayes, DO, 100 W. Main, Union, MO, ph. 314-583-8911
63105, H Walker, Jr., MD, PhD, 138 N. Meramec Ave., St. Louis, MO, ph. 314-721-7227, fax -7247
63122, N. Neeb, DO, 12166 Old Big Bend Rd #104, Kirkwood, MO, ph. 341-984-0033, fax -0020
63127, Generations Health Care, Inc., 9701 Landmark Pkwy. #207, St. Louis, MO, ph. 314-842-4802
63127, Octavio R. Chirino, MD, 9701 Landmark Pkwy. Dr. #207, St. Louis, MO, ph. 314-842-4802
63131, Garry A. Johnson, MD, 1926 Firethorn Dr., Des Peres, MO, ph. 314-821-7616
63136, Russell C. Forbes, DC, 10501 Halls Ferry Road, St. Louis, MO, ph. 314-869-5591, fax 653-2181
63141, Simon M. Yu, MD, 11709 Old Ballas Rd. #202, St. Louis, MO, ph. 314-432-7802, fax -1971

64052, Applewood Med Ctr, Inc., 9120 E. 35th St., Independence, MO, ph. 816-358-2712, fax 229-6696
64052, Terry Nelson, DC, 10704 E. Westport Rd.#300, Independence, MO, ph.816-833-1188
64111, James F. Holleman, DO, 3100 Main St. #201, Kansas City, MO, ph. 816-561-6555, fax -6777
64111, Lisa Humbert, DC, 4301 Main St. #12, Kansas City, MO, ph. 816-531-5645
64114, James Rowland, DO, 8133 Wornall Rd., Kansas City, MO, ph. 816-361-4077
64118, H. Hlth Systems, 8002 N. Oak Trafficway #108, Kansas City, MO, ph. 816-436-9355, fax -1441
64119, C Rudolph, DO, PhD, 2800-A Kendallwood Pkwy., Kansas City, MO, ph 816-453-5940, fax -1140
64804, Ralph D. Cooper, DO, 1608 E. 20 St., Joplin, MO, ph. 417-624-4323
65401, A. Jackson Kessinger, DC, 1210 Hwy 72 East, Rolla, MO, ph.573-341-8292
65401, Elbert Bolsen, ND, 602 W. 6 St., Ste. C, Rolla, MO, ph. 573-364-9386, fax -8078
65711, Doyle B. Hill, DO, 600 N. Bush, Mountain Grove, MO, ph. 417-926-6643
65803, The Shealy Institute, 1328 E. Evergreen, Springfield, MO, ph. 417-865-5940, fax -6111
65803, William C. Sunderwirth, DO, 2828 N. National, Springfield, MO, ph. 417-869-6260
66102, John Gamble, Jr., DO, 1606 Washington Blvd., Kansas City, KS, ph. 913-321-1140
66604, John Toth, MD, 2115 S.W. 10th, Topeka, KS, ph. 913-232-3330, fax -4066
66614, John R. Toth, MD, 5101 SW 34 St., Topeka, KS, ph. 785-273-3330, fax 232-1874
67203, Stanley Beyrle, ND, 1101 N. West St, Wichita, KS, ph. 316-942-2220
67212, Frank Smith, DC, 9505 W. Central #104, Wichita, KS, ph. 316-729-1633
67219, Ctr. Improve Human Funct, 3100 N. Hillside Ave., Wichita, KS, ph. 316-682-3100, fax -5054
67337, J.E. Block, MD, 1501 W. 4th, Coffeyville, KS, ph. 316-251-2400
67601, Roy N. Neil, MD, 105 W. 13th, Hays, KS, ph. 913-628-8341
68114, Jeffrey Passer, MD, 9300 Underwood Ave., #520, Omaha, NE, ph. 402-398-1200, fax -9119
68114, Randall Bradley, ND, 7447 Farnan St., Omaha, NE, ph. 402-391-6714
68144, Eugene C. Oliveto, MD, 10804 Prairie Hills Dr., Omaha, NE, ph. 402-392-0233
68154, Richard J. Holcomb, MD, 248 N. 129th St., Omaha, NE, ph. 402-334-7964, fax 391-6818
68739, SACRAD Heart Clinic, 405 W. Darlene St., Hartington, NE, ph. 402-254-3935, fax -2393
68739, Steve Vlach, MD, 405 W. Darlene St., Hartington, NE, ph. 402-254-3935, fax -2393
68862, Otis W. Miller, MD, 408 S. 14th St., Ord, NE, ph. 308-728-3251
69001, Kenneth W. Ellis, MD, 7 Mashie Dr., McCook, NE, ph. 308-345-4683, fax -4744
70006, Wallace Rubin, 3434 Houma Blvd. #201, Metairie, LA, ph. 504-888-8800, fax -455-6796
70043, Saroj T. Tampira, MD, 800 W. Virtue St. #207, Chalmette, LA, ph. 504-277-8991
70053, Diana Betancourt, MD, 522 3rd St., Gretna, LA, ph. 504-363-0101
70065, Maria Hernandez-Abril, MD, 3814 Williams Blvd., Kenner, LA, ph. 504-443-4306, fax -4547
70112, James Carter, MD, 1430 Tulane Ave., New Orleans, LA, ph. 504-588-5136, fax 584-3540
70118-3761, Janet Perez Chiesa, MD, 360 Millaudon St., New Orleans, LA, ph. 504-484-6655
70121, Charles C. Mary Jr., MD, 1201 S. Clearview Pkwy. #100, Jefferson, LA, ph. 504-737-4636
70448, James Carter, MD, 800 Hwy 3228, Mandeville, LA, ph. 504-626-1985
70471, James P. Carter, MD, 4408 Hwy 22, Mandeville, LA, ph. 504-626-1985, fax -7029
70471, Roy M. Montalbano, MD, 120 Century Oaks Lane, Mandeville, LA, ph. 504-626-1985
70503, Catherine Chastant-Carricut, ND, 217 Oakwood Dr., Lafayette, LA, ph. 318-988-1968
70503, Sydney Crackower, MD, 701 Robley Dr. #100, Lafayette, LA, ph. 318-988-4116
70508, John S. Jester, ND, 3 Flagg Pl. Ste. B-4, Lafayette, LA, ph. 318-984-3770, fax -1202
70560, Adonis J. Domingue, MD, 602 N. Lewis #600, New Iberia, LA, ph. 318-365-2196
70607, Wellness Center, 3501 5th Ave. #A, Lake Charles, LA, ph. 800-566-7360, fax 318-479-2099
70650, Joanie Goss, ND, PO Box 144, Lacassine, LA, ph. 318-588-4249
70809, Chiropractic Sports & Injury Center, 5207 Essen Lane #5, Baton Rouge, LA, ph. 504-766-3031,
70815, Robert Smith, DC, 12235 Brookshire Ave., Baton Rouge, LA, ph.504-272-7100
71315, Andrea Neri, ND, PO Box 12533, Alexandria, LA, ph. 318-443-3322
71357, Joseph R. Whitaker, MD, P.O. Box 458, Newelton, LA, ph. 318-467-5131
71369, Steve Kuplesky, MD, 296 Christine Lane, Simmesport, LA, ph. 318-941-2671
71603-6352, Pine Bluff Allergy Clin., 3900 Hickory St., Pine Bluff, AR, ph. 501-535-8200
71913, William Wright, MD, 1 Mercy Dr. #211, Hot Springs, AR, ph. 501-624-3312
71953, David P. Bowen, MD, 622 Mena St. #A, Mena, AR, ph. 501-394-7570
72201, Norbert J. Becquet, MD, 613 Main St., Little Rock, AR, ph. 501-375-4419
72450, Len Kemp, MD, One Medical Dr., Paragould, AR, ph. 501-239-8504, fax 3204
72601, Carol Chaney, MD, P.O. Box 1254, Harrison, AR, ph. 870-427-6462, fax 741-3949
72645, Melissa Taliaferro, MD, PO Box 400, Leslie, AR, ph. 870-447-2599, fax -2917
72653, Merl B. Cox, DO, 126 South Church, Mountain Home, AR, ph. 501-424-5025
72756, Back to Health Chiropractic, 302 N. 8th St. #1, Rogers, AZ, ph. 501-936-8300
72766, G. Howard Kimball, MD, 900 Dorman, #E, Springdale, AR ph. 501-756-3251, fax -9186
73069, TCM Health Center, 2233 W. Lindsey #118, Norman, OK, ph. 405-579-7888, fax -7890
73102, Paul Wright, MD, 608 N.W. 9th St. #1000, Oklahoma City, OK, ph. 405-272-7494
73109, Charles H. Farr, MD, 5419 S. Western, Oklahoma City, OK, ph. 405-634-7855, fax -7320
73118, Charles D. Taylor, MD, 4409 Classen Blvd., Oklahoma City, OK, ph. 405-525-7751, fax -0303
74012, Michael Leu, ND, 3100 S. Elm Pl., Ste. B, Broken Arrow, OK, ph. 918-449-8343
74012, R. Jeff Wright, DO, 3100 S. Elm, Broken Arrow, OK, ph. 918-455-9400, fax 451-3758
74037, Leon Anderson, DO, 121 S. Second St., Jenks, OK, ph. 918-299-5038, fax -5030

74058, Gordon P. Laird, DO, 304 Boulder, Pawnee, OK, ph. 918-762-3601
74105, Ruth Miller, DO, 1710B E. 51st St., Tulsa, OK, ph. 918-742-1996, fax -5995
74105, Springer Clinic, Inc., 3233 E. 31st St., Tulsa, OK, ph. 918-749-8000, fax 742-6401
74134, Donna S. Hathaway, DC, 3151 S. 129th E. Ave. #R, Tulsa, OK, ph. 918-665-1120
74135, Michael Taylor, DC, 3808 E. 51st St., Tulsa, OK, ph.918-749-4657 .
74136, Planter Naturopathic Clinic, 5711 E. 71st St. #100, Tulsa, OK, ph. 918-488-6100, fax -6112
74764, Ray E. Zimmer, DO, 602 N. Dalton, Valliant, OK, ph. 405-933-4235
75023, Charles W. Sizemore, DDS, 3020 Legacy Dr. #210, Plano, TX, ph. 972-491-1434, fax -1261
75038, Francis, J. Rose, MD, 1701 W. Walnut Hill #200, Irving, TX, ph. 214-594-1111, fax 518-1867
75061, Irving Medical Ctr., 620 N. O'Connor, Irving, TX, ph. 972-259-3541, fax 254-1019
75075, Applied Nutrition Concepts, 2828 W. Parker Rd. #208, Plano, TX, ph. 972-612-5505, fax -5505
75075, Cornelius Matwijecky, MD, 3900 W. 15th St. #305, Plano, TX, ph. 214-964-8889, fax -0026
75075, Linda martin, Do, 1524 Independence #C, Plano, TX, ph. 214-985-1377, fax 612-0747
75150, George Lofgren, ND, 1220 Town East Blvd. #250B, Mesquite, TX, ph. 972-686-0966
75208, James M. Murphy, MS, 400 S. Zang #1218, Dallas, TX, ph. 214-941-3100, fax -1979
75227, Theodore J. Tuinstra, DO, 7505 Scyene Rd. #302, Dallas, TX, ph. 214-275-1141, fax -1370
75231, Donald R. Whitaker, DO, 8345 Walnut Hill Lane #230, Dallas, TX, ph. 214-373-3016
75231, Peter Rivera, MD, 7150 Greenville Ave. #200, Dallas, TX, ph. 214-891-0466
75234, Martha Jo Taylor, 2925 LBJ Freeway, Dallas, TX, ph. 972-488-2533, fax -2533
75234, Natural Wellness Center, 2880 LBJ Freeway #219, Dallas, TX, ph. 972-247-4500, fax -1412
75244, Stephen Sporn, 1`3612 Midway Rd. #333-16, Dallas, TX, ph. 972-490-3703, fax 980-6850
75248, J. Robert Winslow, DO, 5025 Arapaho #550, Dallas, TX, ph. 214-702-99777
75251, Michael G. Samuels, DO, 7616 LBJ Freeway #230, Dallas, TX, ph. 214-991-3977, fax 788-2051
75503, T. Overlock, MD, 2700 Richmond Rd. #14A, Texarkana, TX, ph. 903-832-6565, fax -5120
75956, John L. Sessions, DO, 1609 S. Margaret, Kirbyville, TX, ph. 409-423-2166, fax –5496
75956, John L. Sessions, DO, 1609 S. Margaret, Kirbyville, TX, ph. 409-423-2166, fax -5496
76011, Alan Rader, DC, 2301 N. Collins #190, Arlington, TX 76011, ph. 817-461-6119, fax 226-1162
76012, R.E. Liverman, DO, 1111 San Juan Ct., Arlington, TX, ph 817-469-1266
76017, Dept. Omm, Unthsc-fw, 3500 Camp Bowie Blvd., Ft. Worth, TX, ph. 817-735-2235, fax -2480
76051, Howard J. Lang, DO, 1404 Brown Trail Ste. D, Bedford, TX, ph. 817-268-1171, fax 285-0676
76054, Antonio Acevedo, MD, 729 W. Bedford-Euless Rd., Hurst, TX, ph. 817-595-2580
76095, Nutr. Direction for Total Wellness, P.O. Box 210633, Bedford, TX, ph. 817-685-6304, fax -0078
76107, Gerald Harris, DO, 1002 Montgomery #3-103, Ft. Worth, TX, ph. 817-732-2878, fax -9315
76111, R. Tan, MD, PA, 3220 North Freeway #106, Ft. Worth, TX, ph. 817-626-1993, fax -2310
76112, C. Hawed, DO, 6451 Brentwood Stair Rd. #115, Ft. Worth, TX, ph. 817-446-8416, fax -8413
76112, J. Mahoney, DO, 6451 Brentwood Stair Rd. #115, Ft. Worth, TX, ph. 817-446-8416, fax -8413
76308, Thomas R. Humprey, MD, 2400 Rushing, Wichita Falls, TX, ph. 940-766-4329, fax 767-3227
76801, Larry Doss, MD, 1501 Burnett Dr., Brownwood, TX, ph. 915-646-8541
76903, B. Thurman, MD, 102 N. Magdalen #290, San Angelo, TX, ph. 915-653-3562, fax 994-1162
77027, Kenneth W. O'Neal, MD, 1800 W. Loop S. #1650, Houston, TX, ph. 713-871-8818
77042, Wholistic & Psychosomatic Medicine, 10714 Briar Forest, Houston, TX, ph. 713-789-0133
77055, Jerome L. Borochoff, MD, 8830 Long Point #504, Houston, TX, ph. 713-461-7517
77055, Robert Battle, MD, 9910 Long Point, Houston, TX, ph. 713-932-0552, fax -0551
77057, Moe Kakvan, MD, 3838 Hillcroft #415, Houston, TX, ph. 713-780-7019, fax -9783
77058, Stephen O. Rushing, MD, 16856 Royal Crest Dr., Houston, TX, ph. 713-286-2195, fax -2197
77063, Balanced Bodies Chiropractic 9099 Westheimer #501, Houston, TX, ph. 713-977-0005
77076, Stephen Weiss, MD, 7333 North Freeway #100, Houston, TX, ph. 713-691-0737
77089, Biotech Chiro Clinic, 11003 Resource Parkway #103, Houston, TX, ph. 281-481-9299, fax -9286
77098, Ctr. Integrated Med, 3120 Southwest Freeway #415, Houston, TX, ph. 713-523-4181, fax -4184
77338, John Trowbridge, MD, 9816 Mem. Blvd. #205, Humble Tex. Republic, TX, ph.281-540-2329
77459, Eric K. Tondera, 52 Wellington Ct., Missouri City, TX, ph. 713-988-3223, fax -5643
77480, Elisabeth-Anne Cole, MD, 1002 Brockman St., Sweeny, TX, ph. 409-548-8610, fax -8614
77504, Carlos Nossa, MD, 4010 Fairmont Pkwy. #274, Pasadena, TX, ph. 713-768-3151
77520, Ronald L. Cole, MD, 1600 James Bowie Dr. #C-104, Baytown, TX, ph. 281-422-2229, fax -8064
77536, David Spinks, DO, 4132 Center, Deer Park, TX, ph. 281-479-7088, fax –4188
77706, Rajesh Vyas, ND, 3725 Durwood Dr., Beaumont, TX, ph. 409-896-5466
78028, Candice Jackson, ND, 335 Roundabout, Kerrville, TX, ph. 830-895-1727
78041, Ruben Berlanga, MD, 649-B Dogwood, Laredo, TX, ph. 210-733-0424
78064, Gerald Phillips, MD, 111 Smith St., Pleasanton, TX, ph. 210-569-2118, fax -5958
78229, Pain & Stress Management Clinic, 5282 Medical Dr. #160, San Antonio, TX, ph. 800-669-2256,
78240, J. Archer, DO, 8637 Fredericksburg Rd. #150, San Antonio, TX., ph, 210-697-8445, fax -0631
78240, R. Nelms, DO, 8637 Fredericksburg Rd. #150, San Antonio, TX, ph. 210-697-8445, fax -0631
78550, Robert R. Somerville, MD, 712 N. 77 Sunshine Strip #21, Harlingen, TX, ph. 210-428-0757
78613, Ron Manzanero, MD, 201 S. Bell #104, Cedar park, TX, ph. 512-258-1645, fax -2586
78681, Natural Healing Clinic, 405 Old West Dr., Round Rock, TX, ph. 512-255-3631, fax -3972
78704, The Pain Mgmt. Ctr., 4303 Victory #300, Austin, TX, ph. 512-444-7246, fax -0832
78735, Stephen C. Ahrens, 6108 Highway 290 W., Austin, TX, ph. 512-892-2635, fax -7460

78756, J. William LaValley, MD, 4207 Shoalwood Ave. #13, Austin, TX, ph. 512-467-9396
78757, Vladimir Rizov, MD, 911 W. Anderson Ln. #205, Austin, TX, ph. 512-451-8149, fax -0895
79072, Jan Hamilton, RDLD, 1000 Jefferson, Plainview, TX, ph. 806-296-7953, fax 226-1147
79109, Gerald Parker, DO, 4717 S. Western, Amarillo, TX, ph. 806-355-8263
79109, Health Chiropractic, 6110 Canyon Dr., Amarillo, TX, ph. 806-352-3330, fax 467-0003
79109, John T. Taylor, DO, 4714 S. Western, Amarillo, TX, ph. 806-355-8263
79109, Terry Rudd, ND, 2414 Lakeview #6, Amarillo, TX, ph. 806-359-1003
79119, Roby D. Mitchell, MD, 3501 Soncy Rd. #129, Amarillo, TX, ph. 806-467-9824, fax 354-9823
79410, Mark R. Wilson, MD, 4002 - 21st St. #A, Lubbock, TX, ph. 806-795-9494
79603, William Irby Fox, MD, 1227 N. Mockingbird Lane, Abilene, TX, ph. 915-672-7863
80111, Lori Olaf, ND, 6558 S. Yosemite Circle, Greenwood Village, CO, ph. 303-694-5757
80116, Reiner Kremer, DC, 7601 E.Burning Tree Dr., Franktown, CO, ph.303-688-1111
80122, Milt Hammerly, MD, 5161 E. Arapahoe Rd. #290, Littleton, CO, 303-693-2626, fax 796-8174
80206, Debra Rouse, ND, 255 Detroit St., Denver, CO, ph. 303-322-9294
80206, Jenny Demeaux, ND, 1673 Fillmore St., Denver, CO, ph. 303-331-6919
80206, Kendall Gerdes, MD, 2 Steele St. #200, Denver, CO, ph. 303-377-8837, fax 303-321-3255
80206, Lauren E. Mitchell, DO, 2222 E. 18th St., Denver, CO, ph. 303-333-3733, fax -1351
80206, Scott R. McAdoo, DDS, 201 University Blvd. #203, Denver, CO, ph. 303-393-0039
80218, Philip Incao, MD, 1624 Gilpin St., Denver, CO, ph. 303-321-2100, fax -3737
80228, Frontier Medical Institute, 255 Union St. #400, Lakewood, CO, ph. 303-986-9455, -0892
80231, Jacob Schor, ND, 1181 S. Parker Rd., #101, Denver, CO, ph. 303-337-4884
80231, Rena Bloom, ND, 1181 S. Parker Rd. #101, Denver, CO, ph. 303-337-4884
80246, Thomas Ravin, MD, 45 S. Dahlia St., Denver, CO, ph. 303-331-9339, fax -9338
80301, James Rouse, ND, 3285 30th, Boulder, CO, ph. 303-449-1330
80301, Nancy Rao, ND, 3005 47th St., Ste. F-2, Boulder, CO, ph. 303-545-2021
80302, Arlene Kellman, DO, 2150 Pearl St., Boulder, CO, ph. 303-444-8337, fax -8393
80302, Tara Skye Goldin, ND, 1844 Pearl St., Boulder, CO, ph. 303-443-2206
80303, Erik Flatland, ND, 2885 Aurora Ave. #27, Boulder, CO, ph. 303-447-1339
80303, Jody Shevins, ND, 5353 Manhattan Circle #102, Boulder, CO, ph. 303-494-3713
80304, Johannah Reilly, ND, 2660 13th St., Boulder, CO, ph. 303-541-9600
80304, Michael Z. Zeligs, MD, 1000 Alpine #211, Boulder, CO, ph. 303-442-5492
80401, Michele Loewe, ND, 607 10th St. #105, Golden, CO, ph. 303-215-1669
80401, Terry Grosman, MD, 2801 Youngfield St., Golden, CO, ph. 303-233-4247, fax -4249
80477, Virginia Osborn, ND, PO Box 774135, Steamboat Springs, CO, ph. 970-879-8569
80524, Clare Wykert, ND, 504 S. College Ave., Fort Collins, CO, ph. 970-495-9067
80526, Clinton Pomroy, ND, 2160 W. Drake Rd., Ste. A-1, Fort Collins, CO, ph. 970-484-6390
80631, Pathways, 3211 20th St. #D, Greeley, CO, ph. 970-356-3100, fax -4827
80903, Edith Sucher, ND, 712 S. Tejon St., Colorado Springs, CO, ph. 719-634-0292
80903, Glen Nagel, ND, 104 E. St. Vrain #10, Colorado Springs, CO, ph. 719-635-2050
80903, Mary Frazel, ND, 104 E. St. Vrain #10, Colorado Springs, CO, ph. 719-635-2050
80903, William Nelson, ND 1422 N. Hancock Ave. #5-S, Colorado Springs, CO, ph. 719-635-4776
80903, William Nelson, ND, 1422 N. Hancock Ave., Colorado Springs, CO, ph. 719-635-4776
80904, Ruth Adele, ND, 1625 W. Uintah St., Ste. 1, Colorado Springs, CO, ph. 719-636-0098
80907, James R. Fish, MD, 3030 N. Hancock Ave., Colorado Springs, CO, ph. 719-471-2273
80907, James R. Fish, MD, 3030 N. Hancock, Colorado Springs, CO, ph. 719-471-2273
80910, M. Martin Hine, MD, 303 S. Circle #202, Colorado Springs, CO, ph. 719-632-7003
80918, Carl Osborn, DO, 6050 Erin Park #200, Colorado Springs, CO, ph. 719-260-8122
80918, George J. Juetersonke, DO, 5455 N. Union Blvd. #200, Colorado Springs, CO, ph. 719-528-1960
80918, George Juetersonke, DO, 5455 N Union #200, Colorado Springs, CO, ph. 719-528-1960
81001, Ron Concialdi, DDS, 2037 Jerry Murphy Rd. #202, Pueblo, CO, ph. 719-545-3070, fax -3071
81301, James Massey, ND, 755 E. Second Ave., Ste. C, Durango, CO, ph. 970-259-7979
81301, Louise Edwards, ND, 929 E. Third Ave., Durango, CO, ph. 970-247-2043
81301, Miclene A. Fecteau, DO, 1911 Main Ave. #101, Durango, CO, ph. 970-247-1160
81401, Columbia Naturopathic Health Ctr, 700 E. Main #5, Montrose, CO, ph. 970-240-2082, fax -8677
81501, Rick Jensen, ND, 835 Colorado Ave., Grand Junction, CO, ph. 970-248-9520
81505, William L. Reed, MD, 2700 G Rd. #1-B, Grand Junction, CO, ph. 970-242-1417
81622, Rob Krakovitz, MD, 430 W. Main St., Aspen, CO, ph. 970-927-4394
82001, Jonathan Singer, DO, 1805 E. 19th St. #202, Cheyenne, WY, ph. 307-635-4362
82580, Abram Ber, 5011 N. Granite Reef Rd., Scottsdale, AZ, 602-941-2141, fax -4114
82604, Preventive Health Resources, 2300 Mulberry, Casper, WY, ph. 307-234-2044
82717, Rebecca Painter, MD, 201 West Lakeway, Gillette, WY, ph. 307-682-0330, fax 686-8118
82718, Rebecca Painter, MD, 201 W. Lakeway #300, Gillette, WY, ph. 307-682-0330, fax 686-8118
83440, Dana Miller, DC 19 N. Center St., Rexburg, ID, ph. 208-356-6772, fax -8658
83651, Integrated Medical Arts Ctr., 824 17th Ave. S., Nampa, ID, ph. 208-466-5517, fax -3172
83651, Nampa Chiropractic Center, 1003 7th Street S., Nampa, ID, ph. 208-466-5459
83702, Brent Mathieu, ND, 1412 W. Washington, Boise, ID, ph. 208-338-5590
83705, Karen Erickson, ND, 1509 S. Roberts #101, Boise, ID, ph. 208-383-4833

83814, Todd Schlapfer, ND, 1000 W. Hubbard #120, Coeur d'Alene, ID, ph. 208-664-1644
83864, Alan Miller, ND, 501 S. Lincoln, Sandpoint, ID, ph. 208-265-1342
83864, Gabrielle Duebendorfer, ND, 2023 Sandpoint West Dr., Sandpoint, ID, ph. 208-265-2213
83864, Kathleen Head, ND, 2013 Janelle Way, Sandpoint, ID, ph. 208-263-1337
84047, Meridian Health Ctr, 1225 E. Fort Union Blvd. #200, Midvale, UT, ph. 801-561-4804, fax -5078
84058, Leslie Peterson, ND, 502 S. State St., Orem, UT, ph. 801-224-5780
84058, Ulrich Knorr, ND, 502 State St., Orem, UT, ph. 801-224-5780
84088, Cordell Logan, ND, 9265 S. 1700 W., Ste. A., West Jordan, UT, ph. 801-562-2211
84088, Cordell Logan, PhD, ND, 9265 S. 1700 W #A, West Jordan, UT, ph. 801-562-2211, fax -0063
84098, Kenneth Wolkoff, MD, 3065, W. Fawn Dr., Park City, UT, ph. 801-655-8214
84105, Todd Cameron, ND, 1059 E. 900 S. #100, Salt Lake City, UT, ph. 801-531-7337
84107, Dennis Harper, DO, 5263, S. 300 W #203, Murray, UT, pg. 801-288-8881, fax 262-4860
84107, William Allen Nunn, ND, 345 E. 4500 S., Ste. H, Murray, UH, ph. 801-265-0077
84321, Katherine Ruggeri, ND, 200 E. 500 S., River Heights, UT, ph. 801-753-5987
84604, Dennis Remington, MD, 1675 N. Freedom Blvd. #11-E, Provo, UT, ph. 801-373-8500, fax -3426
84604, Judith S. Moore, DO, 1675 N. Freedom Blvd. #11-E, Provo, UT, ph. 801-373-8500, fax -3426
85008, Michael Cronin, ND, 2524 N. 53 St., Phoenix, AZ, ph. 602-990-7424
85012, Ralph F. Herro, MD, 5115 N. Central Ave., Phoenix, AZ, ph. 602-266-2374, fax 264-2172
85014, Ann Manby, NMD, 3543 N. Seventh St., Phoenix, AZ, ph. 602-222-3578
85014, Dana Keaton, ND, 5333 N. Seventh St. #C-221, Phoenix, AZ, ph. 602-266-4670
85015, Sam Schwart, DO, DSC, 1822 W. Indian School Rd., Phoenix, AZ, ph. 602-277-8911
85016, John Oxley, ND, 6130 N. 16 St., Phoenix, AZ, ph. 602-970-0000
85016, Tilli Williams, ND, 5333 N. Seventh St. #C-221, Phoenix, AZ, ph. 602-266-4955
85018, Bruce H. Shelton, MD, 2525 W. Greenway Rd. #300, Phoenix, AZ, ph. 602-993-1200, fax -0160
85018, Marianna Fisher, ND, 5743 E. Indian School Rd., Phoenix, AZ, ph. 602-994-8474
85018, Royal Orthoped & Pain Rehab, 3610 N. 44th St. #210, Phoenix, AZ, ph. 602-912-4996, fax -5635
85018, S. Olsztyn, MD, 4350 E. Camelback Rd. #B-220, Scottsdale, AZ, ph. 602-840-8424, fax -8545
85022, H.C. Purtzer, DO, 13825 N. 7th St. #H, Phoenix, AZ, ph. 602-942-6944, fax -6945
85027, Larry Abel, ND, 36633 N. 21 St., Phoenix, AZ, ph. 602-595-9358
85032, J Sherman, DO, 1222 Paradise Vill. Pkwy. S. #328-A, Phoenix, AZ, ph. 602-494-1735, fax -1735
85032, Karsten Alexandria, ND, 13832 N. 32 St., Ste. C2-4, Phoenix, AZ, ph. 602-493-2273
85032, Konrad Kail, ND, 13832 N. 32 St., Ste. C2-4, Phoenix, AZ, ph. 602-493-2273
85201, Gracey Chiropractic Clinic, 1530 N. Country Club Drive #18, Mesa, AZ, ph. 602-964-4407
85203, Bruce Davis, ND, 1004 E. Jensen, Mesa, AZ, ph. 602-962-7893
85204, Scott Luper, NMD, 845 S. 21 St., Mesa, AZ, ph. 602-920-0000
85206, William W. Halcomb, DO, 4323 E. Broadway #109, Mesa, AZ, ph. 602-832-3014
85213, Pat Hallman, ND, 2112 E. Lehi Rd., Mesa, AZ, ph. 602-668-0307
85224, Carol Cooper, Lac, 3417 N. Evergreen St. #A, Chandler, AZ, ph. 602-777-9045
85224, Gilberto Leon Jr., ND, 1257 W. Warner, Ste. A-1, Chandler, AZ, ph. 602-857-3484
85224, Rick Chester, ND, 590 N. Alma School Rd. #11, Chandler, AZ, ph. 602-963-4410
85251, Karen Van Der Veer, NMD, 7950 E. Camelback Rd. #206, Scottsdale, AZ, ph. 602-945-8407
85251, Kathleen Dry, MD, 4020 N. Scottsdale Rd. #300, Scottsdale, AZ, ph. 602-947-1545, fax -2392
85251, Serene Wai-Mei Loh, NMD, 6505 E. Osborn Rd. #243, Scottsdale, AZ, ph. 602-990-9635
85251, Stuart Lanson, MD, 7301 E. 2 St. #106, Scottsdale, AZ, ph. 602-994-9512, fax -3773
85251, Theresa Ramsey, ND, 7375 E. Stetson #100, Scottsdale, AZ, ph. 602-945-7770
85253, Chris Beltran, ND, 10301 N. 70 St. #103, Scottsdale, AZ, ph. 602-596-0915
85253, Nicholas J. Meyer, DDS, 7170 E. McDonald Dr. #11, Scottsdale, AZ, ph. 602-948-0560
85254, Louise Gutowski, ND, 13430 N. Scottsdale Rd. #102, Scottsdale, AZ, ph. 602-443-1600
85254, T. Friedmann, MD, 10565 N. Tatum Blvd. #B115, Phoenix, AZ, ph. 602-381-0800, fax 0054
85257, Daniel Rubin, ND, 7502 E. Kimsey Lane, Scottsdale, AZ, ph. 602-481-7683
85257, Ian Bier, ND, 8010 E. McDowell #205, Scottsdale, AZ, ph. 602-970-0000
85258, Allergy Disease Ctr., 9699 N. Hayden Rd. #108, Scottsdale, AZ, ph. 602-951-9090, fax -9270
85258, Christine Madsen, NMD, 8300 N. Hayden Rd. #207, Scottsdale, AZ, ph. 602-596-0671
85258, Clark Hansen, ND, 8040 E. Morgan Trail #23, Scottsdale, AZ, ph. 602-991-5092
85260, Gordon Josephs, MD, 7315 E. Evans Rd., Scottsdale, AZ, ph. 602-998-9232
85260, Jeffrey Feingold, ND, 7227 E. Shea Blvd., Scottsdale, AZ, ph. 602-998-8736
85268, Allyn Krieger-Fiedler, ND, 16650 E. Hawk Dr., Fountain Hills, AZ, ph. 602-816-1600
85271, David Macallan, ND, PO Box 3881, Scottsdale, AZ, ph. 619-490-9860
85271, Kevon Arthurs, ND, PO Box 3881, Scottsdale, AZ, ph. 619-490-9860
85282, Farra Swan, ND, 2435 E. Southern #8, Tempe, AZ, ph. 602-820-0911
85282, Kareen O'Brien, ND, 2140 E. Broadway Rd., Tempe, AZ, ph. 602-858-9100
85282, Nick Buratovich, NMD, 2435 E. Southern Ave #9, Tempe, AZ, ph. 602-831-0717
85282, Paul Mittman, ND, 2140 E. Broadway Rd., Tempe, AZ, ph. 602-858-9100
85297, Alan Christianson, ND, 1402 N. Miller Rd., Ste. F-6, Scottsdale, AZ, ph. 602-425-9224
85301, John Brewer, ND, 5002 W. Glendale Ave. #101, Glendale, AZ, ph. 602-937-4756
85308, Gen. Practice, Assoc., PC, 4901 W. Bell Rd. #2, Glendale, AZ, ph. 602-939-8916, fax 978-2817
85308, Lloyd D. Arnold, 4901 W. Bell Rd. #2, Glendale, AZ, ph. 602-939-8916, fax 978-2817

85331, F. George II, DO, 38425 N. Spur Cross Rd., Cave Creek, AZ, ph. 602-488-6331 fax -0297
85344, S.W. Meyer, DO, 322 River Front Dr. P.O. Box 1870, Parker, AZ, ph. 520-669-8911
85374, Natural Healthcare,12211 West Bell Road #205B, Surprise, AZ, ph. 602-583-9180, fax -9180
85541, Gary E. Gordon, MD, 901 Awasazi Rd., Payson, AZ, ph. 520-472-9086, fax 474-1297
85635, Debbie Jacques, ND, 1858 Paseo San Louis, Ste. H, Sierra Vista, AZ, ph. 520-459-5210
85704, Judy Hutt, ND, 268 E. River Rd. #130, Tucson, AZ, ph. 520-887-4287
85704, Nancy Aton, NMD, 5813 N. Oracle, Tucson, AZ, ph. 520-293-3751
85705, J. Lyn Patrick, ND, 540 W. Prince Rd., Ste. A, Tucson, AZ, ph. 520-293-5400
85705, Stacey Kargman, NMD, 540 W. Prince Rd., Ste. A, Tucson, AZ, ph. 520-293-5400
85711, Autumn Holder, NMD, 1001 N. Swan Rd., Tucson, AZ, ph. 520-323-7133
85712, Alan K. Ketover, MD, 10752 N. 89th Pl. #C-134m, Scottsdale, AZ, ph. 602-880-4700
85712, Gene D. Schmutzer, DO, 2425 N. Alvernon Way, Tucson, AZ. ph. 802-795-0292
85712, Gordon Josephs, MD, 7315 E. Evans Rd., Scottsdale, AZ, ph. 602-998-9232, fax –1528
85712, Jesse Stoff, MD, 2122 N. Cracroft Rd. #112, Tucson, AZ, ph. 520-290-4516, fax -6403
85716, Jorge Badillo-Cochran, ND, 1601 N. Tucson Blvd., Tucson, AZ, ph. 520-322-8122
85716, Lance Morris, ND, 1601 N. Tucson Blvd. #37, Tucson, AZ, ph. 520-322-8122
85718, John V. Dommisse, MD, 1840 E. River Rd. #210, Tucson, AZ, ph. 520-577-1940, fax 1743
85718, Woody R. McGinnis, MD, 3150 Cerrada Los Palitos, Tucson, AZ, ph. 520-529-0658
85737, R.Michael Cessna, DC, 37966 S. Spoon Dr., Tucson, AZ, ph.520 825 0030
85742, Gregg G. Libby, DC, 4811 W. Daphne Lane, Tucson, AZ, ph. 520-579-9775
85747, Teri Davis, ND, 11505 E. Camino Del Desierto, Tucson, AZ, ph. 520-886-7721
85749, Alzheimer's Prev. Found., 11901 E. Coronado, Tucson, AZ, ph. 520-749-8374, fax -2669
85750, Alexander P. Cadoux, MD, 5655 E. River Rd., #151, Tucson, AZ, 520-529-9668, fax -9669
86001, Mark James, ND, 809 N. Humphreys, Flagstaff, AZ, ph. 520-774-1770
86001, Mary Poore, ND, 809 N. Humphreys, Flagstaff, AZ, ph. 520-774-1770
86001, Natureworks Medical Center, 516 N. Humphreys, Flagstaff, AZ, ph. 520-779-1016
86032, Judith Petersen, ND, PO Box 126, Joseph City, AZ, ph. 520-288-3920
86301, Gene Schroeder, MD, 843 Miller Valley Rd. #204, Prescott, AZ, ph. 520-717-0678, fax –0712
86303, Debora Chelson, ND, 315 W. Goodwin St., Prescott, AZ, ph. 520-445-4995
86326, Darrel Parry, DO, 1699 E. Cottonwood St., Cottonwood, AZ, ph. 602-639-2200
86334, Eric D. Bower, NMD, P.O. Box 404, Paulsen, AZ, ph. 520-771-3740
86336, Eric Yarnell, ND, 2081 W. Hwy 89A, Sedona, AZ, ph. 520-282-6909
86336, John J. Adams, MD, 299 Van Deren, #3, Sedona, AZ, ph. 520-282-3014
86336, Lester Adler, MD, 40 Soldiers Pass #12, Sedona, AZ, ph. 520-282-2520, fax –2895
86336, Michael Vesely, NMD, 15 Cindy Lane, Sedona, AZ, ph. 520-203-0807
86336, Silena Heron, ND, 2081 W. Hwy 89A, Sedona, AZ, ph. 520-282-6909
86336, Welch Medical Clinic, 2301 W. Hwy. 89A, Sedona, AZ, ph. 520 282 0609
86351, Cheryl Harter, MD, 80 Raintree Rd., Sedona, AZ, ph. 520-284-9777
86403, Frank Sweet, ND, 1731 Mesquite #5, Lake Havasu City, AZ, ph. 520-453-9525
87110, Ralph Luciani, DO, 2301 San Pedro NE, Albuquerque, NM, ph. 505-888-5995, fax 884-4091
87111, Gerald Parker, DO, 9577 Osuna NE, Albuquerque, NM, ph. 505-271-4800
87111, John T. Taylor, DO, 9577 Osuna NE, Albuquerque, NM, ph. 505-271-4800
87501, Bert A. Lies, Jr., MD, 539 Harkle Road #D, Santa Fe, NM, ph. 505-982-4821
87501, W.A. Shrader Jr., MD, 141 Paseo de Peralta, Ste. A, Santa Fe, NM, ph. 505-983-8890
87504, Shirley B. Scott, MD, P.O. Box 2670, Santa Fe, NM, ph. 505-986-9960
87505, John L. Laird, MD, 1810 Calle de Sebastian #H-4, Santa Fe, NM, ph. 505-989-4690
87532, LaMesilla Clinic, 116 Rt. 399, Esponola, NM, ph. 505-753-4466
87544, Los Alamos Pediatric Clinic, 3917 W. Road #136, Los Alamos, NM, ph. 505-662-9620
88005, Adex Cantu, MD, 301 Perkins Dr., Albuquerque, NM, ph. 505-524-4858
88201, Annette Stoesser, MD, 112 S. Kentucky, Roswell, NM, ph. 505-623-2444, fax -9693
88201, Mark Danforth, DO, 1114 S. Union, Roswell, NM, ph. 505-627-7164
89040, William O. Murray, MD, P.O. Box 305, Overton, NV, ph. 702-397-2677, fax -2420
89102, J. Leandra Even, ND, 2810 W. Charleston Blvd. #F-55, Las Vegas, NV, ph. 702-258-7860
89104, M. Michael Robertson, MD, 1150 S. Eastern Ave., Las Vegas, NV, ph. 702-385-4429, fax -1383
89106, Milne Medical Center, 2110 Pinto Lane, Las Vegas, NV, ph. 702-385-1393, fax -4170
89108, Adelaida V. Resuello, MD, 1808 N. Torrey Pines Dr., Las Vegas, NV, ph. 702-219-8717
89119, Ji-Zhou Kang, MD, 5613 S. Eastern, Las Vegas, NV, ph. 702-798-2992
89121, F. Fuller Royal, MD, 3663 Pecos McLeod, Las Vegas, NV, ph. 702 732-1400
89128, Desert Shores Medical Opt, 2620 Regatta Dr. #211, Las Vegas, NV, ph. 702-360-5000
89410, Frank Shallenberger, MD, 1524 Main St. Hwy 395, Gardnerville, NV, ph. 702-782-4164
89410, Steven Holper, MD, 3233 W. Charleston #2, Las Vegas, NV, ph. 702-878-3510, fax -1405
89501, Donald E. Soli, MD, 708 N. Center Dr., Reno, NV, ph. 702-786-7101
89502, W. Douglas Brodie, MD, 309 Kirman Ave. #2, Reno, NV, ph. 702-324-7071, fax –7639
89509, C. Ibarra-Ilarina, MD, 6490 S. McCarran Blvd. #C24, Reno, NV, ph. 702-827-1444, fax -2424
89509, Michael L. Gerber, MD, 3670 Grant Dr., Reno, NV, ph. 702-826-1900
90006, Hans D. Gruenn, MD, 12732 Washington Blvd., Los Angeles, CA, ph. 310-822-4614
90025, M. Olsen, MD, Inc., 11600 Wilshire Blvd. #306, Los Angeles, CA, ph. 310-473-0911, fax -0311

90025, Yancey R. Rousek, 12021 Wilshire Blvd. #802, West Los Angeles, CA, ph. 310-478-5301
90028, James J. Julian, MD, 1654 Cahuenga Blvd., Hollywood, CA, ph. 213-467-5555
90031, M. R. Rose, MD, 3325 N. Broadway, Los Angeles, CA, ph. 213-221-6121, fax -225-6120
90064, Joseph Sciabbarasi, MD, 2211 Corinth Ave. #204, Los Angeles, CA, ph. 310-477-8151
90064, Murray Susser, MD, 2211 Corinth Ave. #204, Los Angeles, CA, ph. 310-966-9194, fax –9196
90064, R. Grossman, Lac, 11500 West Olympis Blvd. #635, Los Angeles, CA, ph. 310-358-6125
90210, Uzzi Reiss, MD, 414 N. Camden Dr. #750, Beverly Hills, CA, ph. 310-247-1300, fax 205-0164
90211, C. Lippman, MD, 291 La Cienega Blvd. #207, Beverly Hills, CA, ph. 310-289-8430, fax -8165
90212, Larrian Gillespie, MD, 505 S. Beverly Dr. #233, Beverly Hills, CA, ph. 310-471-2375
90247, Takeshi Hayashida, MD, 16204 Orchard Ave., Gardena, CA, ph. 310-532-4535, fax 329-2156
90265, Jesse L. Hanley, MD, 22917 Pacific Coast Hwy. #220, Malibu, CA, ph. 310-456-9393
90272, Joe D. Goldstrich, MD, P.O. Box 306, Pacific Palisades, CA, ph. 310-454-1212
90401, Bridget O'Bryan, ND, 1437 7th St. #301, Santa Monica, CA, ph. 310-458-8020
90401, Cynthia Watson, MD, 530 Wilshire Blvd. #203, Santa Monica, CA, ph. 310-393-0937
90401, David Y. Wong, MD, 1431 7th St. #20, Santa Monica, CA, ph. 310-450-9998
90401, Pamela Durgin, ND, 612 Santa Monica Blvd., Santa Monica, CA, ph. 310-576-6176
90403, Charles Marcus, Lac, 1821 Wilshire Blvd. #570, Santa Monica, CA, ph. 310-586-9737
90403, Holly Castle, ND, 1821 Wilshire Blvd. #300, Santa Monica, CA, ph. 310-453-9591
90403, Joseph Sciabbarrasi, MD, 1502 Wilshire Blvd. #306, Santa Monica, CA, ph. 310-395-2453
90403, Keith DeOrio, MD, 1821 Wilshire Blvd., Santa Monica, CA, ph. 310-828-3096, fax 453-1918
90403, M. Susser, MD, 2730 Wilshire Blvd. #110, Santa Monica, CA, ph. 310-453-4424, fax 828-0261
90403, Santa Monica Well. Ctr, 1137 Second St. #116, Santa Monica, CA, ph. 310-451-7170, fax -4044
90404, Chi H. Yang, MD, 1260-15th St. #1119, Santa Monica, CA, ph. 310-587-2441
90404, Sports Med., 1454 Cloverfield Blvd. #200, Santa Monica, CA, ph. 310-829-1990, fax -5134
90406, Marcus Laux, ND, PO Box 1577, Santa Monica, CA, ph. 310-306-2220
90505, David Y. Wong, MD, 3250 Lomita Blvd. #208, Torrance, CA, ph. 310-326-8625, fax -1735
90680, William Goldwag, MD, 7499 Cerritos Ave., Stanton, CA, ph. 714-827-5180
90804, H. Casdorph, MD, PhD, 1703 Termino Ave. #201, Long Bch, CA, ph. 310-597-8716, fax -4616
90804, Michael E. Lieppman, MD, Inc., 1760 Termino Ave. #10, Long Beach, CA, ph. 562-597-5511
91010, Robert Banever, OMD, Lac, 2961 Royal Oaks Drive, Duarte, CA, ph. 318-514-5756
91024, Keenan Chiropractic, 90 N Baldwin Ave. #2, Sierra Madre, CA, ph. 818-355-9884, fax -9837
91101, Kathleen Power, DC, 151 S. El Molino Ave.#301, Pasadena, CA, ph. 818-793-7161
91107, Carrson M. Morris, DC, 1131 W. Duarte Rd. #12, Arcadia, CA, ph. 626-445-7010
91208, Joseph Lee Filbeck, Jr., MD, 1812 Verdugo Blvd., Glendale, CA, ph. 818-952-2243
91316, I. Abraham, MD, 17815 Ventura Blvd., #'s 111, 113, Encino, CA, ph. 818-345-8721
91324, Richard Creitz, DC, 19401 Parthenia St. #10, Northridge, CA, ph. 818-700-9600, fax -1314
91345, Sion Nobel, MD, 10306 N. Sepulveda Blvd., Mission Hills, CA, ph. 818-361-0155
91361, E. Hanzelik, MD, 1240 Westlake Blvd. #231, Westlake Village, CA, 805-446-4444, fax -4448
91361, J. Horton, MD, 1240 Westlake Blvd. #231, Westlake Village, CA, ph. 805-446-4444, fax -4448
91361, Phillip H. Taylor, MD, Inc., 3180 Willow Lane #104, Thousand Oaks, CA, ph. 805-497-3839
91362, Med Altern & Pain Center, 1864 Orinda Ct., Thousand Oaks, CA, ph. 805-942-1881, fax -1881
91364, Community Chiro. Health Center, 23317 Mulholland Dr., Woodland Hills, CA, ph. 818-591-8847
91401, Salvacion Lee, MD, 14428 Gilmore St., Van Nuys, CA, ph. 818-785-7425
91405, Salvacion M. Lee, MD, 15243 VanOwen #406, Van Nuys, CA, ph. 818-785-7425, fax -7455
91406, Donald Getz, OD, 7136 Haskell Ave. #125, Van Nuys, CA, ph. 818-997-7888, fax -0418
91436, A. L. Klepp, MD, Inc., 16311 Ventura Blvd. #845, Encino, CA, ph. 818-981-5511, 907-1468
91436, Tony Perrone, PhD, 15720 Ventura Blvd. #508, Encino, CA, ph. 818-783-2881, fax -2886
91472, Whitaker Wellness Inst., 4321 Birch St. #100, Newport Beach, CA, ph. 800-340-1550
91505, Douglas Hunt, MD, 2625 W. Alameda #326, Burbank, CA, ph. 818-566-9889, fax -9879
91506, David J. Edwards, MD, 2202 W. Magnolia, Burbank, CA, ph. 800-975-2202
91602, David C. Freeman, MD, 11311 Camarillo St. #103, N. Hollywood, CA, ph. 818-985-1103
91604, Chas. Law Jr., MD, 3959 Laurel Canyon Blvd., Studio City, CA, ph. 818-761-1661, fax –0482
91702, William Bryce, MD, 400 N. San Gabriel Ave., Azusa, CA, ph. 626-334-1407, fax –1116
91723, James Privitera, MD, 105 N. Grandview Ave., Corvina, CA, ph. 818-966-1618, fax -7226
91730, John B. park, MD, 9726 Foothill Blvd., Rancho Cucamonga, CA, ph. 909-987-4262
91780, H.Q. Hoang, MD, 9700 Las Tunas Dr. #340, Temple City, CA, ph. 818-286-3686, fax -9617
91780, Leo Milner, DC, 5814 Temple City Blvd., Temple City, CA, ph. 818-285-4142, fax 291-2017
91786, B. Chan, MD, 1148 San Bernadino Rd. #E-102, Upland, CA, ph. 909-920-3578, fax 949-1238
92008, Cynthia Leeder, DC, 800 Grand Ste. C-2, Carlsbad, CA, ph. 760-434-4615, fax -7191
92008, Mark Drucker, MD, 4004 Skyline Rd., Carlsbad, CA, ph. 619-729-4777
92008, S. Lawrence, DDS, 785 Grand Ave. #206, Carlsbad, CA, ph. 760-729-9050, fax 439-1624
92014, Ronald M. Lesko, DO, 13983 Mango Dr. #103, Del mar, CA, ph. 619-259-2444, fax -8925
92021, William J. Saccoman, MD, 505 N. Mollison Ave. #103, El Cajon, CA, ph. 619-440-3838
92024, Asano Acupuncture Assoc., 543 Encinitas Blvd., Encinitas, CA, ph. 760-753-8857
92024, Bonnie Marsh, ND, 937 S. Coast Hwy 101, Ste. 205, Encinitas, CA, ph. 760-436-3455
92024, Brenna Hatami, ND, 555 Second St. #2, Encinitas, CA, ph. 760-943-9903
92028, Erhardt Zinke, MD, 2131 Winter Warm Rd, Fallbrook, CA, ph. 619-728-4901

92037, Charles A. Moss, MD, 8950 Villa Jolla Dr. #2162, La Jolla, CA, ph. 619-457-1314, fax -3615
92037, Longevity Clinic of LaJolla, 5580 La Jolla Blvd. #113, LaJolla, CA, ph. 619-456-1996, fax -1955
92037, Pierre Steiner, MD, 1550 Via Corona, La Jolla, CA, ph. 619-657-8333
92054, Angela Stengler, ND, 342 Rimhurst Ct., Oceanside, CA, ph. 503-526-8600
92054, Mark Stengler, ND, 342 Rimhurst Ct., Oceanside, CA, ph. 503-526-8600
92069, William C. Kubitschek, DO, 1194 Calle Maria, San Marcos, CA, ph. 619-744-6991
92083, Health & Longevity Inst. 2598 Fortune Way #K, Vista, CA, ph. 760-598-7042, fax 727-4554
92102, Jacqueline Carson, ND, 2496 "E" St. #300, San Diego, CA, ph. 619-236-8285
92102, John L. May, MD, 458 - 26th St., San Diego, CA, ph. 619-685-6900, fax -6901
92105, David Getoff, CNC, 2128 Ridgeview Dr., San Diego, CA, ph. 619-262-2232
92109, Stephen Kaufman, DC, 2443 Wilbur Ave., San Diego, CA, ph. 619-581-1795, fax -9043
92110, The Livingston Found. Med. Ctr., 3232 Duke St., San Diego, CA, ph. 619-224-3515, fax -6253
92111, Dragon West Family Health Center, 4683 Mercury St., San Diego, CA, ph. 619-607-3806
92118, Capt. D.E. Sprague, MD, USS Constellation CV 64, Coronado, CA, ph. 619-545-5655
92121, Jas. Murphy Jr., DO, 5445 Oberlin Dr. #101, San Diego, CA, ph. 619-450-5959, fax 457-0136
92234, Arianne Kloven, ND, 34464 Calle Las Palmas, Cathedral City, CA, ph. 760-328-1070
92262, David C. Freeman, MD, 2825 Tahquitz McCallum #200, Palm Springs, CA, ph. 619-320-4292
92262, Edmund Chien, MD, 2825 Tahquitz Ste. A, Palm Springs, CA, ph. 760-327-8939, fax –0844
92262, Sean Degnan, MD, 2825 Tahquitz McCallum #200, Palm Springs, CA, ph. 619-320-4292
92270, Charles Farinella, MD, 69-730 Hwy. 111 #106A, Rancho Mirage, CA, ph. 619-324-0734
92270, Don H. Wasserman, MD, 26 Dartmouth Dr., Rancho Mirage, CA, ph. 760-770-1122
92313, Hitendra H. Shah, MD, 22807 Barton Rd., Grand Terrace, CA, ph. 909-783-2773, fax –6625
92324, Hiten Shah, MD, 22807 Barton Rd., Grand Terrace, CA, ph. 714-783-2773
92373, Jeannette M. McKee, DC, 1150 Brookside Ave. #L, Redlands, CA, ph. 714-793-5226, fax -2787
92405, First Chiropractic, 1947 N. E. Street, San Bernadino, CA, ph. 909-882-0575, fax -3965
92544, Health and Growth Assoc., 28195 Fairview Ave., Hemet, CA, ph. 909-927-1768, fax -1548
92587, John V. Beneck, MD, 22107 Old Paint Way, Canyon Lake, CA, ph. 909-244-3866, fax -0109
92620, Ronald Wempen, MD, 14795 Jeffrey Rd. #101, Irvine, CA, ph. 714-551-8751, fax –1272
92626, Subhash Gharmalkar, ND, 1530 Baker St., Ste. G, Costa Mesa, CA, ph. 949-437-7710
92646, Francis Foo, MD, 10188 Adams Ave., Huntington Beach, CA, ph. 714-968-3266, fax -6408
92653, D. Calabrese, MD, 24953 Passo De Valencia #3A, Laguna Hills, CA, 714-454-0509, fax -2033
92653, Robert Abell, ND, 24953 Paseo de Valencia, Ste. 16C, Laguna Hills, CA, ph. 949-206-9090
92660, Allen Green, MD, 4019 Westerly Pl. #100, Newport Beach, CA, ph. 714-251-8700, fax -8900
92660, Ctr.Personal Develop, 4299 MacArthur Blvd. #106, Newport Bch, CA, ph. 714-756-1642, fax -8618
92660, J. W.Thompson, MD, 4321 Birch St. #100, Newport Beach, CA, ph. 714-851-1550, fax -9970
92660, Joan Resk, DO, 4063, Birch St. #230, Newport Beach, CA, ph. 714-863-1110
92660, Julian Whitaker, MD, 4321 Birch St. #100, Newport Beach, CA, ph. 714-851-1550
92667, Ntrl Hlth Women, 30100 Town Centre Dr. #U-117, Laguna Niguel, CA, ph. 714-249-1612, fax -4911
92677, Joseph A. Ferreira, MD, 23 Redondo, Laguna Niguel, CA, ph. 714-249-2091, fax -2091
92691, Crown Vlly Chiro, 27652 Crown Valley Pkwy. Mission Viejo, CA, ph. 714-364-1901, fax -4437
92691, David A. Steenbock, DO, 26381 Crown Valley Pkwy. #130, Mission Viejo, CA, ph. 800-300-1063,
92691, Duke D. Kim, MD, 27800 Medical Ctr. Rd. #116, Mission Vijeo, CA, ph. 714-364-6040, -0502
92705, Jeremy E. Kaslow, MD, 720 N. Tustin #102, Santa Ana, CA, ph. 714-565-1032, fax –1035
92706, Felix Praklasam, MD, 415 Brookside Ave., Redlands, CA, ph. 909-798-1614
92708, Prudence Broadwell, ND, 18837 Brookhurst #210, Fountain Valley, CA, ph. 949-965-9266
92708, Robert Broadwell, ND, 18837 Brookhurst #210, Fountain Valley, CA, ph. 949-965-9266
92720, Ronald R. Wempen, MD, 14795 Jeffrey Rd. #101, Irvine, CA, ph. 714-551-8751, fax -1272
92780, Marjorie Moore-Jones, 1034 Irvine Blvd., Tustin, CA, ph. 714-528-0216
92804, Schwartz Chiropractic, 504 S. Brookhurst Street, Anaheim, CA, ph. 714-533-1813
92821, Edgar A. Lucidi, MD, 410 W. Central #101, Brea, CA, ph. 714-256-8458, fax 990-5724
92833, Richard Hansen, DMD, 1031 Rosencrans #104, Fullerton, CA, ph. 714-870-0310, fax –0153
92843, Dr. Jeremy E. Kaslow, 12665 Garden Grove Blvd. #604, Garden Grove, CA, ph. 714-530-5691
92869, James Gordon Vatcher, MD, 872 Cedarwood St., Orange, CA, ph. 714-771-2223
93018, H.J. Hoegerman, MD, 101 W. Arrellaga #D, Santa Barbara, CA, ph. 805-963-1824
93023, Richard Hiltner, MD, 169 E. Roblar, Ojai, CA, ph. 805-646-1495
93023, The Natural Medicine Ctr., 1434 E. Ojai Ave., Ojai, CA, ph. 805-640-1100, fax -8020
93041, Knight Chiro Health, 521 W. Channel Islands Blvd. #4, Port Hueneme, CA, ph. 805-984-1500
93065, Derrick D'Costa, MD, 2816 Sycamore Dr. #101, Simi Valley, CA, ph. 805-522-1344, fax -2074
93101, Kenneth J. Frank, MD, 831 State St. #280, Santa Barbara, CA, ph. 805-730-7420, fax -7434
93101, Luc Maes, DC, ND, 19 E. Mission St., Ste. A, Santa Barbara, CA, ph. 805-563-8660
93103, H.J. Hoegerman, MD, 119 N. Milpas, Santa Barbara, CA, ph. 805-963-1824
93108, Las Aves Fmly Hlth , 1805 D. E. Cabrillo Blvd., Santa Barbara, CA, ph. 805-565-3959, fax -3989
93111, Michael Hergenroet, 5290 Overpass Road #101, Santa Barbara, CA, ph. 805-681-7322
93301, A. Laser & Prev. Med., 500 Old River Rd. #170, Bakersfield, CA, ph. 805-663-3099, fax -3095
93301, Carmelo A. Palteroti, DO, 606 34th St., Bakersfield, CA, ph. 805-327-3756
93301, Ralph G. Seibly, MD, 2123-17th Ave., Bakersfield, CA, ph. 805-631-2000, fax -0914
93313, John B. Park, MD, 6501 Schirra Ct. #200, Bakersfield, CA, ph. 805-833-6562, fax -3498

93401, Zoe Wells, ND, 891 Pismo St., San Luis Obispo, CA, ph. 805-541-2614
93420, Rober J. Thiel, ND, 1248 Grand Ave. Ste. C, Arrogo Grande, CA, ph. 805-489-7188
93465, Richard A. Hendricks, MD, 1050 Las Tablas Rd., Templeton, CA, ph. 805-434-1836
93527, John B. Park, MD, 200 N. G. St., Porterville, CA, ph. 209-781-6224, fax -0294
93534, Mary Kay Michelis, MD, 1739 W. Avenue J, Lancaster, CA, ph. 805-945-4502, fax -4841
93534, Richard P. Huemer, MD, 1739 West Ave. J, Lancaster, CA, ph. 805-945-4502, fax -4841
93551, Vitality Health, 4505 Talento Way, Palmdale, CA, ph. 805-722-0612, fax 943-0792
93727, David J. Edwards, MD, 360 S. Clovis Ave., Fresno, CA, ph. 209-251-5066, -5108
93922, Bruce West, MD, PO Box 22620, Carmel, CA, ph. 408-372-8899, fax –3805
93923, Gerald A. Wyker, MD, 25530 Rio Vista Dr., Carmel, CA, ph. 408-625-0911, fax -0467
93940, Howard Press, MD, 172 Eldorado St., Monterrey, CA, ph. 408-373-1551, -1140
94022, Claude Marquetta, MD, 5050 El Camino Real #110, Los Altos, CA, ph. 415-964-6700
94022, Robert F. Cathcart III, MD, 127 2nd St. #4, Los Altos, CA, ph. 415-949-2822
94022, Women's Hlth Care & Prev. Med, 101 1st St. #441, Los Altos, CA, ph. 415-941-5905, fax -2175
94025, Jeffry L. Anderson, MD, 45 San Clemente Dr. #100-B, Corte Madera, CA, ph. 415-927-7140
94061, Rajan Patel, MD, 1779 Woodwide Rd. #101, Redwood City, CA, ph. 415-365-2969
94061, Springer Homeopathic Care, 1244 Crompton Road, Redwood City, CA, ph. 415-365-2023
94070, Chiro Chiropractic, 1701 Laurel St., San Carlos, CA, ph. 415-508-9111, fax 591-8800
94102, Gary S. Ross, MD, 500 Sutter #300, San Francisco, CA, ph. 415-398-0555
94102-1114, Alan S. Levin, MD, 500 Sutter St. #512, San Francisco, CA, ph. 415-677-0829, fax -9745
94107, Bruce Wapen, MD, P.O. Box 77007, San Francisco, CA, ph. 415-696-4500
94107, Carl Hangee-Bauer, ND, 1615 20th St., San Francisco, CA, ph. 415-643-6600
94109, Gene Pudberry, DO, 2000 Van Ness Ave. #414, San Francisco, CA, ph. 415-775-4448
94114, Larry Forsberg, Lac, 1201 Noe Street, San Francisco, CA, ph. 415-207-9878
94114, Rosemary Rau-Levine, MD, 690 Church St. #1, San Francisco, CA, ph. 414-522-0250, fax -0250
94115, Richard Kunin, M.D., 2698 Pacific Ave., San Francisco, CA, ph. 415-346-2500, fax -4991
94121, Laurens Garlington, MD, 56 Scenic Way, San Francisco, CA, ph. 415-751-9600, fax 750-0466
94127, Denise Mark, MD, 345 W. Portal Ave., San Francisco, CA, ph. 415-566-1000, fax 665-6732
94127, Paul Lynn, MD, 345 W. Portal Ave., San Francisco, CA, ph. 415-566-1000, fax 665-6732
94127, Scott V. Anderson, MD, 345 West Portal Ave., San Francisco, CA, ph. 415-566-1000
94133, Wai-Man Ma, MD, DC, 728 Pacific Ave. #611, San Francisco, CA, ph. 415-397-3888
94134, Leo Bakker, MD, 830 Felton St., San Francisco, CA, ph. 415-239-4954
94306, Connie Hernandez, ND, 4153-B El Camino Way, Palo Alto, CA, ph. 650-857-0226
94306, Marcel Hernandez, ND, 4153-B El Camino Way, Palo Alto, CA, ph. 650-857-0226
94520, Ilene Dahl, ND, 2342 Almond Ave., Concord, CA, ph. 510-602-0582
94520, John P. Toth, MD, 2299 Bacon St. #10, Concord, CA, ph. 510-682-5660, fax –8097
94523, Alternatives in Psychiatry, 1224 Contra Costa Blvd., Concord, CA, ph. 510-945-1447
94523, Ellen Potthoff, DC, ND, 200 Gregory Lane, Ste. B1, Pleasant Hill, CA, ph. 510-603-7300
94533, Edward J. Noa, DC, 3045 Travis Blvd., Fairfield, CA, ph. 707-426-6135, fax -6135
94538, Klein Chiropractic, 39201 Liberty St., Freemont, CA, ph. 510-790-1000, fax -1000
94549, Ezra Clark, MD, 3772 Happy Valley Rd., Lafayette, CA, ph. 510-284-4845, fax -2820
94550, Geraldine P. Donaldson, MD, 1074 Murietta Blvd., Livermore, CA, ph. 510-443-8282
94577, Stephen A. Levine, PhD, 400 Preda St., San Leandro, CA, ph. 510-639-4572, fax 635-6730
94577, Steven H. Gee, MD, 595 Estudillo St., San Leandro, CA, ph. 510-483-5881
94596, Alan Shifman Charles, MD, 1414 Maria Lane, Walnut Creek, CA, ph. 510-937-3331
94609, Thaleia Li'Rain, Lac, 6355 Telegraph Avenue #305, Oakland, CA, ph. 510-848-0937
94705, Wellmed, 3031 Telegraph Ave. #230, Ber Valley, CA, ph. 510-548-7384
94706, Ross Gordon, MD, 405 Kains Ave., Albany, CA, ph. 510-526-3232, fax –3217
94903, Scott V. Anderson, MD, 25 Mitchell Blvd. #8, San Rafael, CA, ph. 415-472-2343
94920, Tiburon Chiro. Wellness Center, 1640 Tiburon Blvd., Tinuron, CA, ph. 415-435-7420, fax -7421
94925, Michael Rosenbaum, MD, 300 Tamal Plaza #120, Corte Madera, CA, ph. 415-927-9450
94925, Sally LaMont, ND, 500 Tamal Plaza #507, Corte Madera, CA, ph. 415-927-7015
95003, Jade Mtn. Health Ctr., 8065 Aptos St., Aptos, CA, ph. 408-685-1800, fax -0108
95008, Carl L. Ebnother, M.D., 621 E. Cambell Ave. #11A, Campbell, CA, ph. 408-378-7970, fax -4908
95032, Cecil A. Bradley, MD, 14981 National Ave. #6, Los Gatos, CA, ph. 408-358-3663
95032, Judy Lee, ND, 455 Los Gatos Blvd. #107, Los Gatos, CA, ph. 408-358-3544
95032, Los Gatos Longevity Inst., 15215 National Ave. #103, Los Gatos, CA, ph. 408-358-8855
95062, Michele Goodwin, ND, 555 Soquel Ave. #260-H, Santa Cruz, CA, ph. 408-459-9206
95070, John C. Wakefield, MD, 18998 Cox Ave. #D, Saratoga, CA, ph. 408-366-0660, fax -0665
95134, F.T. Guiliford, MD, 2674 N. First St. #101, San Jose, CA, ph. 408-433-0923
95202, Luigi Pacini, MD, 1307 N. Commerce St., Stockton, CA, ph. 209-464-7757
95207, Walter S. Yourchek, MD, 4553 Quail Lakes Dr., Stockton, CA, ph. 209-951-1133
95401, Ron Kennedy, MD, DC, 2460 W. third St. #225, Santa Rosa, CA, ph. 707-576-0100, fax -1700
95404, J. Claire Green, ND, 4778 Holly St., Santa Rosa, CA, ph. 707-544-5546
95404, Terri Su, MD, 95 Montgomery Dr. #220, Santa Rosa, CA, ph. 707-571-7560, fax -8929
95405, David Field, ND, 46 Doctors Park Dr., Santa Rosa, CA, ph. 707-576-7388
95405, James Seeba, OMD, Lac, 3861 Montgomery Dr., Santa Rosa, CA, ph. 707-546-9628, fax -0403

95437, Peter Glusker, MD, 442 M. Merherson St., Fort Bragg, CA, ph. 707-964-6624, fax -6624
95567, JoAnn Vipond, MD, 12559 Hwy. 101 N., Smith River, CA, ph. 707-487-3405
95602, Heidi Hook, ND, 6615 Bear River Lane, Auburn, CA, ph. 530-269-2576
95616, Bill Gray, MD, 413 F St., Davis, CA, ph. 916-756-0567, fax -0567
95662, David M. McCann, 8880 Greenback Lane #B, Orangevale, CA, 916-988-7275, fax -0782
95669, William A. Lockyer, MD, P.O. Box 790, Plymouth, CA, ph. 209-267-5620
95678, James Mally, ND, 112 Douglas Blvd., Roseville, CA, ph. 916-782-1275
95816, Priscilla Monroe, ND, 2600 Capital Ave. #213, Sacramento, CA, ph. 916-448-9927
95819, Jon Kvenvolden, ND, 4220 H St., Sacramento, CA, ph. 916-491-5170
95823, Health Associates, 3391 Alta Arden #3, Sacramento, CA, ph. 916-489-4400, fax -1710
95825, Martin Mulders, MD, 3301 Alta Arden #3, Sacramento, CA, ph. 916-489-4400, fax -1710
95825, Michael Kwiker, DO, 3301 Alta Arden #3, Sacramento, CA, ph. 916-489-4400, fax -1710
96001, Bessie Jo Tillman, MD, 2054 Market St., Redding, CA, ph. 916-246-3022, fax -7894
96021, Jeannette Abel, ND, PO Box 1042, Corning, CA, ph. 808-969-7848
96028, Charles K. Dahlg, MD, Hwy. 299, E. Hosp. Annex, Fall River Mills, CA, ph. 916-335-5354
96701, Center for Holistic Med, 99-128 Aiea Heights Dr. #501, Aiea, HI, ph. 808-487-8833, fax -8859
96701, John Turetzky, ND, 99-128 Aiea Hts Dr. #501, Aiea, HI, ph. 808-487-8833
96704, Mary Lynn Garner, ND, PO Box 1152, Captain Cook, HI, ph. 808-334-6294
96732, Kevin Davidson, ND, 444 Hana Hwy #211, Kahului, HI, ph. 808-871-4722
96740, Michael Traub, ND, 75-5759 Kuakini Hwy. #202, Kailua Kona, HI, ph. 808-329-2114
96746, Miles Greenburg, ND, 1420 Kanepoonui Rd., Kapaa, HI, ph. 808-245-2277
96750, Anne-Marie Lambert, ND, PO Box 688, Kealakekua, HI, ph. 808-323-3370
96750, Clifton Arrington, MD, P.O. Box 649, Kealakekua, HI, ph. 808-322-9400
96766, Steven Dubey, ND, 3093 Akahi St., Lihue, HI, ph. 808-245-2277
96767, Laura O'Neal, ND, PO Box 98, Lahaina, HI, ph. 808-661-5432
96768, David Kern, ND, PO Box 567, Makawao, HI, ph. 808-572-6091
96768, Nathan Ehrlich, ND, PO Box 756, Makawao, HI, ph. 808-572-1388
96790, Julie Holmes, ND, 651 Omaopio Rd., Kula, HI, ph. 808-878-3267
96813, Fred M.K. Lam, MD, 1270 Queen Ema St. #501, Honolulu, HI, ph. 808-537-3311, fax -3312
96813, James Howard, ND, 1188 Bishop St. #1408, Honolulu, HI, ph. 808-536-8891
96813, Jason Uchida, ND, 181 S. Kukui #207, Honolulu, HI, ph. 808-545-2093
96814, Hazel Ogawa-Lerman, ND, 1150 S. King St. #404, Honolulu, HI, ph. 808-597-8109
96814, Jack Burke, ND, 615 Piikoi St., Penthouse 2, Honolulu, HI, ph. 808-593-9445
96814, Karen Tan, ND, 615 Piikoi St., Penthouse 2, Honolulu, HI, ph. 808-593-9445
96816, Laurie Steelsmith, ND, 4211 Waialae Ave. #401, Honolulu, HI, ph. 808-737-0414
96816, Linda A. Fickes, DC, 3728 Lurline Dr., Honolulu, HI, ph. 808-377-1811, fax 737-7486
96816, Linda Fickes, DC, 3728 Lurline Dr., Honolulu, HI, ph 808-377-1811, fax 737-7486
96822, Lori Kimata, ND, 1968 Nehoa Pl., Honolulu, HI, ph. 808-537-4144
96826, David Miyauchi, MD, 1507 S. King St. #407, Honolulu, HI, ph. 808-949-8711, fax -988-2188
96826, Wendell K.S. Foo, MD, 2357 S. Beretania St. #A-349, Honolulu, HI, ph. 808-373-4007
97005, Dickson Thom, DDS, ND, 4770 SW Watson Ave., Beaverton, OR, ph. 503-520-8859
97005, George F. Wittkopp, MD, 5040 S W Griffith Dr. #102, Beaverton, OR, ph. 503-643-0049
97005, Jack Daugherty, DC, ND, 12195 SW Allen Blvd., Beaverton, OR, ph. 503-646-0697
97005, Mitchell Stargrove, ND, 4720 SW Watson Ave., Beaverton, OR, ph. 503-526-0397
97005, Ravinder Sahni, DC, ND, 9570 SW Beaverton Hillsdale, Beaverton, OR, ph. 503-641-8503
97006, Chris Meletis, ND, 2708 SW 199 Pl., Aloha, OR, ph. 503-231-1825
97006, David Shefrin, ND, Beaver Creek Business Park, Beaverton, OR, ph. 503-644-7800
97008, Linda Meloche, ND, 8070 SW Hall, Beaverton, OR, ph. 503-643-0156
97009, William Mehan, ND, 27636 SE Haley Rd., Boring, OR, ph. 503-663-0596
97026, Rene Minz, MD, 5909 SE Division, Portland, OR, ph. 503-234-1531
97030, Amber Ackerson, ND, 2204-8 NW Birdsdale, Gresham, OR, ph. 503-661-5401
97030, Corey Resnick, ND, 2204-8 NW Birdsdale, Gresham, OR, ph. 503-661-5401
97030, Jennifer Reid, ND, 657 NE Hood Ave., Gresham, OR, ph. 503-519-4680
97030, Pamela Jeanne, ND, 22400 SE Stark St., Gresham, OR, ph. 503-669-2997
97034, Anna MacIntosh, ND, 545 First St., Lake Oswego, OR, ph. 503-631-8621
97034, Jacob Farin, ND, 560 First St. #204, Lake Oswego, OR, ph. 503-636-2734
97034, Kathleen Germain, ND, 545 First St., Lake Oswego, OR, ph. 503-635-6643
97034, Kenneth Rifkin, ND, 338 SW Second St., Lake Oswego, OR, ph. 503-636-2975
97034, Noel Peterson, ND, 560 First St. #204, Lake Oswego, OR, ph. 503-636-2734
97042, Durr Elmore, ND, PO Box 990, Mulino, OR, ph. 503-829-7326
97080, Victoria Larson, ND, 10000 SE 222 Ave., Gresham, OR, ph. 503-658-7130
97116, Clyde G. Reynolds, ND, PO Box 785, Forest Grove, OR, ph. 800-357-2464, fax 503-359-3825
97124, Kevin Wilson, ND, 150 NE Third Ave., Hillsboro, OR, ph. 503-648-0484
97128, Bruce Dickson, ND, 1900 N. Hwy 99, Ste. A, McMinnville, OR, ph. 503-434-6515
97128, Larry Herdener, ND, 415 E. Third St., McMinnville, OR, ph. 503-434-6170
97201, Catherine Downey, ND, 049 Porter St., Portland, OR, ph. 503-499-4343
97201, Dohn Kruschwitz, MD, ND, 4444 SW Corbett, Portland, OR, ph. 503-224-8476

97201, Erin Lommen, ND, 4444 SW Corbett Ave., Portland, OR, ph. 503-224-4003
97201, Guru Sandesh Khalsa, ND, 049 SW Porter, Portland, OR, ph. 503-499-4343
97201, Jared Zeff, ND, 1099 SW Columbia #300, Portland, OR, ph. 503-221-9974
97201, Kathleen Flewelling, ND, 4444 SW Corbett Ave., Portland, OR, ph. 503-224-8476
97201, OHSU Dept. Surg, 3181 SW Sam Jackson Park Rd., Portland, OR, ph. 503-494-5300, fax -8884
97201, Richard Barrett, ND, 049 SW Porter St., Portland, OR, ph. 503-255-4860
97201, Stanley Jacob, MD, Oregon Health Sciences Univ., Portland, OR, ph. 503-494-8474
97201, Susan Roberts, ND, 4444 SW Corbett Ave., Portland, OR, ph. 503-224-4003
97202, Daniel Beeson, DC, 7215 Southeast 13th Ave., Portland, OR, ph.503-238-7025
97202, Steven Sandberg-Lewis, ND, 6315 SE 15th Ave., Portland, OR, ph. 503-255-7355
97205, Peggy Rollo, ND, 833 SW 11th #612, Portland, OR, ph. 503-223-7067
97209, Michelle Suber, ND, 1915 NW Northrup, Portland, OR, ph. 503-224-4876
97209, Tori Hudson, ND, 2067 NW Lovejoy, Portland, OR, ph. 503-222-2322
97210, Arianna Staruch, ND, 1715 NW 23 Ave., Portland, OR, ph. 503-227-3828
97210, Bradley Bongiovanni, ND, 2515 NW Overton, Portland, OR, ph. 503-255-7355
97210, Samatha Brody, 2606 NW Vaughn, Portland, OR, ph. 503-231-8322
97210, Steven Bailey, ND, 2606 NW Vaughn, Portland, OR, ph. 503-224-8083
97212, Bernie Bayard, ND, 1722 NE Schuyler, Portland, OR, ph. 503-288-9793
97212, Mary Caselli, ND, 1823 NE 13th, Portland, OR, ph. 503-335-8983
97212, Sonja Petterson, ND, 3412 NE Fremont St., Portland, OR, ph. 503-255-7355
97213, Jonna Alexander, ND, 635 NE 78, Portland, OR, ph. 503-256-0931
97213, Lori Von Der Heydt, ND, 4445 NE Fremont, Portland, OR, ph. 503-249-7752
97214, Martin Milner, ND, 1330 SE 39 Ave., Portland, OR, ph. 503-232-1100
97214, Stephen Austin, ND, 1330 SE 39 Ave., Portland, OR, ph. 503-232-1100
97215, Barbara MacDonald, ND, 7735 SE Morrison St., Portland, OR, ph. 503-255-7355
97215, Lowell Chodosh, ND, 1922 SE 42, Portland, OR, ph. 503-231-6476
97215, Mary Scott, ND, 1835 SE 50 Ave., Portland, OR, ph. 503-232-4047
97215, Patricia Timberlake, ND, 1835 SE 50 Ave., Portland, OR, ph. 503-236-1366
97215, Russell Marz, ND, 2002 SE 50 Ave., Portland, OR, ph. 503-233-0585
97216, Alexandra Gayek, ND, 8316 SE Yamhill, Portland, OR, ph. 503-261-9010
97216, J. Stephen Schaub, MD, 9310 S.E. Stark St., Portland, OR, ph. 503-256-9666, fax 253-6139
97216, Joseph Coletto, ND, 10525 SE Cherry Blossom Dr., Portland, OR, ph. 503-254-3566
97216, Nancy Scarlett, ND, 11231 SE Market St., Portland, OR, ph. 503-255-7355
97216, Susan Allen, ND, 8602 SE Taylor St., Portland, OR, ph. 503-257-9754
97217, Gary Weiner, ND, 5833 N. Haight Ave., Portland, OR, ph. 503-224-8476
97217, Sierra Levy, ND, 5247 N. Haight, Portland, OR, ph. 503-335-0292
97220, Elizabeth Collins, ND, 10360 NE Wasco, Portland, OR, ph. 503-252-8125
97220, Jeffrey Tyler, MD, 163 N.E. 102nd Ave., Portland, OR, ph. 503-255-4256
97220, Katherine Zieman, ND, 10360 NE Wasco, Portland, OR, ph. 503-252-8125
97220, Nora Tallman, ND, 10360 NE Wasco, Portland, OR, ph. 503-252-8125
97220, Northwest Ctr. for Environm Med, 177 N.E. 102nd Bldg. V, Portland, OR, ph. 503-261-0966
97220, Rita Bettenburg, ND, 10360 NE Wasco, Portland, OR, ph. 503-252-8125
97220, Suzanne Lawton, ND, 4041 NE 99 Ave., Portland, OR, ph. 503-252-2612
97220, Thomas Abshier, ND, 1414 NE 109, Portland, OR, ph. 503-255-9500
97221, Barbara Betcone Jolley, DC, 4610 SW Beaverton Hillsdale, Portland, OR, ph. 503-245-3444
97222, Joyce Ho, ND, 6501 SE King Rd., Milwaukie, OR, ph. 503-777-9839
97222, Louise Tolzmann, ND, 3436 SE Johnson Creek Blvd., Portland, OR, ph. 503-255-7355
97223, Stacey Raffety, ND, 9830 SW McKenzie, Tigard, OR, ph. 503-639-1712
97224, David Greenspan, ND, 11810 SW King James Pl., Tigard, OR, ph. 503-684-1875
97225, Jacqueline Jacques, ND, 1600 SW Cedar Hills Blvd., Portland, OR, ph. 503-644-4446
97225, Rick Marinelli, ND, 1600 SW Cedar Hills Blvd., Beaverton, OR, ph. 503-644-4446
97232, Beverly Yates, ND, 2161 NE Broadway, Portland, OR, ph. 503-280-1950
97232, Donna Leia Melead, ND, 2119 NE Halsey, Portland, OR, ph. 503-249-2121
97232, Holly Zapf, ND, 1444 NE Broadway, Portland, OR, ph. 503-460-0630
97232, Suzanne Scopes, ND, 316 NE 28, Portland, OR, ph. 503-230-0812
97233, Brian Maccoy, ND, 19125 SW Stark, Portland, OR, ph. 503-491-1067
97233, John Collins, ND, 800 SE 181 Ave., Portland, OR, ph. 503-667-1961
97233, Patricia Meyer, ND, 800 SE 181 Ave., Portland, OR, ph. 503-667-1961
97233, Thomas A. Kruzel, ND, 800 SE 181 Ave., Portland, OR, ph. 503-667-1961, fax 669-4263
97233, Thomas Kruzel, ND, 800 SE 181 Ave., Portland, OR, ph. 503-667-1961
97266, Jan Selliken Bernard, ND, 9350 SE Dundee Ct., Portland, OR, ph. 360-906-1180
97267, Robert Sklovsky, ND, 6910 SE Lake Rd., Milwaukie, OR, ph. 503-654-3938
97292, Dan Carter, ND, PO Box 33961, Portland, OR, ph. 503-255-7355
97301, Alex Serkalow, ND, 859 Medical Center Dr. NE, Salem, OR, ph. 503-588-2333
97301, Andrew Perry, ND, 410 Lancaster Dr. NE, Ste. B, Portland, OR, ph. 503-364-1441
97302, Chiropractic Physicians PC, 705 Ewald SE, Salem, OR, ph. 503-378-0068, fax -0069
97302, James Auerbach, MD, 235 Salem Heights Ave, SE, Salem, OR, ph. 503-363-0524

97302, Linda Taylor, ND, 1447 Liberty St. SE, Salem, OR, ph. 503-910-7771
97302, Paul Anderson, ND, 1115 Liberty St. SE, Salem, OR, ph. 503-365-0377
97304, Terrence Howe Young, MD, 1205 Wallace Rd., N.W., Salem, OR, ph. 541-371-1588
97321, Monty Ross Ellison, MD, 909 Elm Street, Albany, OR, ph. 541-928-6444
97330, Acupuncture Clinic of Corvallis, 2021, NW Grant Ave., Corvallis, OR, ph. 541-753-5152
97333, Michael Jacobs, ND, 804 SW Fourth St., Corvallis, OR, ph. 541-757-7660
97365, I.F. Kelley, DC, 530 NW Third St., Ste. A. Newport, OR, ph. 541-265-5132, fax –8680
97365, K.E. Edmisten, ND, 344 SW Seventh St., Ste. B, Newport, OR, ph. 541-265-6378
97401, Adrienne Borg, ND, 74 E. 18 Ave. #12, Eugene, OR, ph. 503-686-3330
97401, Daniel Hardt, ND, 280 W. 11 Ave., Eugene, OR, ph. 503-683-4404
97401, Elizabeth Dickey, ND, 132 E. Broadway #420, Eugene, OR, ph. 541-465-1155
97401, Stephanie Wilson, ND, 1755 Coburg Rd., Bldg. 2, Eugene, OR, ph. 541-683-9357
97401, Stephen Messer, ND, 400 E. Second St. #105, Eugene, OR, ph. 503-343-2384
97417, James Siegel, DC, Box 375, Canyonville, OR, ph.541-839-4421
97420, Joseph T. Morgan, MD, 1750 Thompson Rd., Coos Bay, OR, ph. 541-269-0333, fax -7389
97424, Julie Parke, ND, 15 S. Sixth St., Cottage Grove, OR, ph. 541-942-8399
97424, Mark Thomas, DC, 500 Whiteaker Ave., Cottage Grove, OR, ph. 541-942-5024
97426, Sharol Marie Tilgner, ND, PO Box 279, Creswell, OR, ph. 541-895-5152
97439, Mark Immel, ND, 1525 12 St. #4B, Florence, OR, ph. 541-997-6255
97487, Joseph Kassel, ND, 25632 Jeans Rd., Veneta, OR, ph. 541-935-3453
97520, Integrated medical Services, 1607 Siskiyou Blvd., Ashland, OR, ph. 541-482-7007, fax -5123
97520, Linda Herrick, ND, 586 Glenwood Dr., Ashland, OR, ph. 541-482-0409
97520, Partners for Health, 3206 Linda Ave., Ashland, OR, ph. 541-488-0478, fax -5509
97520, Ronald L. Peters, MD, 1607 Siskiyou Blvd., Ashland, OR, ph. 541-482-7007, fax –5123
97526, Deborah Frances, ND, 316 SE Eighth St., Grants Pass, OR, ph. 541-474-0503
97527, James Fitzsimmons, Jr., MD, 591 Hidden Valley Rd., Grants Pass, OR, ph. 541-474-2166
97701, Howard Reingold, ND, 365 NE Greenwood #3, Bend, OR, ph. 541-389-6935
97701, John Hahn, ND, 334 NE Irving Ave. #104, Bend, OR, ph. 541-385-0775
97701, Sheila Myers, ND, 711 NE Irving, Bend, OR, ph. 541-385-6249
97702, Mark Cooper, ND, 61555 Parrell Rd., Bend, OR., ph. 541-389-4600
97850, John Winters, ND, 1606 Sixth St., La Grande, OR, ph. 541-963-7289
97914, George Gillson, MD, 915 SW 3rd Ave., Ontario, OR, ph. 541-889-9121, fax -5302
98001, Jonathan V. Wright, MD, 515 W. Harrison, Kent, WA, ph. 253-854-4900, fax 850-5639
98003, Thomas A. Dorman, MD, 929 S. 291 St., Federal Way, WA, ph. 253-859-9009, fax –8660
98004, Bellevue Chiropractic Center, Inc., 1530 Bellevue Way SE, Bellevue, WA, ph. 206-455-2225
98004, David Buscher, MD, 1603 116th Ave., NE #112, Bellevue, WA, ph. 206-453-0288
98004, Elizabeth Freeman, ND, 10603 NE 14 St., Bellevue, WA, ph. 425-454-0908
98004, Paula Baruffi, ND, 9236 SE Shorland Dr., Bellevue, WA, ph. 425-644-6048
98004, Sheila Dunn-Merritt, ND, 2025 112th Ave. NE, Bldg. 2, Bellevue, WA, ph. 425-452-9366
98007, Sigrid Penrod, ND, 14777 NE 40 St. #206, Bellevue, WA, ph. 425-882-2089
98008, Leo Bolles, MD, 15611 Bellevue-Redmond Rd., Bellevue, WA, ph. 425-881-2224, fax –2216
98011, Leanna Standish, ND, 14500 Juanita Dr. NE, Bothell, WA, ph. 425-602-3166
98011, Pamela Snider, ND, 14500 Juanita Dr. NE, Bothell, WA, ph. 206-523-9585
98011, Sarah Ringdahl, ND, 14500 Juanita Dr. NE, Bothell, WA, ph. 425-602-3386
98020, Judyth Reichenberg-Ullman, ND, 131 Third Ave. N., Edmonds, WA, ph. 425-774-5599
98020, Robert Ullman, ND, 131 Third Ave. N., Edmonds, WA, ph. 425-774-5599
98023, Thomas A. Dorman, MD, 515 W. Harrison St. #200, Kent, WA, ph. 206-854-4900
98026, Cheryl Wood, ND, 7614 195th St. SW, Edmonds, WA, ph. 425-778-5673
98026, Craig Baldwin, ND, 23700 Edmonds Way, Edmonds, WA, ph. 425-775-6001
98026, David Wood, ND, 7614 195th St. SW, Edmonds, WA, ph. 425-778-5673
98026, Dean Neary, ND, 21200 72nd Ave. W., Edmonds, WA, ph. 425-775-3717
98026, Kasra Pournadeali, ND, 21701 76th Ave. W. #302, Edmonds, WA, ph. 425-744-1780
98026, Richard Kitaeff, ND, 23700 Edmonds Way, Edmonds, WA, ph. 425-783-2873
98026, The Evergreen Clinic, 22200 Edmonds Way #A, Edmonds, WA, ph. 206-542-5595
98027, Steve MacPherson, ND, 85 NW Alden Pl., Ste. C, Issaquah, WA, ph. 425-391-1080
98032, Davis Lamson, ND, 515 W. Harrison, Kent, WA, ph. 253-854-4900
98032, Jonathan Wright, MD, 515 W. Harrison St. #200, Kent, WA, ph. 206-854-4900, fax 850-5639
98033, Robert Martinez, DC, ND, 11417 124th Ave. NE #103, Kirkland, WA, ph. 425-828-6232
98034, Geoff Lecovin, DC, ND,11919 NE 128 St., Ste. C, Kirkland, WA, ph. 425-820-4148
98034, Jonathan Collin, MD, 12911 120th Ave. NE, Ste. A50, Kirkland, WA, ph. 425-820-0547
98034, Lucinda Messer-Lecovin, ND, 11919 NE 128 St., Ste. C, Kirkland, WA, ph. 425-820-4148
98034, Michelle N. Ramauro, ND, 12040 98th Ave. #205-A, Kirkland, WA, ph. 425-821-3006
98034, Walter Crinnion, ND, 11811 NE 128 St. #202, Kirkland, WA, ph. 415-821-8118
98035, Joni Olehausen, ND, PO Box 1627, Kent, WA, ph. 253-854-4900
98052, Leah Stebbens, ND, 16260 NE 85 St., Redmond, WA, ph. 425-883-6565
98052, Robert Garrison, ND, 16140 NE 87, Redmond, WA, ph. 425-889-8722
98070, Fran Brooks, ND, PO Box 1921, Vashon Island, WA, ph. 206-463-5611

98070, Lisa Ann Azzopardi, ND, 11025 SW 238 St., Vashon Island, WA, ph. 206-938-9890
98102, Cathy Lindsay, DO, 914 E. Miller St., Seattle, WA, ph. 206-325-5430
98102, Sherry Kerchner, ND, 2366 Eastlake Ave. E. #317, Seattle, WA, ph. 206-323-7864
98103, Cathy Rogers, ND, 4649 Sunnyside N. #300E, Seattle, WA, ph. 206-527-5522
98103, James Wallace, ND, 1307 N. 45 St. #200, Seattle, WA, ph. 206-632-0354
98103, Jenifer Huntoon, ND, 1329 N 45 St., Seattle, WA, ph. 206-632-8804
98103, Joanna (Theresa) Forwell, ND, 4800 Phinney Ave. N. #6, Seattle, WA, ph. 206-633-3117
98103, Marie Adams, ND, 3931 Bridge Way N., Seattle, WA, ph. 206-545-1310
98103, Michael Woo, ND, 8500 Linden Ave. N. #103, Seattle, WA, ph. 206-527-5694
98103, Pamela Houghton, ND, 6303 Phinney Ave. N., Seattle, WA, ph. 206-789-4066
98103, R. Wood Wilson, ND, P.O. Box 31205, Seattle, WA, ph. 206-673-2437
98103, Trina Doerfler, DC, ND, 4649 Sunnyside N. #350, Seattle, WA, ph. 206-632-8670
98103, William Wulsin, ND, 753 N 35 St. #302, Seattle, WA, ph. 206-632-0411
98105, Sheryl Kipnis, ND, 5502 34th Ave. NE, Seattle, WA, ph. 206-522-0488
98105, Stephen King, ND, 5502 34th Ave. NE, Seattle, WA, ph. 206-522-0488
98107, Irvin Miller, ND, 1153 NW 51, Seattle, WA, ph. 206-781-4677
98107, Judy Christianson, ND, 1102 NW 64 St., Seattle, WA, ph. 206-782-6521
98107, Marleen Haverty, ND, 1120 NW 63 St., Seattle, WA, ph. 206-632-0354
98109, Barbara Kreemer, ND, 311 Blaine St., Seattle, WA, ph. 206-281-4282, fax 283-1146
98109, Bill Caradonna, ND, 311 Blaine St., Seattle, WA, ph. 206-524-2421
98109, Rebecca Wynsome, ND, 150 Nickerson #211, Seattle, WA, ph. 206-283-1383
98109, Styliani Kondilis, ND, 2225 Queen Anne Ave. N., Seattle, WA, ph. 206-378-1712
98109, William Mitchell, ND, 518 First Ave. N. #28, Seattle, WA, ph. 206-284-6040
98110, C. Brown, MD, 25995 Barber Cut-off Rd NE #B-1, Kingston, WA, ph. 360-297-8700, fax -8777
98112, Felice Barnow, ND, 2705 E. Madison, Seattle, WA, ph. 206-328-7929
98112, Rainbow Natural Health Clinic, 409 - 15th Avenue E., Seattle, WA, ph. 206-726-8450
98112, Richard Posmantur Jr., ND, 2705 E. Madison, Seattle, WA, ph. 206-328-7929
98115, Bruce Milliman, ND, 420 NE Ravena Blvd., Seattle, WA, ph. 206-522-5646
98115, David Bove, ND, 6520 17th Ave. NE, Seattle, WA, ph. 206-526-8384
98115, Douglas Lewis, ND, 9111 Roosevelt Way NE, Seattle, WA, ph. 206-525-8078
98115, Fernando Vega, MD, 420 NE Ravenna Blvd., Seattle, WA, ph. 206-522-5646
98115, Karen Coshow, ND, 8043 Ravenna Ave. N., Seattle, WA, ph. 206-729-0907
98115, Linda Warren, ND, 7746 18th Ave. NE, Seattle, WA, ph. 206-525-5257
98115, Lisa Meserole, ND, 420 NE Ravenna Blvd., Seattle, WA, ph. 206-527-6355
98115, Mylinh Vo, ND, 1815 NE 82 St., Seattle, WA, ph. 206-283-1383
98115, Nancy Mercer, ND, 7114 Roosevelt Way NE, Seattle, WA, ph. 206-526-0203
98115, Ralph T. Golan, MD, 7522 20th Ave. NE, Seattle, WA, ph. 206-524-8966
98115, Robert May, ND, 8029 Brooklyn Ave. NE, Seattle, WA, ph. 206-632-0354
98115, Steven Hall, MD, 420 NE Ravenna #A, Seattle, WA, ph. 206-523-8580, fax 524-5054
98116, Jeana Kimball, ND, 4141 California Ave. SW, Seattle, WA, ph. 206-938-1393
98116, Ralph Wilson, ND, 3419 61st Ave. SW, Seattle, WA, ph. 206-634-3679
98117, Molly Linton, ND, 1409 NW 85 St., Seattle, WA, ph. 206-781-2206
98119, Brad Lichtenstein, ND, 600 W. McGraw, Suite 1, Seattle, WA, ph. 206-285-4625
98119, Christy Lee-Engel, ND, 600 W. McGraw, Suite 1, Seattle, WA, ph. 206-285-4625
98119, Linda Luster, MD, 200 West Mercer #E-114, Seattle, WA, ph. 206-284-6907
98122, Cynthia Phillips, ND, 726 Broadway #301, Seattle, WA, ph. 206-726-0034
98122, Eileen Stretch, ND, 726 Broadway #301, Seattle, WA, ph. 206-726-0034
98122, Jane Guiltinan, ND, 211 Euclid Ave., Seattle, WA, ph. 206-632-0354
98122, John Hibbs, ND, 1523 E. Madison St., Seattle, WA, ph. 206-322-4416
98122, Lise Alschuler, ND, 726 Broadway #301, Seattle, WA, ph. 206-726-0034
98122, Marian Small, ND, 1523 E. Madison, Seattle, WA, ph. 206-322-4416
98122, Que Areste, ND, 1122 E. Pike #806, Seattle, WA, ph. 206-328-2926
98125, Mitchell Marder, DDS, 822-A Northgate Way, Seattle, WA, ph. 206-367-6453, fax -4971
98125, NW Ctr.Compl Med, 10212 5th Ave. NE #200, Seattle, WA, ph. 206-282-6604, fax -9631
98133, Nancy Roberts, ND, 14546 Greenwood Ave. N., Seattle, WA, ph. 206-362-3250
98136, Eva Urbaniak, ND, 5236 California Ave. SW, Ste. D, Seattle, WA, ph. 206-938-9505
98144, Tom Ballard, ND, 2006 19th Ave. S., Seattle, WA, ph. 206-726-0034
98155, Health & Wellness Institute, 3521 NE 148th St., Seattle, WA, ph. 206-440-1526, fax -8511
98166, Kenneth Harmon, ND, 1835 SW 152 St., Seattle, WA, ph. 206-243-5252
98168, Herbert Schuck, ND, 12610 Des Moines Mem. Dr. #202, Seattle, WA, ph. 206-248-0061
98188, Health Balances, 4109 S. 179th St., Seattle, WA, ph. 206-244-1383, fax 244-1383
98201, Dean Howell, ND, 1827 37th St., Everett, WA, ph. 425-252-6066
98201, Laura Martin, ND, 2520 Colby Ave., Everett, WA, ph. 425-257-9713
98208, Barbara Davies, ND, 1809 100th Pl. SE, Ste. B, Everett, WA, ph. 425-337-5004
98208, Corina Going, ND, 1809 100th Pl. SE, Ste. B. Everett, WA, ph. 425-337-5004
98208, Melanie Whittaker, ND, 713 SE Everett Mall Way, Ste. D, Everett, WA, ph. 425-290-5309
98208, Miechelle Poulos, ND, 1809 100th Pl. SE, Ste. B, Everett, WA, ph. 425-337-5004

98221, W. Hunter Greenwod, DC, ND, 1116 17th St., Anacortes, WA, ph. 360-293-6277
98225, Laura Shelton, ND, 1707 F St., Bellingham, WA, ph. 360-734-1560
98225, Mark Steinberg, ND, 1919 Broadway #206, Bellingham, WA, ph. 360-738-3230
98225, Rachelle Herdman, MD, ND, 1919 Broadway #204, Bellingham, WA, ph. 360-734-0045
98236, Brad Weeks, MD, 6456 S. Central Ave., Clinton, WA, ph. 360-341-2303, fax -2313
98249, Robert Jangaard, ND, PO Box 130, Freeland, WA, ph. 360-331-6470
98256, Rhonda Summerland, ND, PO Box 115, Index, WA, ph. 360-793-1033
98273, Gary Bachman, ND, 1910 Riverside Dr. #5, Mt. Vernon, WA, ph. 360-424-3460
98279, Magda Mische, ND, PO Box 22, Olga, WA, ph. 360-376-5454
98335, Mary Griffith, ND, 5122 Olympic Dr. NW #B104, Gig Harbor, WA, ph. 253-851-7550
98335, Steven Davis, ND, 5603 38th Ave. NW, Gig Harbor, WA, ph. 253-857-5544
98349, Mary Wheeler, ND, PO Box 895, Lakebay, WA, ph. 253-884-6116
98362, Richard Marschall, ND, 162 S. Barr Rd., Port Angeles, WA, ph. 360-457-1515
98368, Douwe Rienstra, MD, 242 Monroe St., Port Townsend, WA, ph. 360-385-5658, fax –5142
98368, J. Douwe Rienstra, MD, 242 Monroe St., Port Townsend, WA, ph. 360-385-5658, fax -5142
98370, Jane Bernstein Pearson, ND, PO Box 1664, Poulsbo, WA, ph. 360-697-7070
98382, Mark Swanson, ND, 720 E. Washington St., Sequim, WA, ph. 360-683-1110
98390, Linda Dyson, ND, 17610 49th St. E., Summer, WA, ph. 253-926-2229
98405, Health Enhancement Corporation, 3315 S. 23rd #200, Tocoma, WA, ph. 253-566-1616
98405, Owen Miller, ND, 1530 S. Union #4, Tacoma, WA, ph. 253-752-2558
98406, Paul Reilly, ND, 3620 Sixth Ave., Tacoma, WA, ph. 253-752-4544
98466, Anthony Calpeno, DC, ND, 4111-A Bridgeport Way W., Univ. Place, WA, ph. 253-565-2444
98499, Thomas Young, ND, 8909 Gravelly Lake Dr. SW, Tacoma, WA, ph. 253-584-1144
98501, Dennis Sklar, ND, 3726 Pacific Ave. SE, Ste. A, Olympia, WA, ph. 206-754-8576
98502, Jon Dunn, ND, 2617-B 12th Ct. SW #6, Olympia, WA, ph. 360-352-7880
98506, All Ways Chiropractic Center, 1401 Forth Ave. East, Olympia, WA, ph. 360-351-8896
98506, Robin Moore, ND, 3627 Ensign Rd., Ste. B, Olympia, WA, ph. 360-459-9082
98506, Suzanne Adams, ND, 3627 Ensign Rd., Ste. B, Olympia, WA, ph. 360-459-9082
98516, Jennifer Booker, ND, 6326 Martin Way E., Ste. 205, Olympia, WA, ph. 360-491-2111
98516, Patricia Hastings, ND, 4324 Martin Way, Ste. B, Olympia, WA, ph. 360-438-2882
98577, Pierre Wise, ND, 301 Ocean Ave., Raymond, WA, ph. 360-942-3956
98597, Carol Knowlton, MD, 503 1st St. S. #1, Yelm, WA, ph. 360-458-1061, fax -1661
98597, Elmer M. Cranton, MD, 503 First St. S., Yelm, WA, ph. 360-458-1061, fax -1661
98604, Jill Stansbury, ND, 408 E. Main St., Battle Ground, WA, ph. 360-687-2799
98661, Anne Scott, ND, 316 E. Fourth Plain Blvd., Ste. B, Vancouver, WA, ph. 360-750-4642
98663, Cheryl Deroin, ND, 3606 Main St. #202, Vancouver, WA, ph. 360-695-7699
98663, Kevin Murray, ND, 316 E. Fourth Plain Blvd., Ste. B, Vancouver, WA, ph. 360-750-4642
98663, Richard P. Huemer, MD, 3303 N.E. 44th St., Vancouver, WA, ph. 360-696-4405
98665, Harry C.S. Park, MD, 1412 N.E. 88th St., Vancouver, WA, ph. 360-574-4074
98665, Meed West, ND, 1612 NE 78 St., Vancouver, WA, ph. 360-573-3223
98672, Elyssa Harte, ND, 40 Major Creek Rd., White Salmon, WA, ph. 509-493-3835
98683, Steve Kennedy, ND, 406 S.E. 131st Ave. #202-B, Vancouver, WA, ph. 360-256-4566
98801, Jacqueline Thomas, ND, 1214 Fifth St., Wenatchee, WA, ph. 509-665-0867
98841, Andrea Black, ND, 138 Buzzard Lake Rd., Okanagan, WA, ph. 509-826-1164
98862, Sierra Breitbeil, ND, PO Box 993, Winthrop, WA, ph. 509-996-3970
98902, R S. Wilkinson, MD, 302 S. 12th Ave., Yakima, WA, ph. 509-453-5506, fax 575-0211
99009, High Rond Clinic, 42207 N. Sylvan Dr., Elk, WA, ph. 509-292-2748, fax -2748
99114, Randy Sandaine, ND, 143 Garden Homes Dr., Colville, WA, ph. 509-685-2300
99203, Holistic Family Medicine, 2814 S. Grand Blvd., Spokane, WA, ph. 509-747-2902
99203, William Corell, MD, South 3424 Grand, Spokane, WA, ph. 509-838-5800, fax -4042
99205, Letitia Watrous, ND, W 1137 Garland Ave., Spokane, WA, ph. 509-327-5143
99206, Burton B. hart, DO, E. 12104 Main, Spokane, WA, ph. 509-927-9922, fax -9922
99352, Stephen Smith, MD, 1516 Jadwin, Richland, WA, ph. 509-946-1695
99503, Cary Jasper, ND, 1407 W. 31 Ave. Fourth Floor, Anchorage, AK, ph. 907-276-4611
99503, David Mulholland, DC, 550 E.Tudor Rd., Anchorage, AK, ph.907-562-5366
99503, Mary Minor, ND, 1113 W. Fireweed Lane #200, Anchorage, AK, ph. 907-567-2330
99503, Sandra Denton, MD, 3201 C St. #306, Anchorage, AK, ph. 907-056-3620, fax 561-4933
99503, Torrey Smith, ND, 1407 W. 31 Ave. Fourth Floor, Anchorage, AK, ph. 907-276-4611
99504, Tim Hagney, ND, 3201 C St. #602, Anchorage, AK, ph. 907-563-6200
99518, Robert Rowen, MD, 615 E. 82nd St. #300, Anchorage, AK, ph. 907-344-7775, fax 522-3114
99567, Peters Creek Chiropractic, P.O. Box 367, Chugiak, AK, ph. 907-688-7676
99577, Daniel Young, ND, 10928 Eagle River Rd. #254, Eagle River, AK, ph. 907-694-5522
99577, Madeleine Morrison-Young, ND, 10928 Eagle River Rd., Eagle River, AK, ph 907-694-5522
99577, Omni Medical Ctr., 615 E. 82nd Ave. #300, Anchorage, AK, ph. 704-344-7775
99603, Toby Wheeler, ND, PO Box 2289, Homer, AK, ph. 907-235-5954
99645, D. Lynn Mickelson, MD, 440A W. Evergreen, Palmer, AK, ph. 907-745-3880, fax -2631
99687, Patton Pettijohn, ND, PO Box 878894, Wasilla, AK, ph. 907-276-5077

99687, Robert E. Martin, MD, P.O. Box 870710, Wasilla, AK, ph. 907-367-5284
99701, John Solieau, ND, 222 Front St., Fairbanks, AK, ph. 907-451-7100
99701, Ruth Bar-Shalom, ND, 222 Front St., Fairbanks, AK, ph. 907-451-7100
99801, Emily Kane, ND, 418 Harris St. #329, Juneau, AK, ph. 907-586-3655
99801, Maureen Longworth, MD, 16295 Point Lena Loop, Juneau, AK, 907-789-0266
IN CANADA
B0J 1J0, J.W. LaValley, MD, 227 Central St., Chester, NS, ph. 902-275-4555
K7A 1C3, Clare McNeilly, MD, 33 Williams St. E., Smith Falls, Ontario, ph. 613-283-7703
K8A 5T3, Naturopathic Outreach, 360 Renfrew Street, Pembroke, Ontario, ph. 613-732-9298
L4N 8K2, Barrie Holistic Centre, 127 Golden Meadow Rd, Barrie, Ontario, ph. 705-721-9932
L8N 3Z5, A. Fargas-Babjek, MD, 1200 Main St. W, Hamilton, Ontario, ph. 905-521-2100, fax 523-1224
M1E 3E6, L. Direnfeld, MD, 256 Morningside Ave. #325, W. Hill, Ontario, ph. 416-282-5773
M2N 6L4, Pain Clinic, 5 Park Home #620, North York, Ontario, ph. 416-221-2118
M4K 3T1, Paul Jaconello, MD, 751 Pape Ave, #201, Toronto, Ontario, ph. 416-463-2911, fax 469-0538
M4T 1Y7, K. Kerr, MD, 401 - 1407 Yonge St. #401, Toronto, Ontario, ph. 416-927-9502, fax 929-1424
N0B 2N0, Woolwich Health Ctre, 10 Parkside Drive, Saint Jacobs, Ontario, ph. 519-664-3794
N0M 1H0, Richard W. Street, MD, Bo 100 - Gypsy Lane, Blythe, Ontario, ph. 519-523-4433
N3H 3Y7, Complementary Healing Arts, 401 Laurel St., Cambridge, Ontario, ph. 519-653-3731
N3H 3Y7, Complementary Healing Arts, 401 Laurel St., Cambridge, ON, ph. 519-653-3731
P6B 1R4, Healing Arts Center, 426 Bruce St., Sault Ste. Marie, Ontario, ph. 705-256-8112
T0A `T0, Richard Johnson, MD, Box 96 - 4818 - 51st St., Grand Centre, Alberta, ph. 403-594-7574
T0G 1E0, P.V. Edwards, MD, Box 449, High Prairie, Alberta, ph. 403-523-4501, fax -4800
T0G 1E0, R. Laughlin, MD, Box 449, High Prairie, Alberta, ph. 403-523-4501, fax -4800
T0H 1L0, A Cooper, MD, Box 283, Fairview, Alberta, ph. 403-835-2525
T2G 1A2, F. Logan Stanfield, MD, 206 - 25 12th Avenue SE, Calgary, Alberta, ph. 403-265-6171
T2L 1V9, W.J. Mayhew, MD, 102 - 3604 52 Ave NW, Calgary, Alberta, ph. 403-284-2261, -9434
T3B 0M3, Bruce Hoffman, MD, 202-4411 16th Ave. NW, Calgary, Alberta, ph. 403-286-7311
T5E 1N8, Andrew W. Serada, MD, 10 - 4936 - 87th, Edmonton, Alberta, ph. 403-450-1991, fax -1990
T5E 1N8, Northgate medical Center, 9535-135 Avenue, Edmonton, Alberta, ph. 403-476-3344
T5L 4X5, White Oaks Sqr, 12222 - 137 Ave #116, Edmonton, Alberta, ph. 403-423-9355, fax 473-2856
T5P 4J5, K.B. Wiancko, MD, 205-9509 156 St., Edmonton, Alberta, ph. 403-483-2703, fax 486-5674
T6E 4G6, Tris P. Trethart, MD, 8621 - 104 St., Edmonton, Alberta, ph. 403-433-7401, fax -0481
V0H 2C0, Alex A. Neil, MD, 216 - 3121 Hill Road, Winfield, BC, ph. 604-766-0732
V1R 4C2, Hunt Naturopathic Clinic, 1338A Cedar Avenue, Trail, BC, ph. 250-368-6999, fax -6995
V2A 6J9, Dietrich Wittell, MD, P.O. Box 70, Penticton, BC, ph. 604-492-9849
V2G 1G6, D. Loewen, MD, 177 Yorkston St, #202, Williams Lake, BC, ph. 604-398-7777, fax -7734
V3S 2P1, Zigurts Strauts, MD, 304 - 16088 - 84th Ave., Surrey, BC, ph. 604-543-5000, fax -5002
V4V 1H8, Health Trek Research Inc., 11270 Highway 97, Winfield, BC, ph. 250-766-3633, fax -3633
V6K 2E1, D. Stewart, MD, 2184 W. Broadway #435, Vancouver, BC, ph. 604-732-1348, fax -1372
V6K 3C4, Saul Pilar, 205-2786 W. 16th Avenue, Vancouver, BC, ph. 604-739-8858, fax -8858
V9Y 4T9, John Cline, MD, 3855 - 9 Ave., Port Alberni, BC, ph. 604-723-1434

CHAPTER 15

★

NUTRITION AND CANCER BOOKS

If you cannot obtain these books from your local book store, try the following mail order stores: Tattered Cover Bookstore, Denver, CO, 800-833-9327; or Mail Order books 800-233-5150; or Discount Books 800-833-0702 or the Internet via www.amazon.com.

-Balch, JF, PRESCRIPTION NUTRITIONAL HEALING, Avery, Garden City, NY, 1990
-Bendich, A., and Chandra, RK, MICRONUTRIENTS AND IMMUNE FUNCTION, Annals of New York Academy of Sciences, vol.587
-Boik, J., CANCER & NATURAL MEDICINE, Oregon Medical, Princeton, MN, 1995
-Cilento, R., HEAL CANCER, Hill Publishers, Melbourne, Australia, 1993
-Congress of United States, Office of Technology Assessment, UNCONVENTIONAL CANCER TREATMENTS, U.S. Government Printing Office, Washington, DC, 1990, GPO # 052-003-01208-1, (ph. 800-336-4797)
-Diamond, WJ, et al, DEFINITIVE GUIDE CANCER, Future Med, Tiburon, CA, 1997
-Jacobs, M., VITAMINS AND MINERALS IN THE PREVENTION AND TREATMENT OF CANCER, CRC Press, Boca Raton, FL, 1991
-Kaminski, MV, HYPERALIMENTATION, Marcel Dekker Press, NY, 1985
-Laidlaw, SA, VITAMINS AND CANCER PREVENTION, Wiley, 1991
-Machlin, LJ, HANDBOOK OF VITAMINS, Marcel Dekker, NY, 1991
-Meyskens, FL, and Prasad, KN, MODULATION AND MEDIATION OF CANCER BY VITAMINS, S. Karger Publ., Basel, Switzerland, 1983
-Meyskens, FL, and Prasad, KN, VITAMINS AND CANCER, Humana Press, Clifton, NJ
-National Academy of Sciences, DIET, NUTRITION, AND CANCER, National 1982
-Poirier, LA, et al., ESSENTIAL NUTRIENTS CARCINOGENESIS, Plenum, NY, 1986
-Prasad, KN, and Meyskens, ML, NUTRIENTS AND CANCER PREVENTION, Humana Press, Clifton, NJ, 1990
-Prasad, KN, VITAMINS AGAINST CANCER, Healing Arts Press, Rochester, VT, 1984
-Quillin, P and Williams, RM (eds), ADJUVANT NUTRITION IN CANCER TREATMENT, Cancer Treatment Research Foundation, Arlington Heights, IL, 1994
-Quillin, P, BEATING CANCER WITH NUTRITION, Nutrition Times, Tulsa, OK 1998
-Simone, CB, CANCER AND NUTRITION, Avery Publ., Garden City, NY, 1992
-U.S. DHHS, SURGEON GENERAL'S REPORT ON NUTRITION AND HEALTH, U.S. Government Printing Office (ph. 800-336-4797), 1988
-Werbach, MR, NUTRITIONAL INFLUENCES ON ILLNESS, Third Line, Tarzana, 1996

CHAPTER 16
★
REFERRAL AGENCIES
FOR CANCER TREATMENT

YOU JUST RECEIVED THE DIAGNOSIS OF "CANCER" AND YOUR WHOLE WORLD STARTED SPINNING. There are many emotions that surface after such a diagnosis: why me?, anger, self-pity, stunned silence, depression and much more. All of these emotions are okay. Once you have surfaced from the depths of these emotions, your best strategy is to first get educated. But where do you start? There is so much information out there today! It has been said that getting information in today's information age is "like trying to get a drink from a fire hydrant". Maybe so.

But the following agencies can help to reduce the volume, complexity and confusion of the information available on your particular cancer. I strongly encourage everyone to get a second and third opinion before taking steps that are irreversible, such as surgery, chemotherapy and radiation. As I said at the beginning of this book, the best way for you to beat cancer is to first develop a sense of "can do"; others before you have beat your form of cancer. Secondly, get educated. The following groups can be of great assistance. They charge for their services, but provide a rational and balanced analysis of the therapies that have demonstrated some effectiveness in your cancer.

✓ The Health Resource, 209 Katherine Drive, Conway, AR 72032, (501) 329-5272

✓ CanHelp, 3111 Paradise Bay Rd., Port Ludlow, WA 98365, (360) 437-2291, FAX 437-2272

✓ People Against Cancer, P.O. Box 10, Otho, IO 50569, (515) 972-4444, fax-4415

✓ Center for Advancement in Cancer Education, 300 E. Lancaster Ave. #100, Wynnewood, PA 19096; ph 610-642-5057, fax 896-6339

✓ World Research Foundation, 41 Bell Rock Plaza, Sedona, AZ 86351; ph 520-284-3300

✓ INTERNET USERS: www.healthy.com or www.onhealth.com

INFORMATION SERVICES

Some of the following charge fees for their services, which include providing information on a wide range of unconventional cancer therapies. You should ask at the outset what the total fees are. The value of each service may depend on what you are looking for. Some services run computer searches, and others do in-person or over-the-telephone consultations.

-The Arlin J. Brown Information Center, Inc., P.O. Box 251, Fort Belvoir, VA 22060, (703) 752-9511

-Cancer Control Society, 2043 North Berendo St., Los Angeles, CA 90027, (213) 663-7801

-Cancer Federation, P.O. Box 52109, Riverside, CA 92517, (714) 682-7989

-Foundation for Advancement in Cancer therapy (FACT), P.O. Box 1242, Old Chelsea Station, New York, NY 10113, (212) 741-2790

-International Health Information Institute, 14417 Chase St., Suite 432, Panorama City, CA 91402

-International Holistic Center, Inc., P.O. Box 15103, Phoenix, AZ 85060, (602) 957-3322

-DATIC Health Resources, Inc. (Diagnostic Aides Therapeutic Information Computerized), Apt. 114, 1075 Bernard Ave., Kelowna, British Columbia V1Y 6P7, Canada, (604) 862-3228 or P.O. Box 218, Chilliwack, British Columbia V5P 6J1, Canada, (604) 792-7175

-National Health Federation, 212 West Foothill Blvd., P.O. Box 688, Monrovia, CA 91016, (818) 357-2181

-National Self-Help Clearinghouse, 25 West 43rd St., Room 620, New York, NY 10036

-Nutrition Education Association, Inc., 3647 Glen Haven, Houston, TX 77025, (713) 665-2946

-Patient Advocates for Advanced Cancer Treatments, Inc. (PAACT), 1143 Parmelee NW, Grand Rapids, MI 49504, (616) 453-1477

-Planetree Health Resource Center, 2040, Webster St., San Francisco, CA 94115, (415) 923-3680

INFORMATION AND REFERRALS ON ALTERNATIVE TREATMENTS

-American Assoc. of Orthomolecular Medicine, 7375 Kingsway, Burnaby, British Columbia, V3N3B5 Canada

-American College of Advancement in Medicine, 231 Verdugo Drive, Suite 204, Laguna Hills, CA 92653, Ph# 714-583-7666

-Arlin J. Brown Information Center, PO Box 251, Ft. Belvoir, VA 22060, Ph#703-451-8638

-Cancer Control Society, 2043 N. Berendo St., Los Angeles, CA 90027, Ph# 213-663-7801

-Comm. for Freedom of Choice in Medicine, 1180 Walnut Av., Chula Vista, CA 92011, Ph# 800-227-4473/Fax: 619-429-8004

-European Institute for Orthomolecular Sciences, PO Box 420, 3740 A.K., Baarn, Holland

-Found. for Advancement in Cancer Therapy, Box 1242, Old Chelsea Sta., New York, NY 10113, Fax: 212-741-2790
-Gerson Institute, PO Box 430, Bonita, CA 91908, Ph# 619-267-1150/Fax: 619-267-6441
-Intl. Academy of Nutrition and Preventive Medicine, PO Box 18433, Asheville, NC 28814, Ph# 704-258-3243/Fax: 704-251-9206
-Intl. Assn. of Cancer Victors & Friends, 7740 W. Manchester Ave., No.110, Playa del Rey, CA 90293, Ph#213-822-5032/Fax: 213-822-5132
-We Can Do!, 1800 Augusta, Ste.150, Houston, TX 77057, Ph# 713-780-1057

PSYCHONEUROIMMUNOLOGY (mental, spiritual) READING LIST
General
-Dossey, L., Meaning & Medicine, New York, Bantam, 1991
-Anderson, G., The Cancer Conquerer, Kansas City, Andrews & McMeel, 1988
-LeShan, L., Cancer as a Turning Point
Imagery
-Epstein, G., Healing Visualizations: Creating Health Through Imagery, New York, Bantam, 1989
Relaxation/Meditation
-Keating, T., Open Mind, Open Heart: The Contemplative Dimension of the Gospel, New York, Amity House, 1986
-LeShan, L., How to Meditate, New York, Bantam, 1974
Forgiveness
-Casarjian, R., Forgiveness: A Bold Choice for a Peaceful Heart, New York, Bantam, 1992
Healing
-Borysenko, J., Minding the Body, Mending the Mind, New York, Bantam, 1987
-Simonton, O.C., & Henson, R., The Healing Journey, New York, Bantam, 1992
-Myss, C., Why People Don't Heal and How They Can, Harmony, NY 1997
-Moyers, B., Healing the Mind, New York, Bantam Doubleday, 1993
Thought, Attitude, and Negativity
-Benson, H., Your Maximum Mind: Changing Your Life by Changing the Way You Think, New York, Random House, 1987
-Cousins, N., Head First: The Biology of Hope, New York, E.P. Dutton, 1989
-Martorano, J.T. & Kildahl, J., Beyond Negative Thinking: Reclaiming Your Life Through Optimism, New York, Avon, 1989
-Pennebaker, J.W., Opening Up: The Healing Power of Confiding in Others, New York, Avon Books, 1990
-Seligman, M.E.P., Learned Optimism: How to Change Your Mind and Your Life, New York, Pocket Books, 1990
Spirituality
-Borysenko, J., Fire in the Soul, New York, Warner, 1993

NOTES

IMMUNOPOWER pills

EACH PACKET CONTAINS 12 pills consisting of:

1 capsule containing:
Garlic, (Kyolic)	600 mg

1 capsule containing:
Probiotics	1.5 billion bacteria

1 capsule containing:
Mixed digestive enzymes:	520 mg

1 capsule containing:
lipoic acid	33 mg
lycopene	3 mg
ellagic acid	100 mg
quercetin	167 mg
L-carnitine	100 mg
methyl sulfonyl methane	250 mg
ascorbyl palmitate	10 mg

1 capsule containing:
Coenzyme Q-10	100 mg
Thymic concentrate	300 mg
Spleen concentrate	300 mg

2 capsules containing:
OPC	50 mg
Silymarin (milk thistle)	140 mg
Echinecea (purpurea)	80 mg
Curcumin (curcuma longa)	50 mg
Ginkgo biloba (24%)	40 mg
Astragalus (membranaceus)	167 mg
Panax ginseng (8%)	167 mg
Green tea polyphenols	67 mg
Cruciferous 400	80 mg
Cat's claw, 3:1	200 mg
Maitake D-fraction	33 mg
L-glutathione	100 mg

Lipids (in soft gelatin capsules)
Cod liver oil	1 gram
vitamin A	2500 iu
vitamin D	270 iu
Evening primrose oil (2)	2600 mg
Shark oil (1 capsule)	1 gram
Conjugated linoleic acid	1 gram

IMMUNOPOWER powder

Each 22 gm scoop (about 3 T) contains:

Vitamins
betacarotene (betatene)	15 mg,	25,000 iu
E (2/3 succinate, 1/3 natural)		400 iu
K (menadione)		100 mcg
C total		2500 mg
ascorbic acid		1000 mg
sodium ascorbate		1500 mg
B-1 (thiamine mononitrate)		10 mg
B-2 (riboflavin)		10 mg
B-3 (hexanicotinate)		500 mg
B-5 (D-calcium pantothenate)		20 mg
B-6 total		50 mg
P-5-P		3.3 mg
pyridoxine HCl		46.6 mg
B-12 (cyanocobalamin)		1 mg
Folic acid		200 mcg
Biotin		50 mcg

Minerals
Calcium (aspartate)	150 mg
Magnesium (aspartate)	150 mg
Potassium (citrate)	333 mg
Zinc (chelate)	10 mg
Iron (chelate)	3.3 mg
Copper (chelate)	1 mg
Iodine (potassium iodide)	50 mcg
Manganese (chelate)	1.67 mg
Chromium (GTF niacinate)	200 mcg
Selenium (selenomethionine)	200 mcg
Molybdenum (chelate)	167 mcg
Vanadium (vanadyl sulfate)	33 mcg
Nickel (sulfate)	3.3 mcg
Tin (chloride)	3.3 mcg

Accessory Factors
Aloe powder	167 mg
Dimethylglycine	16.7 mg
Bovine cartilage (VitaCarte)	3 gm
Nucleic acid (DNA)	500 mg
Nucleic acid (RNA)	500 mg
FOS, fructo-oligosaccharides	1 gm
Tocotrienols	20 mg
Medium chain triglycerides	1 gm
Lecithin powder	1500 mg
Genistein (from 6 gm soy)	6 mg
L-glycine	1 gm
Glucaric acid (cal D glucarate)	500 mg
vanilla flavoring	